WALr
NOR⸀

t
o
r
f

Nᴏ
___

........ᵣorders of Fluid and Electrolyte Balance

....

....

....

....

..2.

.... .

✓

Disorders of Fluid and Electrolyte Balance

R. N. Walmsley MB BS FRCPath MCB MAACB

Director of Clinical Biochemistry,
Flinders Medical Centre, Adelaide.
Visiting Consultant (Chemical Pathology),
Repatriation General Hospital, Adelaide.
Honorary Senior Lecturer in Clinical Biochemistry,
The Flinders University of South Australia

and

M. D. Guerin MB BS BSc(Hons) MAACB

Medical Clinical Chemist,
Institute of Medical and Veterinary Science, Adelaide.
Affiliate Registrar in Medicine,
Royal Adelaide Hospital

WRIGHT

1984   Bristol

Published by:
John Wright & Sons Ltd,
823–825 Bath Road,
Bristol BS4 5NU, England

ISBN 0 7236 0758 3

Library of Congress
Catalog Card Number:
83-62857

*British Library Cataloguing in
Publication Data*

Walmsley, R. N.
   Disorders of fluid and electrolyte balance.
   1. Water-electrolyte imbalance
   I. Title   II. Guerin, M.D.
   616.3'9   RC630

Typeset and printed in Great Britain by
John Wright & Sons (Printing) Ltd
at The Stonebridge Press, Bristol BS4 5NU

Preface

Most patients on admission to hospital, or at some period during their stay, will have their plasma electrolytes estimated, and many of them will have abnormal values. However, the evaluation and management of fluid-electrolyte and acid–base disorders is often a difficult, and sometimes incomprehensible, area for most medical students and junior hospital doctors. The general unfamiliarity with this subject usually reflects inadequate instruction and limited exposure to case material during the student's clinical years. There is no doubt that confidence in the diagnosis and therapy of these disorders can only be gained from bedside instruction, but the prevailing teaching methods, and lack of opportunity to deal with patients, force students to rely on textbook knowledge.

This book, prepared with medical students, junior doctors and clinical biochemists in mind, does not pretend to replace the 'hands on' clinical instruction approach. It is offered as a short didactic course in fluid and electrolyte disorders woven around a logical approach to the subject, and reinforced by descriptions of actual cases. Where feasible, patterns of common electrolyte disorders are reinforced, rather than effects on one analyte.

This text covers three aspects of fluid-electrolyte and acid–base metabolism: (1) normal homeostasis, (2) an approach to evaluation and management of disordered homeostasis, and (3) illustrated examples in the form of case material from our own hospitals. We believe that this latter section may aid the reader in getting a 'feel' for laboratory result values as he works through the case examples, instead of being presented with the unsatisfactory 'increased', 'greatly decreased' approach found elsewhere.

We have endeavoured to cover most of the commonly encountered clinical and laboratory problems in this area. However, due to space restraints, important sections, e.g. parenteral nutrition, dialysis and paediatric problems, have been left out. These are well presented in a variety of texts which specialize in these subjects.

Many of the investigations recommended throughout this book, e.g. urinary electrolytes, are not necessary for the diagnosis and evaluation of suspected fluid and electrolyte disorders in every patient. However, in the occasional patient, whose plasma electrolyte pattern and clinical features are unhelpful, or equivocal, these extra investigations often provide valuable clues to the underlying pathophysiology. We therefore suggest that readers new to this area should familiarize themselves with these tests, and the values found in various pathophysiological states. This can be achieved, not by reading books on the subject, but only by requesting the appropriate tests of the laboratory, and studying the results in parallel with the patient's clinical presentation.

Such a practice, although frowned at by laboratory directors, is the only way to get the 'feel' of laboratory values so that when they may be necessary in difficult diagnostic situations they can be interpreted with confidence.

The reference ranges used throughout this text are peculiar to our laboratories; they should not be applied to laboratory values available in the reader's particular institution as reference values vary from laboratory to laboratory depending on the local population and the analytical methods used.

We wish to thank Dr Graham White and Mr Peter McCarthy for reading the manuscript, and helpful suggestions and criticisms.

Acknowledgements

We are indebted to Blackwell Scientific Publications Pty Ltd for their kind permission in allowing us to reproduce *Figs.* 5.7 5.8, 5.9, 9.2 and 9.3 from Walmsley R. N. and White G. H. (1983) *A Guide to Diagnostic Clinical Chemistry.* Melbourne, Blackwell Scientific.

Contents

Abbreviations

[ ]	Concentration
AAS	Atomic absorption spectrophotometer
AcAc	Acetoacetic acid
ACE	Angiotensin converting enzyme
ACTH	Adrenocorticotropic hormone
ADH	Antidiuretic hormone
AG	Anion gap
$AHCO_3$	Actual bicarbonate
Alb	Albumin
Aldo	Aldosterone
AP	Alkaline phosphatase
AST	Aspartate aminotransferase
ATN	Acute tubular necrosis
ATP	Adenosine triphosphate
Ca^{2+}	Calcium ion
Ca	Total calcium
CAT	Carnitine acyl transferase
CCF	Congestive cardiac failure
Cl	Chloride
CMO	Corticosterone methyl oxidase
CNS	Central nervous system
COAD	Chronic obstructive airway disease
Creat	Creatinine
CRF	Chronic renal failure
DHCC	1,25-dihydroxycholecalciferol
DKA	Diabetic ketoacidosis
2,3-DPG	2,3-diphosphoglyceric acid
e.c.f.	Extracellular fluid
ECV	Extracellular volume
EDTA	Ethylenediamine tetra-acetate

ix

FE_x	Renal fractional excretion of x
FFA	Free fatty acids
GFR	Glomerular filtration rate
Glob	Globulins
Glu	Glucose
H^+	Hydrogen ion
Hb	Haemoglobin
HCMA	Hyperchloraemic metabolic acidosis
Hg	Mercury
HCO_3	Bicarbonate
i.c.f.	Intracellular fluid
IDDM	Insulin-dependent diabetes mellitus
i.m.	Intramuscular
i.v.	Intravenous
i.v.v.	Intravascular volume
K	Potassium
LRH	Low renin hypertension
Mg	Magnesium
Na	Sodium
NIDDM	Non-insulin-dependent diabetes mellitus
β-OHB	β-hydroxybutyric acid
o.p.	Osmotic pressure
Osmol	Osmolality
P_{CO_2}	Partial pressure of carbon dioxide
PCV	Packed cell volume
P_{O_2}	Partial pressure of oxygen
PO_4	Inorganic phosphate
PRA	Plasma renin activity
PRU	Prerenal uraemia
PTH	Parathyroid hormone
i-PTH	Immunoreactive PTH
RBF	Renal blood flow
RR	Reference range
RTA	Renal tubular acidosis
SHH	Syndrome of hyporeninaemic hypoaldosteronism
SIAD	Syndrome of inappropriate antidiuresis
SIADH	Syndrome of inappropriate secretion of ADH
TA	Titratable acidity
TB_x	Total body content of x
TCA	Tricarboxylic acid cycle
TP	Total protein

Conversion factors for SI units

Analyte	SI units	Conversion (×)	Traditional units
PLASMA			
Albumin	g/l	0·1	g/dl
Bicarbonate	mmol/l	1	mEq/l
Blood gases			
P_{CO_2}	kPa	7·5	mmHg
P_{O_2}	kPa	7·5	mmHg
Calcium	mmol/l	4	mg/dl
Chloride	mmol/l	1	mEq/l
Cortisol	nmol/l	0·036	µg/dl
Creatinine	mmol/l	11·3	mg/dl
Glucose	mmol/l	18	mg/dl
Lactate	mmol/l	9	mg/dl
Magnesium	mmol/l	2·4	mg/dl
Osmolality	mmol/kg	1	mosmol/kg
Phosphate	mmol/l	3·1	mg/dl
Potassium	mmol/l	1	mEq/l
Protein (total)	g/l	0·1	g/dl
Sodium	mmol/l	1	mEq/l
Urate	mmol/l	16·8	mg/dl
Urea	mmol/l	6	mg/dl
URINE			
Calcium	mmol/24 h	40	mg/24 h
Creatinine	mmol/24 h	113	mg/24 h
Creatinine clearance	ml/s	60	ml/min
Phosphate	mmol/24 h	31	mg/24 h
Urea	mmol/24 h	0·06	g/24 h

1

Introduction—basic principles

When interpreting plasma electrolyte values it is necessary to keep in mind some notion of what is meant by a normal (or reference) range; and what a particular analyte value means in terms of the laboratory's ability to measure it.

Reference Range
Reference ranges (or 'normal' values) can be estimated by a variety of methods—none of them being completely satisfactory. Every laboratory should calculate its own reference range to suit the local population and the analytical methods used. Thus the ranges will vary from laboratory to laboratory.

The commonest method used is the mean, plus/minus two standard deviations, of a number of so-called 'normal' people. By definition this method includes only 95% of this population within its range and, therefore, in any investigation of a given 'normal' population 5 people in each 100 (1 in 20) will have a result outside of the reference range, i.e. 1 person in 20 'normals' will have a value considered abnormal.

It is also necessary to bear in mind that a 'reference range' covers a fairly wide range of values (e.g. plasma $[Na^+]$ of 132–144 mmol/l), and a patient may have a 'normal' result which is abnormal for him, e.g. using this range for plasma sodium, a patient, whose plasma sodium concentration is normally ~ 132 mmol/l, would probably have an abnormal value if his level was 144 mmol/l.

The reference ranges used throughout the following text are those of the authors' laboratories and should not be applied to patient values from other laboratories.

Precision of a Test
This term, now often called imprecision, is a measure of a laboratory's ability to achieve the same value for a particular analyte if it is re-analysed. For a given test the imprecision is calculated by analysing the same sample a number of times and calculating the analytical error. This error may be expressed in percentage or absolute units, e.g. the analytical error of a sodium method may be 2% or 3 mmol/l. This means that a reported value of 140 mmol/l has a value somewhere between 137 and 143 mmol/l (140 ± 3 mmol/l). This value has important implications when

1

following the results of therapy, e.g. a patient who is receiving active therapy for hypernatraemia may show, in the course of treatment, a plasma sodium concentration fall from 160 to 156 mmol/l. If the error of the test is 3 mmol/l then:

1.   Estimated value of 160 mmol/l = value of 157–163 mmol/l
2.   Estimated value of 156 mmol/l = value of 153–159 mmol/l

The overlap between values (1) and (2) suggest that it is possible there is no improvement. On the other hand if the sodium fell to 153 mmol/l (150–156 mmol/l) then an improvement is probable.

Table 1.1 shows the errors of various tests in the authors' laboratory. These values will not be the same as values from other laboratories. If these values are not available a useful 'rule of thumb' is: for inorganic ions (Na^+, K^+, Ca^{2+}, etc.) allow 2% error; for organic substances (urea, creatinine, etc.) allow 5%; and for enzymes allow 10%.

Table 1.1. Examples of some analytical errors

Plasma/analyte	Error	Plasma analyte	Error
Na	3 mmol/l	Mg	0·03 mmol/l
K	0·1 mmol/l	Ca	0·07 mmol/l
Cl	2 mmol/l	PO_4	0·04 mmol/l
HCO_3	2 mmol/l	TP	2 g/l
Urea	0·5 mmol/l	Alb	2 g/l
Creatinine	0·02 mmol/l	AP	10 u/l
Anion gap	4 mEq/l		

TP, plasma total protein; Alb, plasma albumin; AP, plasma alkaline phosphatase.

Assessment of Plasma Electrolyte Results

The diagnosis and evaluation of possible fluid and electrolyte disorders must always be approached, at the outset, from the point of view of the clinical picture and the possible pathophysiology. A knowledge of the relevant pathophysiology, and its manifestations in terms of plasma (and/or urine) electrolyte values, enables the medical attendant to make certain assumptions which can be acted on with reasonable confidence. For example, a patient presenting with diabetic ketoacidotic coma will usually be depleted of water, sodium and potassium. He will therefore require, in addition to insulin, an infusion of saline followed later by potassium, and perhaps bicarbonate, supplements.

If the patient's clinical picture is unfamiliar, or unhelpful, or equivocal, then the evaluation of possible electrolyte problems can be difficult. In these cases the simplest approach is to attempt a clinical assessment of the patient's fluid and electrolyte status (e.g. dehydration, overhydration, etc.), and then evaluate the plasma electrolyte pattern. In the case of the latter a useful approach is to keep in mind some simple check-lists similar to those outlined below.

1.   Common causes of individual plasma electrolyte abnormalities
2.   Causes of common electrolyte patterns

Common Causes of Plasma Electrolyte Abnormalities

Sodium

High
Hypertonic dehydration—decreased fluid intake

Low
1. Decreased water excretion
  a. 'Stress' and intravenous therapy (e.g. 'surgical hyponatraemia')
  b. Syndrome of inappropriate antidiuresis
2. Diuretic therapy
3. Specimen taken from a 'drip arm'

Potassium

High
1. Haemolysis/unseparated plasma in contact with red cells for > 4 h
2. Renal failure
3. Diabetic acidosis

Low
1. Diuretic therapy
2. Vomiting/diarrhoea

Bicarbonate

High
1. Metabolic alkalosis
  a. Diuretic therapy
  b. Vomiting
2. Respiratory acidosis—chronic lung disease

Low
1. Metabolic acidosis
  a. Renal failure
  b. Diabetic ketoacidosis
  c. Compensation of respiratory alkalosis

Anion Gap

High
1. Renal failure
2. Diabetic ketoacidosis

Low (uncommon)
1. Laboratory error
2. Multiple myeloma

Urea/Creatinine

High
1. Renal failure
2. Severe hypovolaemia (dehydration)

Low
Overhydration

Calcium

High
1. Malignant hypercalcaemia
2. Primary hyperparathyroidism

Low
1. Hypoalbuminaemia (nephrosis, cirrhosis)
2. Chronic renal failure
3. EDTA contamination

Common Plasma Electrolyte Patterns

Hyponatraemia and Hyperkalaemia ($\downarrow$ [Na$^+$] and $\uparrow$ [K$^+$])
1. Diabetic ketoacidosis
2. Addison's disease

Hypokalaemic Metabolic Alkalosis ($\downarrow$ [K$^+$] and $\uparrow$ [HCO$_3{}^-$])
1. Diuretic therapy
2. Vomiting
3. Mineralocorticoid excess (ectopic ACTH syndrome)

Hyperkalaemic Metabolic Acidosis ($\uparrow$ [K$^+$] and $\downarrow$ [HCO$_3{}^-$])
1. Renal failure
2. Diabetic ketoacidosis

Hypokalaemic Metabolic Acidosis ($\downarrow$ [K$^+$] and $\downarrow$ [HCO$_3{}^-$])
1. Diarrhoea
2. Carbonic anhydrase therapy (acetazolamide)
3. Renal tubular acidosis

Hypercalcaemia and Hypophosphataemia ($\uparrow [Ca^{2+}]$ and $\downarrow [PO_4^{2-}]$)
1.　Malignant hypercalcaemia
2.　Primary hyperparathyroidism

Hypocalcaemia and Hyperphosphataemia ($\downarrow [Ca^{2+}]$ and $\uparrow [PO_4^{2-}]$)
1.　Chronic renal failure
2.　Hypoparathyroidism

Hypocalcaemia and Hypophosphataemia ($\downarrow [Ca^{2+}]$ and $\downarrow [PO_4^{2-}]$)
Secondary hyperparathyroidism—vitamin D deficiency, malabsorption syndrome

Should the above approach prove unhelpful further investigation should be along the lines suggested in the following text in the sections on diagnosis/ evaluation.

Assessment of Dehydration
Traditionally the severity of dehydration has been described as mild, moderate or severe; and these degrees have been allotted the following amounts of water loss relative to body weight.

Mild $\sim 4\%$ (approx. 3 litres in 70 kg)

Moderate 5–8% (approx. 4–6 litres in 70 kg)

Severe 8–10% (approx. 7 litres in 70 kg)
The ability to assess the degree of dehydration only comes from bedside experience and practice. Mild dehydration is characterized by thirst, dry tongue and other mucous membranes, low urine output with a high osmolality. Severe dehydration, on the other hand, is associated with loss of skin turgor, sunken eyeballs, profound oliguria (<20 ml/h), and compromised cardiovascular function (rapid pulse with low pulse volume, hypotension).
The assessment of the dehydrated patient should include particular attention to the following areas:

History
A good history is valuable and will give some indication of the underlying disorder, e.g. projectile vomiting suggests loss of water, salt, potassium and H^+ (metabolic alkalosis).

Clinical Examination
Specific features that should be noted are thirst, dryness of mucous membranes, loss of skin turgor, hypotension, postural hypotension, pulse rate and pressure, cyanosis, jugular venous pressure.

Urine Output

Providing renal function is intact and diabetes insipidus has been excluded dehydration is usually associated with a low output of concentrated urine (urine osmolality > plasma osmolality). Outputs of less than 20 ml/h indicate severe dehydration.

Weight

The loss of 1 litre of fluid results in a 1-kg weight loss. In adults, however, the body weight is usually a poor guide to the hydration status because of the uncertainty of the patient's normal weight.

Laboratory Assessment

Although a knowledge of the patient's plasma and urine electrolytes values is helpful in the assessment of fluid and electrolyte abnormalities, it is never necessary to withhold therapy until the laboratory results have been examined. The laboratory parameters which may be helpful are haemoglobin (Hb), packed cell volume (PCV), plasma albumin (Alb), and plasma and urinary electrolytes.

Hb, PCV and Alb

In dehydration there is haemoconcentration and the values of these three parameters rise. Unfortunately they are not always helpful guides to volume status as the patient's pre-dehydration levels are not usually known, e.g. if the levels were originally low, due to some other disorder, haemoconcentration may only result in 'normal' levels. A high plasma albumin level invariably indicates haemoconcentration (only common cause of a high level), but a low or normal level does not exclude this diagnosis.

Plasma Urea and Creatinine

A high urea level indicates a decreased glomerular filtration rate (GFR) which may be due to renal disease, or to decreased renal blood flow (RBF) to an otherwise normal kidney (e.g. dehydration, shock). In the presence of a normally functioning kidney a decreased RBF rarely causes the plasma urea level to rise above 20 mmol/l. Levels greater than this usually indicate severe intrinsic renal disease (or postrenal obstruction), or decreased blood flow to an already compromised kidney, e.g. the elderly patient who 'normally' has a low GFR due to the nephron 'dropout' of the aged kidney. Plasma creatinine levels provide similar information to the plasma urea levels. However, it must be remembered that the creatinine level is a function of the patient's muscle mass and that some patients (infants, elderly females) may normally have a low level (< 0·06 mmol/l). In these cases a compromised GFR, due to decreased RBF, may only raise the level to adult 'normal' levels (0·06–0·12 mmol/l).

Plasma Sodium

The plasma sodium concentration only indicates the ratio of the amount of extracellular sodium to that of the extracellular water; it gives no indication of the total extracellular sodium content (*see* p. 22). Its value lies in the classification of the type of dehydration (hyponatraemic, normonatraemic, hypernatraemic), and has a direct bearing on subsequent therapy in terms of the quality of fluid to be infused.

Plasma Potassium
Like plasma sodium estimations, the plasma potassium concentration does not indicate the total body content although hypokalaemia, if severe, is usually associated with a body deficit. However, hypokalaemia and hyperkalaemia may themselves have serious consequences and the plasma potassium estimation is an essential investigation in all patients with possible fluid and electrolyte disorders.

Principles of Management of Fluid and Electrolyte Disorders

Common Intravenous Solutions
A wide range of intravenous fluid preparations are available from commercial manufacturers. However, it is only necessary to be familiar with a few of the more common varieties in order to be able to devise an intravenous programme (*Table* 1.2).

Table 1.2. Some fluids commonly used for intravenous therapy

	Sodium (%)	mmol/l	Chloride (mmol/l)	Glucose (g/l)	Tonicity (mmol/kg)
Normal or physiological saline	0·9	153	153	—	Isotonic ~306
One-half normal saline in 2·5% glucose	0·45	77	77	25	Isotonic ~300
One-quarter normal saline in 3·75% glucose	0·225	38	38	37·5	Isotonic ~300
One-fifth normal saline in 4·3% glucose	0·18	31	31	43	Isotonic ~300
Twice normal saline	1·8	308	308	—	Hypertonic ~600
5% glucose	—	—	—	50	Isotonic ~300

The selection of an intravenous fluid depends on the patient's requirements with respect to water and sodium. If the patient requires both water and sodium in physiological quantities (e.g. isotonic dehydration) then normal saline will be the fluid of choice. Normal in the context of intravenous saline solutions means that it is physiologically normal, or has an osmolality approximating the plasma level (~ 300 mmol/kg).

In a patient requiring more water relative to sodium (e.g. hypernatraemic dehydration, *see* p. 27) the solution of choice will be an isotonic (osmolality ~ 300 mmol/kg) glucose solution with, or without, added sodium chloride (one-half normal saline in 2·5% glucose, 5% glucose). The glucose in these solutions, after infusion, is metabolized leaving behind pure water (infusion of 5% glucose is tantamount to infusing pure water). It is recommended that infused solutions not be hypotonic (one-half normal saline, one-fifth normal saline) because of the possibility of local haemolysis.

In the case of patients requiring more sodium than water (e.g. hypo-natraemic dehydration, p. 37) hypertonic saline solutions are available, e.g. $2 \times$ normal saline. These solutions should be infused slowly because (*a*) they may cause clotting at the infusion site, and (*b*) a rapid increase in a patient's extracellular osmolality may cause undesirable cell water shifts (e.g. rapid cellular dehydration, *see* p. 19).

Bicarbonate Supplements
The commonly available sodium bicarbonate solutions are:
    1·4% 167 mmol/l—isotonic
    2·8% 334 mmol/l—hypertonic, $2 \times$ normal
    8·4% 1000 mmol/l—hypertonic, $6 \times$ normal
    When supplementing a patient's i.v. fluids with sodium bicarbonate two points must be kept in mind:
1.   For each mmol of HCO_3^- given, 1 mmol of Na^+ is also introduced, i.e. large amounts of infused bicarbonate may result in sodium overload.
2.   The resulting decrease in extracellular acidaemia encourages K^+ to move into the cells and this may result in severe hypokalaemia, especially if the plasma $[K^+]$ is initially low.

Potassium Supplements
As well as preparations of saline and glucose solutions containing potassium (e.g. 5% glucose containing 40 mmol/l of KCl), potassium is also available in vials of concentrated KCl, e.g. 10% or 1 g/10 ml. Each gram of KCl contains ~ 13 mmol of K^+. When adding K^+ to i.v. fluids it is recommended, in the interest of precluding severe hyperkalaemia, that the patient does not receive it at a concentration greater than 40 mmol/l or at a rate greater than 20 mmol/h.

Other Supplements
Calcium, magnesium and phosphate are considered in Chapter 6.

In addition to the above fluids there are also available complex solutions containing ions other than sodium and chloride, e.g. Ringer's solution (NaCl, Ca^{2+}), Hartmann's solution (NaCl, Ca^{2+}, lactate—converted to HCO_3^- after infusion), electrolyte replacement solutions (e.g. 'plasmalyte'). These solutions, and others containing amino acids and lipids, etc., are used mainly in long term i.v. therapy, e.g. parenteral nutrition. This area is outside the range of this book and texts on parenteral nutrition should be consulted on the use of these solutions.

Normal Daily Requirements

If we assume that a hypothetical patient requiring intravenous therapy has normal renal function, no fluid or electrolyte deficit, is not losing body fluids from other than normal routes, is not stressed, and will only be on i.v. therapy for a short period (i.e. calories not a major consideration), then his daily requirements will be as follows.

Water

30–35 ml/kg or 2000–2500 ml for a 70-kg patient.

This volume allows for the following losses from the body:
1.   Skin: 500–750 ml
2.   Respiration: 500–750 ml
3.   Renal: 500–1000 ml

The minimal urinary output required to clear the blood of waste products is around 500 ml, i.e. approximate urinary osmol output by a normal adult is 600 mmol; maximal renal concentration ability is around 1200 mmol/kg ($600/1200 = 0.5$ litres). Thus the amount of fluid infused should be sufficient to give a urine output of at least 500 ml/day. In practice the urine output should be kept at around 750–1000 ml/day.

Sodium

~1 mmol/kg (0·8–1·2)

50–100 mmol for 70-kg patient

Potassium

1 mmol/kg (0·8–1·0)

50–80 mmol for 70-kg patient

These requirements can be given as:
1.   ~2 litres of 5% glucose + ~1 litre of 0·9% ('normal') saline, or
2.   ~3 litres of 0·18% (one-fifth 'normal') NaCl in 4% glucose *plus* potassium supplements, e.g. 2 g of KCl (~26 mmol) into each litre of fluid.

During therapy it is important, and necessary, (*a*) to keep a careful fluid balance chart, (*b*) to keep a regular check on the plasma electrolytes, and (*c*) to monitor for signs of fluid overload (increasing jugular venous pressure, pulmonary oedema, dependent oedema, etc.).

Additional Requirements

In practice the above regimen will invariably have to be modified to suit the circumstances of the patient, e.g. excessive body fluid losses due to fever, vomiting, diarrhoea, fistulas, etc. will have to be calculated and added to the above requirements.

The Postoperative Patient

The postoperative patient, who requires i.v. therapy, differs from the above 'normal' patient in that the stress reaction to the operation modifies his homeostatic mechanisms. The main features of this reaction, in terms of fluid and electrolyte balance, are retention of water and sodium, and increased renal excretion of potassium. These events are due to stress-induced release of antidiuretic hormone, aldosterone and cortisol.

Therefore in the postoperative situation a careful fluid balance chart should be kept, and the plasma electrolytes estimated regularly to prevent any fluid and electrolyte imbalance. (Dilutional hyponatraemia is a common problem in postoperative patients as they tend to be 'over watered and under salted'.)

The stress reaction lasts from 24 to 72 h. Recovery is heralded by diuresis, especially if the patient has been water-overloaded during the stress period.

Management of Dehydration

The therapeutic aim in the dehydrated patient is the restoration of the body fluids to normal volume and composition. The amount and type of fluid, and the rate of infusion, depend on:
1.   Severity of dehydration
2.   Type of dehydration (tonicity)
3.   Any ongoing losses

Severity of Dehydration

In any dehydrated patient the first consideration must be the status of the circulatory system. A patient with, or with impending, circulatory collapse must have his circulating volume restored as the first priority. This may be achieved with rapid infusion of 'normal' saline or, in the more severe cases, whole blood, plasma or plasma expanders. In the case of shock other measures, e.g. isoprenaline infusion, may be necessary if the patient does not respond to fluid therapy. Once the patient's blood pressure has been stabilized, and urine output has increased, then attention can be given to the selection of the most suitable i.v. fluid for the patient.

Type of Dehydration

The three types of dehydration, isotonic, hyponatraemic and hypernatraemic, theoretically require infusions of normal saline, hypertonic saline and hypotonic saline respectively. Management of these disorders are discussed further on pp. 47, 37 and 27. An important point to bear in mind in respect to hypertonic and hypotonic dehydration is that rehydration and correction of any body sodium deficit should be carried out slowly (over 12–24 h) in order to preclude sudden cell water shifts.

Ongoing Losses

In planning an intravenous regimen for any patient the following factors must be considered:

1. Patient's basal requirements (*see above*)
2. Patient's presenting fluid and electrolyte deficits
3. Any ongoing losses

Fluids lost from the body during i.v. therapy, e.g. gastric suction, should be carefully measured, added to the fluid balance chart and appropriate corrections made to the i.v. infusion.

Calculation of Requirements

Estimation of Water Requirements

It is usually convenient to plan a patient's 24-h requirements with the object of giving one-third to one-half, depending on the state of hydration, over the first 6 h and the remainder over the next 18 h. If there is severe hypertonicity or hypotonicity rehydration should be gradual over 24–48 h. The 24-h requirement may be calculated as follows:

a. Basal requirement: 25–35 ml/kg ($\sim$2·5 litres for 70-kg patient)
b. Deficit due to dehydration: calculate deficit as a percentage of body weight (mild dehydration $\sim$4%, moderate $\sim$6%, severe $\sim$8%), e.g. moderate dehydration in a 70-kg patient $=\sim$4 litres.

$a+b$ = 24-h total, i.e. for the above 70-kg patient with $\sim$6% dehydration = 6–7 litres.

Any abnormal losses incurred during the period of rehydration should be measured and appropriate adjustments made to the infusion volume.

Estimation of Sodium Requirements

This is difficult to estimate and it is better to 'titrate' the patient over the period of infusion therapy.

With isotonic dehydration the deficit can be made up with isotonic (0·9%) saline, e.g. the above 70-kg patient will require 4–4·5 litres of isotonic saline (4 litres for deficit and 0·5 litre for basal requirement). The remainder may be given as 5% dextrose or as one-fifth normal (0·18%) saline in 4% glucose.

In the case of hypertonic dehydration less sodium than the above will be required and the deficit may be given as one-fifth normal saline or 5% dextrose (*see* p. 27).

If there is hypotonic dehydration the patient will require more sodium than the above example. This may be made up of normal saline (e.g. 5–6 litres for the above example) or if necessary a hypertonic saline solution (*see* p. 37).

Estimation of Potassium Requirements

Again this is difficult to estimate and titration of the patient with potassium supplements is the usual method used in practice. This approach is satisfactory providing certain precautions are taken:

1. Do not give potassium therapy unless renal function is seen to be adequate.
2. Do not give i.v. potassium at a concentration greater than 40 mmol/l or at a rate in excess of 20 mmol/h. Rates and concentrations greater than these may result in dangerous hyperkalaemia.
3. Mix the container when adding potassium supplements to intravenous infusion solutions.
4. Check the plasma potassium concentration regularly, e.g. every 6–12 h or sooner if large quantities are being given i.v.

Estimation of Bicarbonate Requirements

Many clinicians will treat a metabolic acidosis with bicarbonate infusions if the pH is less than 7·1–7·2, with the aim of raising the plasma $[HCO_3^-]$ to ~ 15 mmol/l. A rule of thumb for the calculation of the amount of HCO_3^- required is:

Assume the 'bicarbonate space' to be 50% of the body weight (35 litres in a 70-kg subject) and calculate the HCO_3^- (mmol) required to raise the $[HCO_3^-]$ to 15 mmol/l, e.g. 70-kg patient with a plasma $[HCO_3^-]$ of 5 mmol/l.

$$HCO_3^- \text{ required} = 35 \times 10 = 350 \text{ mmol.}$$

In practice, however, such equations generally overestimate the HCO_3^- requirements, and the usual method of bicarbonate therapy is 'titration' of the patient. As noted above, it is important to remember that for each mmol of HCO_3^- infused 1 mmol of Na^+ also enters the body and sodium overload may occur if large amounts are given.

Overhydration

From the clinical point of view three types of overhydration may be recognized: oedematous states, acute overhydration, chronic overhydration.

Oedematous States

A discussion of this area is outside the scope of this text except to note that they may be associated with hyponatraemia (p. 35); and that diuretic therapy of these conditions may result in various electrolyte and fluid imbalances (p. 256).

Acute Overhydration

This condition, often iatrogenic in nature, may take the form of (a) severe dilutional hyponatraemia due to infusion of hypotonic fluids, (b) hypernatraemia due to salt gain (p. 26) or (c) isotonic water and salt excess due to over infusion of normal saline. The clinical features and management of these conditions are discussed in Chapter 2.

Chronic Overhydration

In this situation, usually associated with an inability of the kidney to excrete 'free' water normally, the usual presenting feature is hyponatraemia. Clinical features that may be associated with acute water intoxication (confusion, disorientation, cerebral oedema, etc.) are usually absent unless there is severe hyponatraemia (e.g. plasma sodium concentration $<115\,\text{mmol/l}$). *See* p. 33.

2
Sodium and water

Definitions

Dehydration
This is a misleading term because it superficially infers a water deficit without a sodium deficit. This in fact is a rare situation because most patients with a water loss also have some degree of sodium depletion. In the following discussion the term dehydration will be used to describe any situation where there is loss of water from the body, with or without sodium loss.

For the purposes of evaluation and management dehydration may be classified as:

Isotonic
Loss of sodium and water from the body in the ratio of 140 mmol of sodium to every 1000 ml of pure water (140 mmol/l being the average extracellular concentration of sodium).

Hypernatraemic (Hypertonic)
Loss of water in excess of sodium (i.e. for each litre of water lost there is a loss of < 140 mmol of sodium).

Hyponatraemic (Hypotonic)
Depletion of sodium in excess of water (i.e. for each litre of water lost the loss of sodium is > 140 mmol).

Hypernatraemia
Plasma sodium concentration greater than the upper reference limit (> 145 mmol/l).

Hyponatraemia
Plasma sodium concentration below the lower reference limit (< 132 mmol/l).

14

Fractional Excretion (FE_x)

The renal fractional excretion of a substance (x) is the amount excreted in the urine expressed as a percentage of the amount filtered by the glomeruli. It is calculated from the following equation on the assumption that creatinine clearance is equivalent to the glomerular filtration rate.

$$FE_x = \frac{\text{amount of x excreted/min}}{\text{amount of x filtered/min}}$$

$$\text{x excreted/min} = Ux \times V \, (\text{l/min})$$

$$\text{x filtered/min} = GFR \, (\text{l/min}) \times Px$$

$$= \text{creatinine clearance} \times Px$$

$$= \frac{Ucr \times V \, (\text{l/min})}{Pcr} \times Px$$

therefore

$$FE = \frac{Ux \times V \, (\text{l/min})}{1} \times \frac{Pcr}{Ucr \times V \, (\text{l/min})} \times \frac{1}{Px}$$

$$= \frac{Ux}{Ucr} \times \frac{Pcr}{Px}.$$

Where Ux = urinary concentration of x (mmol/l); V = volume of urine (e.g. litres/min); Px = plasma concentration of x (mmol/l); Ucr = urinary concentration of creatinine (mmol/l); Pcr = plasma concentration of creatinine (mmol/l); GFR = glomerular filtration rate.

The estimation can be made using a 'spot' urine collected at the same time as the blood sample taken for the plasma analytes.

Osmolality

The osmolality of a fluid is a measure of the total number of particles (ions, molecules) present in solution expressed as mmol/kg of water. For plasma, or the extracellular fluid, the main osmotically active particles are Na^+, K^+, Cl^-, HCO_3^-, urea and glucose. In the laboratory the osmolality is usually measured by freezing point depression (osmometry). However, since Na^+ is the major cation present in the extracellular fluid its osmolality can be roughly estimated from the following equation:

Calculated osmolality (mmol/kg) = $2 \times [Na^+]$ mmol/l
$\qquad\qquad + [\text{urea}]$ mmol/l + $[\text{glucose}]$ mmol/l.

Osmolal Gap

The difference between the measured osmolality and the calculated osmolality is normally < 10 mmol/kg. If the plasma contains large quantities of substances other than electrolytes, urea or glucose (i.e. unmeasured analytes) then the measured osmolality will be much greater than the calculated osmolality.

Substances that may cause this gap include ethanol, methanol and drugs, e.g. patient with acute alcohol intoxication:

Plasma Na	144 mmol/l
K	3·6 mmol/l
Cl	100 mmol/l
HCO_3	24 mmol/l
Urea	2·8 mmol/l
Glucose	5·0 mmol/l
Ethanol	63 mmol/l
Osmolality	370 mmol/kg

calculated osmol (disregarding the ethanol) = 296 mmol/kg

osmolal gap = 74 mmol/kg.

Tonicity (effective osmolality)

Since urea and a number of other small molecules (ethanol, methanol) are able to cross cell membranes freely they do not exert an osmotic force and therefore do not cause water movement in or out of cells. The tonicity, or effective osmolality, of the plasma (or extracellular fluid) may be calculated from the following:

$$tonicity\ (mmol/kg) = 2 \times [Na^+]\,mmol/l + [glucose]\,mmol/l$$

or

$$= measured\ osmolality - [urea]\,mmol/l$$

For example, a patient having the following results:

Plasma Na	142 mmol/l
K	4·5 mmol/l
Cl	107 mmol/l
HCO_3	22 mmol/l
Urea	50 mmol/l
Glucose	5·5 mmol/l
Osmolality	343 mmol/l

has (*a*) a calculated osmolality of 339 mmol/kg

and (*b*) a tonicity of 293 mmol/kg which will not cause water movement out of cells

Water Homeostasis

Distribution

The approximate total body water and its distribution between the main body compartments in a healthy young adult male is shown in *Table* 2.1.

The amount of body water and its compartmental distribution varies according to age (decrease in extracellular water with age) and sex (females have a lower total body water than males due to relatively more adipose tissue), *Table* 2.2.

Normally the day-to-day fluctuations in the total body water are very small (<0·2%), due to a fine balance between input, controlled by the thirst mechanism, and output, controlled mainly by the renal-ADH system.

Table 2.1. Approximate compartmental distribution of water in a healthy young adult male

	Litres	% of body weight
Total	~42	~60
Intracellular	~23	~33
Extracellular	~19	~27
interstitial	~16	~23
plasma	~3	~4

Table 2.2. Total body water content according to age

	Total body weight (% body weight)
Infants	~75
Young males	~60
females	~54
Elderly males	~50
females	~45

Input

The daily water intake (*Fig.* 2.1) varies considerably depending on body losses (urine, skin, lungs) and various psychosocial factors. Thirst is the most important factor influencing intake, and it is controlled by the thirst centre situated in the hypothalamus.

The main factors stimulating the thirst centre are:
1. Hypertonicity of the ECF
2. Decreased blood volume
3. Pain, stress

Output

Although a certain amount of water is lost from the skin, lungs and gastrointestinal tract (*Fig.* 2.1) the major organ controlling fluid output is the kidney which is in turn under the influence of antidiuretic hormone (ADH).

Renal Excretion

The kidney has the ability to excrete large quantities of dilute urine. For example, an adult male is able to drink up to 20–25 litres of water a day and not become water overloaded. On the other hand, the kidney is able to decrease water excretion to less than 500 ml a day if the intake is low.

Renal concentration depends on:
1. Normal delivery of fluid to the diluting segment of the nephron (ascending limb of the loop of Henle).
2. Normal reabsorption of NaCl in the ascending limb of the loop of Henle (diluting segment).

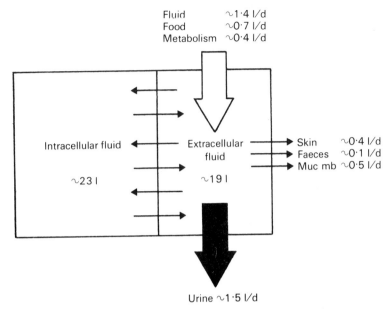

Fig. 2.1. Water balance in an adult. Muc mb, mucous membranes.

3.   Presence of circulating ADH and collecting ducts responsive to ADH.

Renal dilution requires:
1.   Normal delivery of fluid to the diluting segment, i.e. normal GFR and proximal reabsorption.
2.   Normal NaCl reabsorption and thus dilution of the urine (to <100 mmol/kg) in the diluting segment.
3.   Absence of circulating ADH.

Antidiuretic Hormone (ADH)
This hormone is a small peptide (9 amino acids) which is synthesized in the supraoptic and paraventricular nuclei of the hypothalamus. It is transported along nerve axons to the posterior pituitary and released into the systemic circulation in response to various stimuli. It acts on the renal collecting ducts to increase the permeability of the duct cells to water, resulting in water reabsorption and concentration of the urine.
       The two main factors controlling ADH synthesis and release are:
1.   Tonicity of the extracellular fluid (osmoreceptors located in the hypothalamus): ↑ tonicity ⟶ ↑ ADH release; ↓ tonicity ⟶ ↓ ADH release.
2.   Blood volume (baroreceptors located in the right atrium and carotid sinus): ↓ blood volume ⟶ ↑ ADH and ↑ volume ⟶ ↓ ADH.
       The sensitivity of this control mechanism is such that an increase in extracellular tonicity of around 2% stimulates ADH synthesis and release whereas a fall in blood volume of around 10% is required to affect secretion.

Other factors that may stimulate ADH secretion are:
1. Stress—pain, trauma, surgical operations
2. Drugs—opiates, barbiturates, nicotine, clofibrate, chlorpropamide, tolbu-
    tamide, vincristine, vinblastine, carbamazepine
3. Nausea
    The rate of ADH secretion is controlled by the sum of the stimulating and
inhibiting forces acting at the hypothalamic level, e.g. the inhibitory effect of hypo-
osmolality may be overridden by the stimulatory effect of hypovolaemia.

Intracellular/extracellular Distribution
The intracellular water content varies with, and is controlled by, the
extracellular tonicity (*Fig.* 2.2), i.e. an increased extracellular tonicity draws water

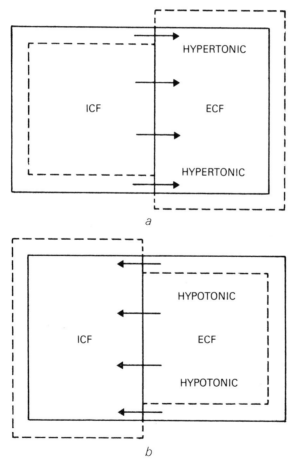

a

b

Fig. 2.2. Body water distribution in response to (*a*) hypertonic extracellular fluid, (*b*) hypotonic extracellular fluid. ICF, intracellular fluid;
ECF, extracellular fluid; ———, original volume; – – –, volume after fluid
redistribution.

out of the cells producing cellular dehydration, whilst a decreased extracellular tonicity allows water to flow into cells, causing cellular overhydration.

As the tonicity of the extracellular fluid is related to the sodium concentration (sodium salts comprise most of the extracellular solute) it follows that the extracellular volume is dependent on the extracellular sodium content, i.e.

1.   ↑ Extracellular sodium content ⟶ ↑ extracellular tonicity ⟶
  a.   ↑ Thirst (increased water intake)
  b.   ↑ ADH secretion (increased renal water reabsorption)
  c.   Water shift from intracellular to extracellular compartment
        a + b + c ⟶ ↑ extracellular volume (and ↓ intracellular volume)
2.   ↓ Extracellular sodium content ⟶ ↓ extracellular tonicity ⟶
  a.   ↓ Thirst (decreased water intake)
  b.   ↓ ADH secretion (increased renal water loss)
  c.   Water shift from extracellular to intracellular compartment
        a + b + c ⟶ ↓ extracellular volume

Therefore it can be said that *total body sodium* (major portion of sodium is in the extracellular fluid) *determines* the *extracellular volume* and, as shall be seen below, the *extracellular volume controls* renal sodium excretion and therefore the *extracellular sodium content.*

Sodium Homeostasis

Distribution (*Table* 2.3)
Some 80–90% of the total body sodium is located in the extracellular compartment, where it influences the volume of the extracellular fluid.

Table 2.3. Body distribution of sodium

	Total sodium (mmol)	Concentration (mmol/l)
Total body	~3150	—
Intracellular	~250	~10
Extracellular	~2900	~140
Plasma	~400	~140

Input
The adult daily intake of sodium, from a Western diet, is of the order of 100–200 mmol/d (6–12 g). Sodium, unlike water, the intake of which is regulated by a thirst mechanism, does not appear to have a similar control centre for intake. Instead, sodium intake appears to be dictated by habit rather than need.

Output
In order to maintain a constant total body sodium content, any losses from the body (sweat, faeces, urine) have to balance the dietary input. Although a small

amount of sodium is lost in the sweat (<10 mmol/d) and faeces (<10 mmol/d) the major organ controlling excretion, and therefore sodium balance, is the kidney.

Renal Sodium Excretion

Each day approximately 25 000 mmol of sodium are filtered by the glomeruli but due to renal tubular reabsorption less than 1% of this amount (100–200 mmol/d) appears in the urine.

Proximal Tubule

Approximately 50–70% of the filtered sodium is reabsorbed in this section of the nephron by an energy-dependent process. Water is reabsorbed iso-osmotically with the sodium, so that the fluid entering the loop of Henle has an osmolality similar to that of the plasma.

Loop of Henle

In the thick ascending limb (diluting segment) 20–30% of the filtered sodium is reabsorbed. This section of the nephron is unique in that:

a.   Sodium ions are thought to be reabsorbed as a consequence of active chloride ion reabsorption.

b.   The tubule cells are impermeable to water, which results in dilute urine (50–100 mmol/kg) entering the distal nephron. The sodium reabsorbed in this area enters, and is trapped in, the renal medullary interstitial tissue. This increases the medullary tonicity and thus allows reabsorption of water from the dilute urine of the collecting ducts (providing ADH is present).

Distal Convoluted Tubule

Approximately 5–10% of filtered sodium is reabsorbed in this segment, which is under the influence of aldosterone (*see below*).

Collecting Ducts

In the context of sodium balance the collecting ducts play the role of a 'fine tuner', i.e. this portion of the nephron, under the influence of aldosterone and possibly natriuretic hormone (*see below*), can increase or decrease the amount of sodium reabsorbed in order to maintain the delicate balance required between dietary intake and renal excretion.

Control of Renal Sodium Excretion

Sodium balance is mainly dependent on renal sodium excretion rate and this rate is determined in the first instance by the intravascular volume (i.v.v.), i.e.

$$\uparrow \text{i.v.v.} \longrightarrow \uparrow \text{renal sodium excretion}$$

and

$$\downarrow \text{i.v.v.} \longrightarrow \downarrow \text{renal sodium excretion}$$

At the kidney level the excretion of sodium is influenced by three factors:

Glomerular filtration rate (GFR)—'first factor'
Aldosterone—'second factor'
Natriuretic hormone—'third factor'

GFR

The amount of sodium presented to the tubules depends on the amount filtered by the glomeruli (approximately 25 000 mmol/d in a normal adult). There is some evidence that the GFR influences the tubular reabsorption of sodium (e.g. ↓ GFR is associated with ↑ tubular reabsorption and low urine sodium output). However the mechanism and its importance in renal sodium excretion is unclear.

Aldosterone

If the renal blood flow (RBF) is decreased (e.g. dehydration, shock) there is an increased renal secretion of renin with a consequent increased production of angiotensin II and secretion of aldosterone (*see* p. 240 for a full description). The reverse also applies (i.e. ↑ RBF ⟶ ↓ aldosterone). Aldosterone acts on the distal nephron (distal convoluted tubules, collecting ducts) and causes increased sodium reabsorption, it also increases K^+ (and H^+) secretion by the distal convoluted tubule but although there is a loose relationship between Na^+ reabsorption and K^+ secretion they are not exchanged in a 1 : 1 ratio. For example, it has been shown that Na^+ is mainly reabsorbed in the proximal part of the distal tubule, whereas K^+ is secreted mainly in the distal portion. Also the amount of sodium reabsorbed is usually greater than the amount of K^+ plus H^+ secreted.

'Third Factor'

It has been shown experimentally that there is a third factor, independent of GFR and aldosterone, controlling Na^+ excretion. This factor has been termed by some investigators the natriuretic hormone. It is thought to be secreted by the central nervous system in response to an increase in the extracellular fluid volume (or i.v.v.), and to act on the proximal convoluted tubule and/or the collecting ducts, causing a decrease in sodium reabsorption.

Plasma Sodium Concentration

The tonicity, and therefore the sodium concentration of the extracellular fluid, is dependent on the external water balance, i.e.

Positive balance ⟶ ↓ $[Na^+]$

and

Negative balance ⟶ ↑ $[Na^+]$

Negative Water Balance/Hypernatraemia

The most important defence against the development of hypernatraemia is thirst. Even in the absence of ADH (e.g. diabetes insipidus) a patient can still drink sufficient water (up to 20 litres daily) to maintain a normal sodium concentration.

It therefore follows that a negative water balance resulting in hypernatraemia is nearly always due to decreased intake rather than an increased output.

Causes of a decreased intake are:
1. Too old, too young, too sick to drink
2. Obstructive lesions of the gullet
3. Access to water denied
4. Lesions of the thirst mechanism

Positive Water Balance/Hyponatraemia

Since an adult can drink up to 20 litres of water a day, and still excrete sufficient water via the kidney to maintain normonatraemia, it follows that positive water balance will usually only occur if there is a defect in renal excretion. Decreased renal excretion of water, and a positive balance producing hyponatraemia, may occur in the following conditions:
1. ↑ ADH secretion despite hypotonicity of ECF
   a. Hypovolaemia
   b. Drugs (*see* p. 35)
   c. Stress (physical, e.g. surgical operations; psychogenic, e.g. severe depression, schizophrenia)
   d. Syndrome of inappropriate secretion of ADH (SIADH—*see* p. 41)
2. Renal failure

Hypernatraemia

Consequences

Extracellular hypertonicity, due to any cause, is accompanied by cell water loss to the extracellular space until there is osmotic equilibrium between the two compartments. The resultant cellular contraction probably explains many of the clinical features associated with hypertonicity (lethargy, coma, muscle weakness, thirst, etc.). The brain is particularly vulnerable to shrinkage because of its vascular attachment to the rigid bony calvarium (i.e. haemorrhage may occur if the brain shrinkage is of a sufficient degree to tear away these vascular attachments).

There is evidence from both clinical and experimental studies that after initial shrinkage the brain will return to its normal size within hours or days, depending on the material causing the extracellular hypertonicity (glucose—hours; sodium—days). This rehydration of the brain is due to an increase in the intracellular tonicity. About 50% of this gain in tonicity is due to an increased level of intracellular sodium ions in the case of hypernatraemia and a rise in glucose level in the case of hyperglycaemia. The rest of the increased tonicity results from substances of uncertain origin and composition (some are amino acids, e.g. taurine). These undefined substances have been called 'idiogenic osmols'.

It is not known how rapidly these idiogenic osmols disappear following rehydration, and therefore there is a danger of cerebral oedema if the patient's extracellular fluid is rapidly normalized by the administration of hypotonic solutions, i.e. hypertonicity should be corrected slowly over 1–2 days.

The clinical features of hypernatraemia and intracellular dehydration are usually vague and undefined, but may include thirst, clouding of the consciousness, muscle weakness and convulsions. Other features will depend on the initial illness and the volume status of the patient. If there has been fluid loss the features of dehydration may be present (dry mucous membranes, decreased tissue turgor, sunken eyes, tachycardia, hypotension, decreased urine output, etc.). On the other hand, in the case of salt gain, features of fluid overload may be apparent (raised jugular venous pressure, pulmonary oedema).

Causes

It is important to realize that hypernatraemia does not necessarily indicate extracellular sodium excess. Except in the rare case of pure salt gain hypernatraemia usually occurs in association with a depletion of both extracellular water and sodium, the water loss being relatively greater than that of sodium. As stated above, hypernatraemia usually only occurs if the patient's water intake is inadequate, i.e. too old, too young, or too sick to drink, or the patient has no access to water or there is an inadequate intake due to a lesion of the thirst centre.

For the purpose of diagnosis and evaluation it is convenient to classify hypernatraemia (*Table* 2.4) under the following three headings: Pure Water Depletion; Hypotonic Fluid Depletion; Salt Gain.

Table 2.4. Causes of hypernatraemia

Pure water depletion
   Extrarenal loss
      inadequate water intake
      mucocutaneous loss: fever, thyrotoxicosis
   Renal loss
      diabetes insipidus: neurogenic, nephrogenic

Hypotonic fluid loss
   Extrarenal loss
      gastrointestinal: vomiting, diarrhoea
      skin: excessive sweating
   Renal loss
      osmotic diuresis: glucose, urea

Salt gain
   Iatrogenic: i.v. $NaHCO_3$, i.v. hypertonic saline
   Salt ingestion: intentional, accidental ingestion of sea water
      mineralocorticoid excess syndromes (p. 243)

Diagnosis/Evaluation

From the pathophysiological and clinical aspect there are important differences between the above three groups:

Pure Water Depletion

The cell membranes are freely permeable to water, and therefore in pure water depletion the water will be lost from the intracellular and extracellular compartments in proportion to their respective volumes, i.e. if we assume a total body water of 42 litres, an intracellular volume of 23 litres, an extracellular volume of 19 litres and a plasma volume of 3 litres, then a loss of 3 litres of pure water will result in:

a.   Intracellular loss of: $23/42 \times 3000 = 1643$ ml
b.   Extracellular loss of: $19/42 \times 3000 = 1357$ ml
c.   Plasma loss of: $3/42 \times 3000 = 214$ ml
d.   Plasma tonicity increase of: $\sim 214/3000 = \sim 7\%$

Pure water depletion therefore results in an increased extracellular tonicity (and sodium concentration) but a minimal decrease in plasma volume, i.e. peripheral circulatory collapse due to hypovolaemia is uncommon unless the volume loss is severe.

Hypotonic Fluid Loss

Hypotonic fluid can be considered to consist of two components:
1.   Isotonic fluid
2.   Pure water

For example, 3 litres of fluid with a tonicity of one-third of the extracellular fluid can be thought of as:
1.   1000 ml of isotonic fluid
2.   2000 ml of pure water

Therefore, using the above example a loss of 3 litres of fluid with one-third the tonicity of extracellular fluid will result in:
1.   Loss of 2000 ml of pure water $\longrightarrow$
  a.   Intracellular loss of: $23/42 \times 2000 = 1095$ ml
  b.   Extracellular loss of: $19/42 \times 2000 = 905$ ml
  c.   Plasma loss of: $3/42 \times 2000 = 143$ ml
2.   Isotonic fluid will be lost from the extracellular compartment only and causes no change in the intracellular : extracellular osmotic gradient. Thus a loss of 1000 ml of isotonic fluid results in:
  a.   Extracellular loss of: 1000 ml
  b.   Plasma loss of: $3/19 \times 1000 = 158$ ml

Therefore $(1) + (2) \longrightarrow$
  a.   Intracellular loss of: 1095 ml
  b.   Extracellular loss of: 1905 ml
  c.   Plasma loss of: 301 ml
  d.   Plasma tonicity (and [Na$^+$]) increase of: $\sim 143/3000 = 4 \cdot 7\%$

Thus a patient with hypotonic fluid loss (compared with a pure water loss of the same volume) will have:
1.   Smaller increase in plasma tonicity (and [Na$^+$])
2.   Larger decrease in plasma volume

That is, these patients, as well as having hypertonicity, will tend towards vascular collapse because of the depleted extracellular volume.

Note: If a patient loses 3 litres of isotonic fluid from the extracellular space only, the decrease in plasma volume will be:

$$3/19 \times 3000 = 474 \, \text{ml}.$$

Salt Gain

In pure salt gain the increase in extracellular sodium results in withdrawal of water from the intracellular compartment, and therefore extracellular expansion and cellular dehydration. The extracellular expansion may result in pulmonary oedema but in most cases it is accompanied by a diuresis which will mitigate the effects of the extracellular expansion.

From the above examples it can be seen that hypernatraemia can be further classified according to the patient's volume status:
1.   Hypovolaemic = hypotonic fluid loss
2.   Hypervolaemic = salt gain
3.   Normal or near normal volume (euvolaemic) = pure water depletion

The *evaluation* of a patient with hypernatraemia is conveniently approached in the following manner (*see also Fig.* 2.3).

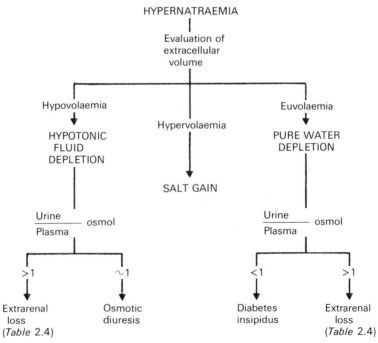

Fig. 2.3. Suggested scheme for the evaluation of hypernatraemia.

1. Suspect type of disturbance from the history, e.g. vomiting suggests hypotonic fluid loss
2. Evaluate patient's extracellular volume, i.e. hypervolaemic, hypovolaemic, euvolaemic
3. Collect a spot urine and estimate the urine/plasma osmolality ratio. This step is usually not necessary as sufficient information for evaluation can be obtained from the clinical picture

Principles of Management

The following discussion concentrates on the problem of hypernatraemia and hypertonicity. However, patients present with a variety of disease processes, and some of these may require intervention before applying the therapeutic principles outlined below. It is important, when treating fluid and electrolyte disorders with intravenous infusions, to check regularly the plasma analytes. It is better to do this too often than too late.

Pure Water Depletion

Water loss without loss of sodium is a fairly rare condition as most patients with the disorders listed under 'pure water depletion' in *Table* 2.4 will also have some depletion of their body sodium (e.g. continual urinary loss). It is probably better to refer to this condition as 'predominant water depletion'.

Management depends to a large extent on the clinical condition of the patient. If the patient can tolerate water orally then tap water can be given to drink. Otherwise an intravenous infusion of a hypotonic solution, e.g. 5% glucose or 4% glucose in one-fifth normal saline should be given. The glucose content of these solutions is metabolized to water and carbon dioxide on entering the body cells, so such an infusion is tantamount to giving pure water or one-fifth normal saline. (Normal saline in the context of intravenous fluids refers to isotonic saline or 0·9% saline solution which has an osmolality of about 300 mmol/kg.)

The major problem with intravenous infusions is 'how much, how soon?' A useful rule of thumb is to estimate roughly the water deficit and give 50% of this over the first 6–12 h. The rest can be given slowly over the next 1–2 days while keeping in mind the possibility of developing cerebral oedema (*see* 'idiogenic osmols', p. 23). The calculated normal daily requirements of fluid (to replace losses from skin, lungs, urine, etc.) should be added to the above volumes.

Calculate the water deficit as follows:

1. Assume
    a. Total body water (TBW) = 60% of body wt
    b. Total body solute has not changed, i.e. TBW × plasma osmolality (Posmol) is constant, then

$$TBW(normal) \times Posmol(normal) = TBW(new) \times Posmol(new)$$

2. As plasma sodium concentration. $P[Na^+]$, is directly related to the osmolality, then $P[Na^+]$ can be substituted for Posmol (assume normal

$P[Na^+] = 140\,mmol/l$), therefore

$$TBW\,(new) = \frac{TBW\,(normal) \times P[Na^+]\,(normal)}{P[Na^+]\,(new)}$$

$$= 0\cdot6 \times body\,wt\,(kg) \times 140/P[Na^+]\,(new)\,litres$$

and

water deficit $=$ TBW (normal) $-$ TBW (new) litres

Hypotonic Fluid Depletion

In this situation there is a significant extracellular volume depletion as well as hypernatraemia. Management should be aimed, in the first instance, at preventing peripheral vascular collapse rather than at reducing the hypertonicity. Normal saline (0·9%), or, if necessary, whole blood or plasma, should be infused rapidly to restore the circulating volume and preserve renal function. After this has been achieved hypotonic fluid replacement aimed at correcting the hypernatraemia, in the same way as for pure water depletion described above, should be instituted.

Salt Gain

Treatment of this condition depends on its severity. If the extracellular volume expansion is severe and there is a danger of pulmonary oedema, it may be necessary to remove salt with a potent diuretic (e.g. frusemide). In this case the diuretic will cause the excretion of more water relative to sodium and thus exaggerate the hypertonicity, so at the same time 'hypotonic fluid' (5% glucose) should be infused. In severe and difficult cases (e.g. renal failure) dialysis may be required.

Case Examples

Pure Water Depletion: Inadequate intake

A 72-year-old female who lived alone was found in an unconscious state at home, 2 days after a cerebrovascular accident. On admission to hospital she had a dry tongue, decreased tissue turgor, a blood pressure of 140/80 and a pulse rate of 100. Her admission plasma electrolyte values and those on the following days after infusion of 3 litres of 5% glucose over the first 12 h, and then 3 litres of 4% glucose in one-fifth normal saline daily are shown below.

Date		12/2	13/2	15/2	
Time (h)		1700	0800	0800	
Plasma	Na	169	156	144 mmol/l	(132–144)
	K	3·4	3·2	3·3 mmol/l	(3·2–4·8)
	Cl	124	120	105 mmol/l	(98–108)
	HCO_3	28	27	27 mmol/l	(23–33)
	Urea	37·5	26·0	9·0 mmol/l	(3·0–8·0)
	Creat	0·28	0·24	0·15 mmol/l	(0·06–0·12)
	Osmol	392	344	302 mmol/kg	(281–295)
Urine	Na	<10	—	30 mmol/l	
	Osmol	670	—	280 mmol/kg	

Comment
This patient was predominantly water depleted due to water deprivation for about 2 days during hot climatic conditions. The admission electrolytes show many of the features of this condition:
1. Hypernatraemia and hypertonicity
2. Moderate to severe hypernatraemia without severe hypovolaemia (absence of severe peripheral vascular collapse)
3. Increased plasma levels of creatinine and urea: due to hypovolaemia, which results in a decreased renal blood flow and a decreased GFR (p. 46)
4. A high (>1) urine:plasma osmolality ratio indicating an appropriate concentration of the urine in response to increased secretion of ADH
    The low urinary sodium level (<10 mmol/l) and the high urinary osmolality (urine osmol > plasma osmol) indicates intact renal tubular function.
    Her response to the treatment regimen has been satisfactory in that there is a slow decrease in the extracellular tonicity and improved renal function (decrease in the plasma creatinine level). The fall in the urinary osmolality indicates that the rehydration has been successful and that the patient is beginning to dilute her urine in response to the decrease in the extracellular tonicity.

Pure Water Depletion: Diabetes insipidus
A 61-year-old man was admitted to hospital following a motor vehicle accident in which he sustained a fracture to the base of his skull. The fluid balance chart over the first day in hospital indicated a negative balance with a urine output of some 5 litres. Traumatic diabetes insipidus was suspected and his fluid intake was increased. Two days later his plasma sodium concentration began to fall and his urine output decreased. He died the following day.

Date		23/12	24/12	26/12	
Time (h)		1200	1100	0800	
Plasma	Na	140	164	124 mmol/l	(132–144)
	K	3·4	3·8	4·7 mmol/l	(3·2–4·8)
	Cl	105	124	97 mmol/l	(98–108)
	HCO$_3$	25	24	19 mmol/l	(23–33)
	Urea	4·0	6·1	4·7 mmol/l	(3·0–8·0)
	Creat	0·11	0·13	0·07 mmol/l	(0·06–0·12)
	Osmol	—	350	261 mmol/kg	(281–295)
Urine	Na	—	<5	65 mmol/l	
	Osmol	—	144	842 mmol/kg	

Comment
The diagnosis of diabetes insipidus made on 24/12 was based on:
1. Negative fluid balance
2. Plasma hypertonicity and hypernatraemia
3. A urine osmolality which was inappropriately low in the presence of a high plasma osmolality (urine:plasma = <1)
    Some patients with traumatic diabetes insipidus go through three phases of fluid and electrolyte disturbance:

1. An early phase of diabetes insipidus with copious dilute urine produced due to the sudden lack of ADH
2. A second phase in which there is a release of stored ADH, resulting in fluid retention, extracellular hypotonicity (and hyponatraemia) and an inappropriately concentrated urine (urine : plasma osmolality = > 1)
3. A third phase in which there is a return of the diabetes insipidus; this usually resolves but may be permanent

This patient's plasma and urine analyte concentrations on 26/12 suggests that the second phase occurred just prior to death.

Hypotonic Fluid Loss: Vomiting

A 56-year-old male was admitted to hospital after 3 days of vomiting due to pyloric obstruction (malignant). He looked severely ill, 'dry', had a pulse rate of 120 and a supine blood pressure of 90/40. He was rehydrated over the first day with 5 litres of normal saline and on the following day with 3 litres of 5% glucose. Potassium chloride was added to the infusion solutions.

Date		24/10	25/10	26/10	
Plasma	Na	154	148	143 mmol/l	(132–144)
	K	2·8	3·2	4·4 mmol/l	(3·2–4·8)
	Cl	96	89	105 mmol/l	(98–108)
	HCO$_3$	>40	>40	30 mmol/l	(23–33)
	Urea	6·9	6·0	5·6 mmol/l	(3·0–8·0)
	Creat	0·22	0·14	0·10 mmol/l	(0·06–0·12)
	Osmol	331	—	298 mmol/kg	(281–295)
Urine	Na	100	—	— mmol/l	
	Osmol	666	419	320 mmol/kg	

Comment

As noted earlier, for a given level of hypernatraemia, a hypotonic fluid loss results in a more severe degree of extracellular hypovolaemia than does pure water loss. This patient's tachycardia and low blood pressure indicates a moderate to severe hypovolaemia.

The vomiting in this patient, which was from above the pylorus, resulted in loss of hydrogen ion (gastric juice) and therefore a metabolic alkalosis ($\uparrow$ [HCO$_3$$^-$], p. 111), consequently a massive amount of bicarbonate is being presented to the renal tubules by the glomerular filtrate, which floods the bicarbonate reabsorptive mechanism causing some to be lost in the urine. The excreted bicarbonate ions carry sodium ions out with them and result in a high 'spot' urinary sodium concentration (> 10 mmol/l). Thus a high urinary sodium concentration in the presence of hypovolaemia and a raised plasma creatinine level does not necessarily mean acute tubular necrosis (p. 187). In the above case the high urine : plasma osmolality ratio (> 1) indicates that tubular function is intact.

The hypokalaemia in this patient represents potassium depletion due to loss in (*a*) the vomitus (minimal), and (*b*) the urine (p. 209).

Treatment of the above fluid and electrolyte disorder involves fairly rapid re-expansion of the depleted extracellular volume with normal saline, and then a relatively slow normalization of the hypernatraemia with hypotonic fluids. Potassium should be added to the infusions at an early stage of rehydration to prevent the development of severe hypokalaemia.

Hypotonic Fluid Loss: Osmotic diuresis

A 73-year-old female was admitted to hospital in a semi-comatosed state with a 6-week history of weight loss, polyuria and malaise. On admission she was clinically dehydrated, had a supine blood pressure of 95/50 and a pulse rate of 130. A diagnosis of hyperosmolar diabetic coma was made on the basis of the history and admission plasma biochemistry values. She was treated in the first instance with an infusion of normal saline and insulin (2 units/h). When the plasma glucose fell below 20 mmol/l she was changed to an infusion of 4% glucose in one-fifth normal saline.

Date		11/5	12/5	13/5	
Time (h)		2100	0400	0800	
Plasma	Na	158	170	143 mmol/l	(132–144)
	K	4·3	4·1	4·2 mmol/l	(3·2–4·8)
	Cl	120	>130	110 mmol/l	(98–108)
	HCO_3	28	27	27 mmol/l	(23–33)
	Urea	16·0	12·0	5·0 mmol/l	(3·0–8·0)
	Creat	0·16	0·11	0·08 mmol/l	(0·06–0·12)
	Glu	39·0	8·1	6·8 mmol/l	(3·0–5·5)
	Osmol	379	—	307 mmol/kg	(281–295)

Comment

Hyperosmolar (non-ketotic) diabetic coma often occurs in elderly people who have not been previously diagnosed as diabetic. This condition has an insidious onset over a period of days or weeks with an increasing plasma glucose level and an osmotic diuresis (renal loss of sodium and water). As the illness proceeds these patients often lapse into coma and, with the subsequent fall in their fluid intake, hypernatraemia occurs.

In this disorder the major contribution to extracellular hypertonicity is made by glucose, which has the effect of drawing water out of the cells and trapping it in the extracellular compartment. Thus the normal constituents of plasma, including sodium, will be diluted. When insulin is administered the glucose that subsequently enters the cells will be accompanied by water, resulting in extracellular water depletion and a further rise in the plasma sodium concentration.

The true plasma sodium concentration (i.e. the plasma $[Na^+]$ which would prevail if the glucose level was instantly returned to normal and the water moved back into the cells) can be roughly calculated from the following empirically derived formula:

$$\text{True plasma } [Na^+] = \text{present plasma } [Na^+] + \text{glucose (mmol/l)}/4$$

In the above case the true plasma $[Na^+]$ would be:

$$158 \text{ mmol/l} + 39/4 = 168 \text{ mmol/l}$$

This calculated value is very near the value found in the patient on 12/5 (5 h after the commencement of insulin infusion). N.B. There are a number of formulae available for the estimation of the 'true' [Na$^+$] value all of which are empirically derived and result in similar corrected values.

These patients usually require very little insulin to lower their blood glucose levels, and if too much is given too early a severe hypernatraemia may ensue. In these patients the hypovolaemia and hypertonicity should be treated with infusions of normal saline before any insulin is given because a reduction in the extracellular tonicity is often associated with improved endogenous insulin release.

Salt Gain: Intravenous sodium bicarbonate

A female aged 48 years was admitted to hospital after an overdose of salicylate (plasma level on admission was 55 mg/dl). An intravenous infusion of sodium bicarbonate was administered in an attempt to render the urine alkaline in order to increase the renal excretion of salicylate. She received approximately 200 mmol (as a 8·4% solution) of sodium bicarbonate in the 3 h prior to venepuncture for plasma electrolytes at 0700 h on 27/7.

Date		26/7	27/7	
Time (h)		1230	0700	
Plasma	Na	144	149 mmol/l	(132–144)
	K	3·9	3·5 mmol/l	(3·2–4·8)
	Cl	104	102 mmol/l	(98–108)
	HCO$_3$	20	38 mmol/l	(23–33)
	Urea	15·0	11·0 mmol/l	(3·0–8·0)
	Creat	0·22	0·09 mmol/l	(0·06–0·12)
Urine	Na	<10	75 mmol/l	

Comment

One of the complications associated with a rapid sodium bicarbonate infusion is that of sodium overload and increased extracellular volume (withdrawal of water from the cells). Although this patient's plasma [Na$^+$] and extracellular volume increased with bicarbonate therapy she did not develop severe symptoms of overload (raised jugular venous pressure, pulmonary oedema), and she rapidly excreted the excess sodium in her urine (i.e. sodium diuresis). It is important to remember that in sodium diuresis due to salt overload (or during diuretic therapy) the urinary water loss is relatively greater than the sodium loss (urinary concentration of sodium is always less than the plasma concentration). Therefore, unless the patient takes in extra hypotonic fluid during this process, the hypernatraemia and extracellular tonicity will increase in severity.

Salt Gain: Mineralocorticoid excess

A 55-year-old male with a known carcinoma of the bronchus presented with muscle weakness, tiredness and general malaise. On examination he showed an Addisonian type of pigmentation, but there was no evidence of dehydration other than a dry, coated tongue. A random plasma cortisol level was requested. His results on admission were as follows:

Plasma	Na	148 mmol/l	(132–144)
	K	1·8 mmol/l	(3·2–4·8)
	Cl	95 mmol/l	(98–108)
	HCO_3	>40 mmol/l	(23–33)
	Urea	6·5 mmol/l	(3·0–8·0)
	Creat	0·08 mmol/l	(0·06–0·12)
	Osmol	295 mmol/kg	(281–295)
	Cortisol	1665 nmol/l	(170–690)

Subsequently the patient's plasma ACTH level was found to be elevated and a diagnosis of the ectopic ACTH syndrome was made.

Comment
In this condition there is excessive mineralocorticoid activity due either to the mineralocorticoid action of the massive amount of circulating cortisol, or to an increased secretion of deoxycorticosterone from the hyperplastic adrenal cortex (p. 248).

Mineralocorticoids increase sodium reabsorption (and K^+ secretion) in the distal renal tubule; this in turn increases the extracellular sodium content and indirectly the extracellular volume (i.e. ↑ sodium reabsorption ⟶ ↑ extracellular $[Na^+]$ ⟶ ↑ extracellular tonicity ⟶ ↑ADH secretion ⟶ ↑ renal water reabsorption).

As water is retained in parallel with sodium the plasma sodium concentration usually does not increase to hypernatraemic levels, but is usually at the upper limit of, or just above, the reference range. However, should there be inadequate fluid intake the patient will readily become hypernatraemic (this was probable in this case as this patient's plasma $[Na^+]$ fell to 142 mmol/l after a short stay in hospital).

This patient's muscle weakness was due to the potassium deficiency (he responded to potassium and spironolactone therapy), and the pigmentation is due to the circulating β-lipotropin (secreted by the tumour along with ACTH) which is thought to have melanocyte-stimulating properties.

Hyponatraemia

Consequences
Sodium salts comprise most of the extracellular solute, and for this reason hypotonicity of the extracellular fluid is always associated with hyponatraemia. On the other hand, hyponatraemia is not always associated with hypotonicity, and may occur in the presence of a normal or even high extracellular tonicity (e.g. hyperglycaemia).

In the case of extracellular hypotonicity, water flows into the cells, causing cellular overhydration (oedema). The organ most at risk of damage is the brain as it is enclosed in a rigid bony cavity, and the increased water content may result in a dangerous increase in intracranial pressure.

The clinical features of extracellular hypotonicity depend on the aetiology of the condition and on the magnitude and rapidity of the decrease in tonicity. In the acute situation, which is a medical emergency with a high mortality rate, symptoms may begin to develop when the plasma sodium concentration has fallen to below 125 mmol/l. If the hypotonicity develops slowly over a period of days rather than hours, symptoms may be absent until the plasma sodium falls below about 115–117 mmol/l.

The clinical picture that is associated with hypotonicity and cerebral oedema is vague and non-specific. There may be nausea, vomiting, muscle weakness, lethargy and delirium. In severe cases coma and seizures have been described, but often the only clue may be impaired mentation.

Causes

Hyponatraemia does not always indicate a depletion of body as it can also occur in association with both a normal and an increased total body sodium.

If the occasional case of pseudohyponatraemia (*see below*) is excluded, hyponatraemia reflects a relative excess of extracellular water over total extracellular sodium (i.e. sodium dilution). This may occur in two situations:

1. Increased extracellular water as a result of an increased extracellular solute (e.g. hyperglycaemia) so that there has been a dilution of plasma constituents by a movement of water from the intracellular space to the extracellular compartment
2. Positive water balance
    In the case of positive water balance the relative excess of extracellular water is usually due to decreased renal excretion, rather than increased input.

The inability to excrete a dilute urine in the presence of hyptonicity may be due to:

1. Decreased delivery of fluid to the renal diluting segments, e.g. hypovolaemia causing an increased proximal tubular reabsorption of salt and water
2. Defective function of the diluting segment (ascending limb of loop of Henle), e.g. loop diuretics (frusemide), renal disease
3. Continued secretion of ADH despite hypotonicity of the extracellular fluid:
    a. Hypovolaemia
    b. Stress
    c. Drugs (*Table* 2.5)
    d. SIADH (syndrome of inappropriate secretion of ADH)

From the evaluation and management point of view patients with hyponatraemia (*Table* 2.6) can be divided into:

1. Pseudohyponatraemia
2. Hyponatraemia with plasma hypertonicity
3. Hyponatraemia with plasma hypotonicity

Table 2.5. Drugs associated with hyponatraemia

Increased ADH Secretion
  Hypnotics: barbiturates
  Narcotics: morphine
  Hypoglycaemics: chlorpropamide, tolbutamide
  Anticonvulsants: carbamazepine
  Antineoplastic: vincristine, vinblastine, cyclophosphamide
  Miscellaneous: clofibrate, isoprenaline, nicotine derivatives

Potentiation of ADH Action
  Chlorpropamide
  Paracetamol
  Indomethacin

Diuretics
  Thiazides
  Frusemide

Table 2.6. Classification of hyponatraemia

Pseudohyponatraemia
  Hyperlipidaemia
  Hyperproteinaemia

Hyponatraemia and plasma hypertonicity
  Hyperglycaemia

Hyponatraemia and plasma hypotonicity
  Hypovolaemia (low ECV and low TB_{Na^+})
    Extrarenal:
      Gastrointestinal (vomiting, diarrhoea)
    Renal:
      Skin (burns)
      Diuretic therapy
      Salt-losing nephritis
      Addison's disease
  Euvolaemia (normal, or near-normal, ECV and TB_{Na^+})
    Acute water overload
      Increased fluid intake in presence of:
        Hypovolaemia: haemorrhage, burns
        Drugs: *see Table* 2.5
        Stress: post-surgery, psychogenic
        Endocrine: hypothyroid, cortisol deficiency
        Renal insufficiency
    Chronic water overload
      SIADH (p. 42)
      Drugs (*Table* 2.5)
      Chronic renal failure
      Endocrine: hypothyroid, glucocorticoid deficiency
  Oedematous states (increased ECV and TB_{Na^+})
    Congestive cardiac failure
    Cirrhosis of the liver
    Nephrotic syndrome

ECV: extracellular volume; TB_{Na^+}: total body sodium.

Pseudohyponatraemia

Sodium ions are present only in the plasma water which makes up some 93% of normal plasma. However, the concentration of sodium in plasma is measured in an aliquot of whole plasma and therefore the concentration is expressed in terms of plasma volume (i.e. mmol per litre of whole plasma). If the percentage of water present in plasma is decreased (e.g. increased plasma lipid or protein) then the amount of sodium present in an aliquot of plasma will also be decreased, even though its concentration in plasma water may be normal. This pseudohyponatraemia can be seen in hyperlipidaemia (plasma triglyceride > 50 mmol/l) and very occasionally in hyperproteinaemia (total plasma proteins > 150 g/l). The measurement of plasma osmolality is helpful in determining the sodium content of the plasma water. If the measured osmolality is normal, and providing the plasma urea and glucose levels are not high, then the plasma water sodium concentration is most likely to be normal. Pseudohyponatraemia is also an example of an osmolar gap, i.e. measured osmolality much greater than calculated osmolality. For example, lipaemic plasma from a patient with a primary hyperlipidaemia.

Plasma	Na	119 mmol/l	(132–144)
	K	4·2 mmol/l	(3·2–4·8)
	Cl	86 mmol/l	(98–108)
	HCO_3	21 mmol/l	(23–33)
	Urea	6·0 mmol/l	(3·0–8·0)
	Glu	7·0 mmol/l	(3·0–5·5)
	Cholesterol	19 mmol/l	(2·5–7·2)
	Triglyceride	5·5 mmol/l	(0·3–1·7)
	Osmol	296 mmol/kg	(281–295)

Calculated osmolality = 251 mmol/kg

Diagnosis/evaluation

A logical approach to the diagnosis and evaluation of a patient with hyponatraemia is suggested below (*see also* Fig. 2.4). However, in many cases the diagnosis will be readily evident from the clinical picture and an inspection of the plasma and urine biochemistry results.

1. Suspect the disturbance from the clinical presentation
2. Has the patient pseudohyponatraemia? i.e. normal plasma osmolality associated with a severe hyperlipidaemia (plasma triglycerides > 50 mmol/l) or hyperproteinaemia (total plasma proteins > 150 g/l)
3. Is the patient's extracellular fluid hypertonic? e.g. high plasma levels of glucose, mannitol
4. If the answer to (2) and (3) is 'no' then what is the patient's extracellular volume status—hypovolaemia (dehydration), euvolaemia, hypervolaemia (oedema)?
5. Take a spot urine and estimate:
    a. Urine : plasma osmolality ratio
    b. Urinary sodium concentration

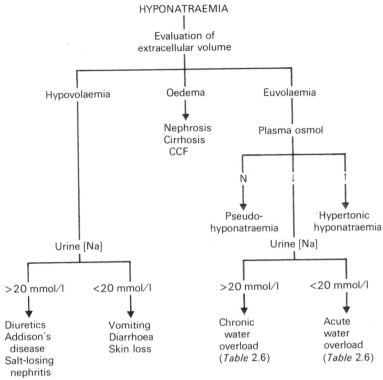

Fig. 2.4. Suggested scheme for the evaluation of hyponatraemia.

Principles of Management

Patients with hyponatraemia, regardless of its cause, can present with a wide range of diseases and the treatment of these may have to take precedence over treatment directed at an electrolyte disorder. The specific therapy for hyponatraemia depends on the immediate cause of the low sodium concentration, and thus it is especially important to understand the pathophysiology of the process before attempting to manipulate the patient's electrolytes.

Pseudohyponatraemia

The importance of this condition lies in its quick recognition, so that it does not confuse the diagnosis, and treatment, of the primary disorder.

Hypertonic Hyponatraemia

In practice the majority of patients with this condition have either diabetes mellitus or been infused with hypertonic glucose solutions (e.g. parenteral nutrition). It is important to calculate the 'true' plasma sodium concentration (*see below*), as this figure will indicate what the sodium level will be after the blood glucose concentration has fallen to normal, e.g. after insulin therapy. If the calculation indicates that hypernatraemia will occur then a hypotonic fluid infusion may be required following restitution of the circulating volume. As most of these patients are volume depleted (due to osmotic diuresis) they will initially require volume repletion with normal saline or other volume expanders.

Hypotonic Hyponatraemia with Low ECV and TB_{Na^+}

The main problem in the majority of these cases is that of hypovolaemia (i.e. a compromised circulating volume) and not the hypotonicity. Such patients should initially be infused fairly rapidly with normal saline until the plasma volume depletion is corrected (i.e. until urinary output has increased and pulse rate and blood pressure have been returned towards normal). Administration of hypertonic saline solutions to correct the hypotonicity is rarely required because with the normal saline infusion and improved renal function the electrolyte picture usually returns towards normal.

Hypotonic Hyponatraemia with Normal ECV and TB_{Na^+}

1. Acute Water Overload

In cases of acute water intoxication (water overload over a period of hours) there occurs a rapid cellular overhydration which may result in cerebral oedema. This is a dangerous situation which should receive prompt treatment. The aim of therapy, in the first instance, is to increase the extracellular tonicity and thus prevent water movement into the cells. It is usually recommended that the plasma $[Na^+]$ be raised, by use of hypertonic saline (e.g. $2 \times$ normal), to a level which lies approximately half-way between the initial level and normal (140 mmol/l) within 8–12 h. The patient should be observed closely for any signs of severe extracellular hypervolaemia, e.g. cardiac failure, pulmonary oedema. If this occurs it may be necessary to increase the renal excretion of water by the administration of a potent diuretic, e.g. frusemide.

2. Chronic Hyponatraemia

In the situation of chronic water overload where the condition (hyponatraemia) has been present for some time (e.g. SIADH) the urgency of treatment depends on whether the patient has any of the signs and symptoms of hyponatraemia. In most cases these patients are only mildly symptomatic and all that is required is to restrict fluid intake (e.g. to less than 1000 ml/d). If the patient does not respond, or there is a problem with compliance, therapy with demeclocycline or lithium carbonate, both of which have been used for the treatment of SIADH, may be tried. In more severe cases the infusion of hypertonic saline and frusemide therapy (as for acute water overload) may be necessary.

Hypotonic Hyponatraemia with Increased ECV and TB_{Na^+}

The patients who have hyponatraemia associated with oedema are notoriously difficult to treat, and have a poor prognosis. The problems associated with their management are complex and outside the range of a text of this kind.

Case Examples

Hypertonic Hyponatraemia: Hyperglycaemia (diabetes mellitus)

A 72-year-old female presented at the casualty department with a history of malaise and polyuria. Her urinalysis showed 4+ for glucose. The plasma electrolyte and glucose levels on admission were:

Plasma			
	Na	121 mmol/l	(132–144)
	K	4·1 mmol/l	(3·2–4·8)
	Cl	85 mmol/l	(98–108)
	HCO$_3$	20 mmol/l	(23–33)
	Urea	10·5 mmol/l	(3·0–8·0)
	Creat	0·19 mmol/l	(0·06–0·12)
	Osmol	315 mmol/kg	(281–295)
	Glu	43 mmol/l	(3·0–5·5)

Comment

Excessive extracellular non-sodium solute, in this case glucose, increases the extracellular tonicity, which in turn draws water out of the cells and dilutes the extracellular constituents. This excess water will return to the cells when the ECF glucose level is returned to normal after insulin is given.

Several formulae have been devised to calculate the 'true' plasma sodium concentration in conditions of hyperglycaemia (i.e. the sodium concentration that would be present if the excess glucose and water were removed from the extracellular fluid). Examples of such formulae are: adding 1·6 mmol/l of sodium for each 5·5 mmol/l the glucose concentration is above 5·5 mmol/l; dividing the glucose level (mmol/l) by 4 and adding the result to the measured sodium concentration. In the above case the 'true' or corrected plasma sodium concentration, using the first formula, is approximately:

$$121 \text{ mmol/l} + 11 \text{ mmol/l} = 132 \text{ mmol/l.}$$

Hypotonic Hyponatraemia with Low ECV and TB$_{Na^+}$: Vomiting and diarrhoea

Date		21/12	22/12	23/12	
Time (h)		2200	0800	0900	
Plasma	Na	116	129	136 mmol/l	(132–144)
	K	3·3	3·1	4·2 mmol/l	(3·2–4·8)
	Cl	74	95	107 mmol/l	(98–108)
	HCO$_3$	27	23	24 mmol/l	(23–33)
	Urea	19·3	14·5	6·8 mmol/l	(3·0–8·0)
	Creat	0·17	0·11	0·08 mmol/l	(0·06–0·12)
	Osmol	268	288	292 mmol/kg	(281–295)
Urine	Na	<10	30	52 mmol/l	
	Osmol	650	400	280 mmol/kg	

A 56-year-old female presented with a 3-day history of severe gastroenteritis. On examination she was 'dry' and moderately volume-depleted as evidenced by decreased skin turgor, dry mucous membranes, a pulse rate of 128/min and supine blood pressure of 110/70. She was infused with normal saline at the rate of 4 litres in the first 12 h and then 4 litres in the following 24 h. Potassium chloride was added to the infusion solutions when the urine volume increased. The admission electrolytes and those of the following 2 days are shown on previous page.

Comment
A patient who loses gastrointestinal fluid is depleted of hypotonic fluid (all body secretions have a sodium concentration less than that of extracellular fluid), and therefore the expected electrolyte pattern would be one of hypernatraemia. However, in many cases including the above, two mechanisms act to produce a hypotonic state:
1.   ↓ Intravascular volume ⟶
   A.   ↑ ADH secretion ⟶ ↑ renal water reabsorption ⟶
      a. Water retention
      b. Concentrated urine (urine : plasma osmolality > 1)
   B.   Thirst
2.   These patients are usually thirsty but too sick to take food (salt), they therefore drink tap water but do not take in sodium

   (1)+(2) ⟶ extracellular water proportionally greater than extracellular sodium ⟶ hypotonicity and ↓ plasma $[Na^+]$.

   This patient's clinical picture and admission electrolytes suggests:
a.   Hypovolaemia: clinical picture and ↑ plasma [creat] i.e. ↓ ECV ⟶ ↓ renal blood flow ⟶ ↓ GFR ⟶ ↑ plasma [creat].
b.   Hypotonicity: ↓ plasma osmol, ↓ plasma $[Na^+]$
c.   ADH is being secreted despite the hypotonicity (volume stimulus): urine : plasma osmolality > 1
d.   Functional kidney: avid retention of sodium (urine $[Na^+]$ = < 10 mmol/l), concentration of the urine (urine : plasma osmolality > 1)
The fluid and electrolyte therapy in this case has been successful, as shown by:
1.   Decreasing plasma [creat] and decreasing urine : plasma osmolality, suggesting volume repletion with increasing GFR and decreasing ADH secretion
2.   Return of plasma $[Na^+]$ and plasma osmolality towards normal

Hypotonic Hyponatraemia with Low ECV and TB_{Na^+}: Addison's disease
A 70-year-old female presented in a semi-comatose condition with a vague history of being 'unwell' for 2 months and vomiting over the previous 2 days. On examination she had a typical Addisonian type of pigmentation and a blood pressure of 80/40. A provisional diagnosis of Addison's disease (later confirmed) was made and she was treated with i.v. hydrocortisone and an infusion of normal saline (8 litres in 24 h). Electrolyte results on admission and on the following 2 days were:

Date		12/10	13/10	14/10	
Time (h)		1630	1000	0800	
Plasma	Na	109	115	128 mmol/l	(132–144)
	K	7·1	7·1	4·9 mmol/l	(3·2–4·8)
	Cl	87	90	99 mmol/l	(98–108)
	HCO$_3$	16	20	20 mmol/l	(23–33)
	Urea	12·5	11·3	6·5 mmol/l	(3·0–8·0)
	Creat	0·14	0·09	0·09 mmol/l	(0·06–0·12)
	Osmol	245	258	279 mmol/kg	(281–295)
Urine	Na	64	—	— mmol/l	
	Osmol	570	—	— mmol/kg	

Comment

The electrolyte and fluid abnormalities of Addison's disease are due to a decreased Na$^+$ reabsorption and decreased K$^+$ secretion by the distal renal tubule because of the mineralocorticoid deficiency. This produces, in the first instance, hypotonicity and a suppression of ADH secretion. Water will then be lost from the kidney, bringing the extracellular osmolality back towards normal. However, the sodium loss is continuous, and therefore more water is lost until the resulting hypovolaemic state stimulates ADH secretion, even though there is an extracellular hypotonicity. At this point water is retained by the kidney (urine:plasma osmolality >1) resulting in a hypovolaemic, hypotonic hyponatraemia. The hyperkalaemia reflects the decreased distal tubular potassium excretion.

The appropriate treatment in the above situation is:

1. Rapid infusion of normal saline (or other plasma expanders) to increase the plasma volume and preclude circulatory collapse
2. Appropriate steroid therapy

Hypotonic Hyponatraemia with Normal ECV and TB$_{Na^+}$: Syndrome of inappropriate secretion of ADH (SIADH)

A male aged 70 years with a known carcinoma of the bronchus presented at casualty with a history of general malaise and mental depression for 1 week. Examination showed nothing specific. His admission electrolytes suggested SIADH, and therefore his fluid intake was restricted to 500 ml per 24 h. The electrolyte picture on admission and 2 days later after fluid restriction are shown below.

Date		22/09	24/09	
Time (h)		0930	0950	
Plasma	Na	119	125 mmol/l	(132–144)
	K	4·2	4·3 mmol/l	(3·2–4·8)
	Cl	78	90 mmol/l	(98–108)
	HCO$_3$	29	28 mmol/l	(23–33)
	Urea	3·0	4·3 mmol/l	(3·0–8·0)
	Creat	0·07	0·09 mmol/l	(0·06–0·12)
	Osmol	248	268 mmol/kg	(281–295)
Urine	Na	64	52 mmol/l	
	Osmol	488	596 mmol/kg	

Comment

The plasma and urinary electrolyte features of SIADH are a consequence of the continued secretion of ADH (or ADH-like substances) despite an extracellular hypotonicity (inappropriate secretion), i.e.

$$\uparrow \text{ADH} \longrightarrow \uparrow \text{renal water retention} \longrightarrow$$

1. $\uparrow$ ECV
2.   Hypotonicity and hyponatraemia
3.   Urine : plasma osmolality > 1

The high urinary sodium concentration (> 20 mmol/l) is due to:

1. $\uparrow$ ECV $\longrightarrow$ $\uparrow$ renal sodium excretion
2.   Highly concentrated urine

A syndrome with similar biochemical features to the above can be associated with the following conditions:

1.   Antidiuretic drugs (*see Table* 2.5)
2.   Thiazide diuretics
3.   Hypothyroidism
4.   Glucocorticoid deficiency

As these syndromes have similar features to SIADH it is probably better to refer to all of these conditions (including SIADH) as the *Syndrome of inappropriate antidiuresis (SIAD)*.

For a definitive diagnosis of SIADH the following criteria should be satisfied:

1.   Decreased plasma osmolality
2.   Urine osmolality inappropriately high for the prevailing plasma osmolality. Although the urine osmolality is usually higher than the plasma osmolality this is not necessary for diagnosis, i.e. a urine osmolality > 200 mmol/kg in the face of a low plasma osmolality suggests an inappropriate antidiuresis
3.   High urine sodium concentration (> 20 mmol/l)
4.   Absence of renal, adrenal, pituitary, thyroid and cardiac disease
5.   Absence of hypovolaemia
6.   Absence of therapeutic agents
7.   Increased plasma ADH concentration
8.   Response to water restriction

The seventh condition, that of an increased plasma ADH level, is usually difficult to satisfy because an ADH assay is usually not readily available. However, a urine osmolality greater than the plasma level is *prima facie* evidence for ADH action.

SIADH may occur in association with:

1.   Malignancy: bronchus, renal, brain, lymphoma
2.   Cerebral disorders: infection, trauma, neoplasia
3.   Pulmonary disorders: tuberculosis, pneumonia, abscess, pneumothorax
4.   Miscellaneous: Guillain–Barré syndrome, acute intermittent porphyria

The treatment of SIADH depends on the severity of the hyponatraemia. In mild cases fluid restriction is usually sufficient. In more severe and refractory cases demeclocycline may be tried or it may be necessary to increase the tonicity of the extracellular fluid by infusion of hypertonic saline and at the same time encouraging water excretion by frusemide.

Hypotonic Hyponatraemia with Normal ECV and TB_{Na^+}: Post-surgical operation

A female aged 44 years had a cholecystectomy and postoperatively was infused with 6 litres of 5% glucose and 2 litres of 4% glucose in one-fifth normal saline over the following 3 days. Following examination of the electrolyte pattern on 08/01 the i.v. infusion was ceased and the patient was allowed only 500 ml of water orally over the next 24 h.

Date		08/01	09/01	
Time (h)		1300	0800	
Plasma	Na	122	130 mmol/l	(132–144)
	K	4·8	4·0 mmol/l	(3·2–4·8)
	Cl	92	100 mmol/l	(98–108)
	HCO$_3$	21	24 mmol/l	(23–33)
	Urea	3·5	3·4 mmol/l	(3·0–8·0)
	Creat	0·07	0·08 mmol/l	(0·06–0·12)
	Osmol	263	275 mmol/kg	(281–295)
Urine	Na	<10	— mmol/l	
	Osmol	465	— mmol/kg	

Comment

The stress reaction (surgical operation) often results in the secretion of ADH and aldosterone which will cause:

1.   Renal retention of water (urine : plasma osmolality > 1)
2.   Renal retention of sodium (urine [Na$^+$] < 10 mmol/l)

If these patients (above case) receive intravenous infusions of salt-poor fluids they will develop a hyponatraemia and hypotonicity that is associated with a high urine osmolality (urine : plasma osmolality > 1), and a low urine sodium concentration (<10 mmol/l), i.e. they are over-watered and under-salted.

Therapy should be aimed at prevention (close attention to the sodium and water needs of the patient), rather than treatment after the development of hyponatraemia. Should this situation develop all that is usually necessary is the restriction of fluid intake.

The biochemical features of the above case are similar to those of SIADH (previous case), except for the low urinary sodium concentration. Because of this similarity many of these cases are misdiagnosed as SIADH.

Hypotonic Hyponatraemia with Increased ECV and TB_{Na^+}: Cirrhosis of the liver

A 45-year-old male with a history of alcoholic cirrhosis presented with jaundice, ankle oedema and ascites. His plasma albumin level on admission was 19 g/l; his plasma and urinary electrolyte values are shown below. Prior to admission he had not been on any medication.

Plasma	Na	124 mmol/l	(132–144)
	K	3·4 mmol/l	(3·2–4·8)
	Cl	90 mmol/l	(98–108)
	HCO$_3$	27 mmol/l	(23–33)
	Urea	2·5 mmol/l	(3·0–8·0)
	Creat	0·14 mmol/l	(0·06–0·12)
	Osmol	269 mmol/kg	(281–295)
Urine	Na	<10 mmol/l	
	Osmol	239 mmol/kg	

Comment

The commonest cause of hyponatraemia in oedematous states (nephrosis, cirrhosis, cardiac failure) is diuretic therapy. However, a number of non-treated oedematous patients will present, usually in the early terminal stage of their disease, with hypotonic hyponatraemia.

In the cases of cirrhosis or nephrosis the primary cause of the hyponatraemia is thought to be due to a decreased intravascular volume as a consequence of hypoalbuminaemia, i.e.

A.   ↓ [albumin] ⟶ ↑ fluid loss to the extravascular space (↓ oncotic pressure) ⟶ ↓ intravascular volume (i.v.v.) ⟶
 1.   ↑ ADH secretion
 2.   ↑ Renal sodium reabsorption
B.   ↓ i.v.v. ⟶ ↑ sodium and water reabsorption in the proximal renal tubule ⟶ ↓ delivery of sodium and water to the renal diluting segment ⟶ ↓ free water generation.

(A) + (B) ⟶ ↑ renal reabsorption of sodium and water and, for reasons that are not clear, water retention is relatively greater than sodium retention.

In the above patient, who was on an unrestricted diet, the sodium retention is reflected by the low urine sodium concentration, and the renal water retention by the urine osmolality which is inappropriately high for the low plasma osmolality (i.e. in normal function a low plasma osmolality should result in a urine osmolality of less than 100 mmol/kg).

In the case of congestive cardiac failure the suggested mechanism of hyponatraemia is:

↓ Cardiac output ⟶ ↓ effective arterial volume (underfilled vascular space) ⟶ ↑ ADH (↑ renal water retention) and ↑ renal sodium reabsorption.

N.B. The term 'effective arterial volume' refers to the central arterial blood volume and infers that the vascular space is 'underfilled'. The majority of patients with oedema (nephrosis, cirrhosis, cardiac failure) actually have an increased blood volume, but because of concomitant peripheral vasodilatation (cause unknown) there is an 'underfilling' of the vascular space.

Isotonic Dehydration

Consequences

In isotonic fluid depletion the loss is from the extracellular compartment and, as there is no change in extracellular tonicity, there is no movement of water to or from the intracellular space. The clinical manifestations of this condition are therefore a reflection of the fall in the circulating blood volume, i.e. circulatory collapse with tachycardia, hypotension and oliguria. The main danger is the development of renal shutdown (acute tubular necrosis, ATN, p. 187) and so treatment should be prompt and aimed at restoring the circulating volume.

Causes

All body fluids (gastrointestinal, urine, sweat, etc.) have sodium concentrations much lower than the extracellular fluid and thus loss of any of them will, in the first instance, be associated with hypernatraemia and hypertonicity (loss of plasma is an exception, e.g. burns). The isotonic (normonatraemic) situation occurs when the patient retains sufficient water (oral intake, increased renal reabsorption) to balance the remaining extracellular sodium, i.e. sufficient water to produce a ratio of 1 litre of water to 140 mmol of sodium. Therefore any condition associated with a loss of sodium and water from the body can result in isotonic dehydration (*Table* 2.7). However, in practice it is most commonly associated with gastrointestinal fluid loss, i.e. vomiting and diarrhoea.

Table 2.7. Causes of isotonic dehydration

Skin loss
  Burns
  Sweat

Gastrointestinal loss
  Vomiting
  Diarrhoea
  Fistula

Renal loss
  Diuretic therapy
  Osmotic diuresis
  Salt-losing nephritis

Third space accumulation
  Ileus
  Pancreatitis
  Peritonitis
  Crush injury

Diagnosis/evaluation

The evaluation of a patient with isotonic fluid depletion should include both a clinical examination and an inspection of laboratory data.

A clinical assessment of the approximate amount of fluid loss and the status of the circulatory system should be carried out, e.g. a mild to moderate (3–5% loss) dehydration is characterized by dry mucous membranes and a low urine output, whereas severe dehydration (5–10% loss) can additionally be associated with hypotension, loss of skin turgor and anuria.

Laboratory data are useful in the assessment of:
1.   Degree of volume depletion
2.   Aetiology
3.   Renal function

Degree of Volume Depletion

Loss of extracellular fluid results in haemoconcentration (increased haemoglobin and/or packed cell volume, increased plasma total protein concentration), and decreased renal blood flow ($\downarrow$ GFR $\longrightarrow$ $\uparrow$ plasma creatinine and urea concentration). However, these parameters may be misleading because analytes such as plasma protein and haemoglobin might have been low prior to the dehydration. Likewise for plasma creatinine (low in people of small muscle mass) and plasma urea which may be low because of decreased protein intake. The plasma urea level may have also been initially high because of pre-existing renal disease.

Aetiology

The cause of the disorder is usually obvious clinically, but in the case of comatosed patients some useful biochemical indicators are plasma glucose levels (diabetes mellitus), and blood gas results (metabolic alkalosis in vomiting, metabolic acidosis in diarrhoea, etc.).

Renal Function

In dehydration that is associated with significant volume depletion and a rising plasma urea and/or creatinine concentration, the decrease in renal function can be due to either the fall in renal blood perfusion (prerenal uraemia, PRU) or to renal shutdown (acute tubular necrosis, ATN). For differentiation of these two disorders there are several useful biochemical tests available. They are all based on the fact that renal tubular function is normal in PRU but compromised in ATN (*Table* 2.8).

The most reliable of the tests listed in *Table* 2.8 is the FE_{Na^+}; however, it is important to remember that both the FE_{Na^+} and urinary $[Na^+]$ can also be increased in conditions other than ATN, e.g.
1.   Chronic renal failure
2.   Obstructive nephropathy
3.   Diuretic therapy
4.   Vomiting with renal loss of HCO_3^-

Fig. 2.5 illustrates a simple approach to the biochemical evaluation of isotonic dehydration.

Table 2.8. Laboratory diagnosis of acute renal failure

	PRU	ATN
Urine:plasma osmolality	>1·3	<1·3
Urine:plasma creatinine	>20	<14
Urine [Na$^+$] (mmol/l)	<20	>20
FE$_{Na}$(%)	<1	>1

PRU: prerenal uraemia;
ATN: acute tubular necrosis;
FE$_{Na}$: renal fractional excretion of sodium.

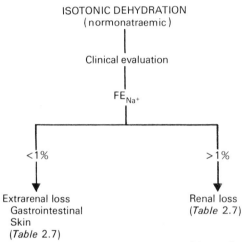

Fig. 2.5. Suggested scheme for the evaluation of isotonic dehydration. FE$_{Na+}$, renal fractional excretion of sodium.

Principles of Management

The management of isotonic dehydration will, as for all other fluid and electrolyte disorders, depend on the aetiology, the severity of the hypovolaemia and the status of both acid–base and potassium homeostasis. The initial goal of treatment is to restore the circulating volume as quickly as possible so as to prevent sudden circulatory collapse or renal shutdown. This is accomplished by the intravenous infusion of normal saline or other plasma expanders (whole blood, plasma, etc.), the choice and rate of infusion depending on the severity of the disorder. A rough estimation of the amount of fluid loss (e.g. ∼5%, ∼10%) should be made, and approximately half of the calculated deficit should be replaced in 3–6 h, and the rest over the next 12–24 h.

During a rapid infusion of fluid replacement the jugular venous pressure should be monitored to warn of hypervolaemia. The efficacy of the therapy should be followed by a regular assessment of the blood pressure, urine output, plasma and urinary electrolyte values, and general clinical status of the patient.

Case Examples

Isotonic Dehydration: Small gut obstruction

A male aged 52 years was admitted complaining of cramping abdominal pain, nausea and vomiting for 3 days. On examination he had a pulse rate of 110, a blood pressure of 115/65 and dry skin and mucous membranes. His urine output was estimated to be 4–5 ml/h. He was given a provisional diagnosis of gut obstruction and infused with 4 litres of normal saline in the first 6 h. The i.v. therapy was then changed to 3 litres of 4% glucose in one-fifth normal saline given over the next 24 h. The electrolyte picture on admission and 9 h later is shown below.

Date		19/20	20/20	
Time (h)		2300	0800	
Plasma	Na	140	138 mmol/l	(132–144)
	K	4·2	4·6 mmol/l	(3·2–4·8)
	Cl	104	100 mmol/l	(98–108)
	HCO_3	25	26 mmol/l	(23–33)
	Urea	22·5	9·0 mmol/l	(3·0–8·0)
	Creat	0·19	0·10 mmol/l	(0·06–0·12)
	Osmol	302	293 mmol/kg	(281–295)
Urine	Na	<10	34 mmol/l	
	Creat	4·8	— mmol/l	
	Osmol	515	320 mmol/kg	
U/P	Osmol	1·7	1·1	
FE_{Na^+} (%)		<0·2	—	

Comment

Isotonic loss of fluid with consequent hypovolaemia and decreased circulating volume results in:

1. ↓ GFR ⟶ ↑ plasma [urea] and [creatinine]
2. ↑ Renal sodium reabsorption ⟶ ↓ urine [Na^+] (<20 mmol/l) and FE_{Na^+} < 1%
3. ↑ ADH ⟶ ↑ renal water reabsorption ⟶ ↑ urine osmolality (U/P osmol > 1)

On admission this patient showed the typical features of PRU due to dehydration. The electrolyte pattern after 9 h of i.v. therapy shows that the rehydration therapy was successful (plasma [creat] ⟶ 0·1 mmol/l and urine osmolality ⟶ 320 mmol/kg).

Isotonic Dehydration: Vomiting (pyloric stenosis)

A male aged 48 years presented after 2 days of vomiting. On admission he had a dry skin and tongue, decreased skin elasticity, a pulse of 110 and a supine blood pressure of 115/65. He was treated with gastric suction, and intravenous normal saline (5 litres in the first 12 h) which was supplemented with potassium chloride. His electrolytes on admission and 18 h after the commencement of therapy are shown below. He was later found to have a carcinoma involving the pylorus of the stomach.

Date		17/12	17/12	
Time (h)		0130	1950	
Plasma	Na	143	142 mmol/l	(132–144)
	K	2·9	4·4 mmol/l	(3·2–4·8)
	Cl	94	105 mmol/l	(98–108)
	HCO$_3$	>40	30 mmol/l	(23–33)
	Urea	15·2	10·5 mmol/l	(3·0–8·0)
	Creat	0·21	0·09 mmol/l	(0·06–0·12)
	Osmol	310	296 mmol/kg	(281–295)
Urine	Na	119	56 mmol/l	
	K	39	— mmol/l	
	Creat	16·1	— mmol/l	
	Osmol	806	305 mmol/kg	
FE$_{Na^+}$ (%)		1·04	—	(<1)
U/P	Osmol	2·6	1·03	

Comment

Vomiting from above the pylorus results in a characteristic electrolyte picture due to the loss of fluid and HCl, i.e.

1.   Fluid loss $\longrightarrow$ hypovolaemia
2.   HCl loss $\longrightarrow$ metabolic alkalosis ($\uparrow$ plasma [HCO$_3^-$])

The increased plasma bicarbonate level results in increased amounts of bicarbonate being filtered by the glomeruli. If the quantity of bicarbonate presented to the proximal tubule floods the capacity of the reabsorptive mechanism then HCO$_3^-$ will appear in the urine as NaHCO$_3$. This results in a high urinary sodium concentration (>20 mmol/l) and often a high FE$_{Na^+}$ (>1%). This situation could be misdiagnosed in the laboratory as acute tubular necrosis (ATN). However, an inspection of the patient's urine : plasma osmolality ratio (>1·3) indicates intact tubular function. The absence of renal damage is confirmed by the fall in plasma [creat] on rehydration.

The hypovolaemia in this patient results in:

1. $\uparrow$ ADH release $\longrightarrow$ $\uparrow$ concentration of the urine
2. $\uparrow$ Aldosterone secretion $\longrightarrow$ $\uparrow$ renal potassium secretion $\longrightarrow$ potassium depletion and hypokalaemia (extracellular alkalosis also increases renal potassium secretion, *see* p. 54)
3. $\uparrow$ Proximal renal tubule HCO$_3^-$ reabsorption which helps to maintain the alkalosis (*see* p. 112).

Patients with a metabolic alkalosis due to vomiting respond to volume expansion with normal saline by an increased renal excretion of bicarbonate and normalization of their plasma electrolytes (*see* Saline responsive metabolic alkalosis, p. 113). As they have a potassium deficit due to the increased renal excretion of this ion they should have their intravenous infusion supplemented with potassium chloride.

Isotonic Volume Depletion: Haemorrhage

A male aged 22 years was involved in a motor vehicle accident in which he sustained multiple injuries and considerable blood loss. There was a delay in transporting him to hospital, where on admission his pulse rate was 140 and his systolic blood pressure was 55 mmHg. He was transfused with 6 units of blood prior to and during a surgical procedure. The electrolyte results on admission and 24 h later are shown below. During this period in hospital his urine output averaged 6 ml/h.

Date		10/05	11/05	
Time (h)		0700	0800	
Plasma	Na	133	138 mmol/l	(132–144)
	K	4·9	5·3 mmol/l	(3·2–4·8)
	Cl	106	107 mmol/l	(98–108)
	HCO_3	18	14 mmol/l	(23–33)
	Urea	30·6	34·0 mmol/l	(3 0–8·0)
	Creat	0·30	0·56 mmol/l	(0·06–0·12)
	Osmol	296	322 mmol/kg	(281–295)
Urine	Na	35	62 mmol/l	
	Creat	3·8	4·2 mmol/l	
	Osmol	315	340 mmol/kg	
FE_{Na+} (%)		2·06	5·99	(<1)
U/P	Osmol	1·06	1·05	

Comment

Although haemorrhage/shock is not strictly classified as isotonic dehydration this patient's plasma and urine biochemical results are an example of the features of renal shutdown (ATN) (*see Table* 2.8), i.e.

1. Rising plasma urea and creatinine concentrations
2. High urinary sodium concentration (> 20 mmol/l)
3. High FE_{Na+} (> 1%)
4. Low urine : plasma osmolality ratio (< 1·3)

Further Reading

Berl T. et al. (1976) Clinical disorders of water metabolism. *Kidney Int.* **10**, 117–132.
Miller M. and Moses A. M. (1976) Drug induced states of impaired water excretion. *Kidney Int.* **10**, 96–103.
Moses M. and Natman D. D. (1982) Diabetes insipidus and syndrome of inappropriate antidiuretic hormone secretion (SIADH). *Adv. Intern. Med.* **27**, 73–100.

3
Potassium

Homeostasis

Input
Potassium occurs in most omnivorous diets, particularly in meat, fish and fruit. The approximate daily intake in a Western diet is of the order of 20–200 mmol/d. Absorption by the small bowel is passive, so that luminal concentration approaches that of plasma.

Distribution
Total body potassium estimates range from 31 to 57 mmol/kg (70 mmol/kg lean body mass). Of the 4500 mmol present in the body, approximately 80 mmol are in the extracellular space and, in direct contrast to sodium, over 4400 mmol are located intracellularly. Potassium is the major intracellular cation (*Fig.* 3.1).

Output
The various body fluids contain differing concentrations of potassium (*Table* 3.1), and significant loss of any of these fluids may result in K^+ depletion. Urinary excretion of the ion varies considerably, being 50–100 mmol/d in the normal adult. Faecal loss averages 10–20 mmol/d. In severe depletion, however, urine potassium levels may fall to less than 10 mmol/d, whereas the faecal loss continues at around 10 mmol/d, and may worsen the potassium depletion.

Control of Homeostasis
The distribution of potassium and the maintenance of the plasma K^+ level depend on two major factors:
1. Control of extracellular–intracellular distribution of K^+
2. Control of renal potassium excretion
A number of other factors are known to have effects, but their actions are mediated by these two factors.

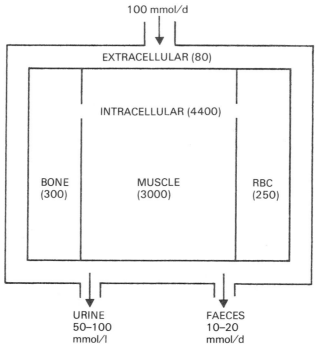

Fig. 3.1. Approximate distribution of body potassium (mmol). The remaining intracellular potassium (i.e. outside of bone, RBCs and muscle) is mainly located in liver, epithelial tissue and connective tissue. RBC, erythrocytes.

Table 3.1. Approximate electrolyte composition of body fluids. N.B. Urinary electrolyte concentrations vary with dietary intake

	Concentration (mmol/l)			
	Na^+	K^+	Cl^-	HCO_3^-
Plasma	140	4	100	25
Saliva	60	15	30	40
Gastric juice	80	10	150	—
Bile	150	10	50	30
Pancreatic juice	110	10	40	100
Succus entericus	140	5	110	25
Diarrhoea fluid	60	40	v	v
Urine	100	50	80	—

v = variable.

Extracellular–Intracellular Distribution

Sodium–Potassium Pump

Potassium is the major intracellular cation (140 mmol/l, extracellular $[K^+]$ of approximately 4 mmol/l), whereas sodium is the major extracellular cation (140 mmol/l, intracellular $[Na^+]$ of approximately 10 mmol/l). This high concentration gradient of sodium and potassium maintained across the cell membrane is the result of an active transport process involving a magnesium-dependent ATPase (Na/K ATPase). The functions of this enzyme may be summarized as:

1. Response to chronic sodium/potassium loads by acting as an adaptive enzyme, the activity of which is regulated by extracellular potassium and intracellular sodium levels
2. Secondary active transport processes, i.e. the movement of molecules (e.g. Ca^{2+}) against a gradient, by mechanisms in some way linked to Na/K ATPase
3. Renal sodium reabsorption—approximately 50% of sodium reabsorption in the kidney is linked to Na/K ATPase, with the major activity occurring in the distal tubule and collecting duct
4. Potassium secretion from the cell—Na/K ATPase activity is stimulated by increased aldosterone, and by extracellular potassium concentrations

Overall, the major stimulators of Na/K ATPase activity appear to be increased concentrations of:

1. Extracellular potassium
2. Intracellular sodium
3. Intracellular ATP

Other factors are known to affect the activity of this complex enzyme, including a number of local membrane factors, and possibly an endogenous compound with a structure similar to digoxin.

Acid–Base Status

Changes in acid–base balance commonly result in variations of the plasma potassium concentration. This effect is the result of redistribution across the cell membrane. In acidosis, for example, the cellular uptake of hydrogen ions, for buffering, leaves electrostatically unbalanced anions behind in the ECF. Consequently, potassium (and sodium) leaves the cell to maintain electrostatic neutrality. A decrease in pH of 0·1 results in an increase in plasma $[K^+]$ of approximately 0·6 mmol/l.

In lactic acidosis, however, the lactate ion is freely permeable across the cell membrane. Since this ion is able to follow H^+, no electrostatic imbalance occurs when H^+ moves across the cell membrane, and thus potassium does not shift out into the ECF.

A decrease in renal potassium excretion occurs initially in acidosis, in favour of increased renal excretion of hydrogen ion. Paradoxically, in chronic acidoses of either metabolic or respiratory origin, increased renal excretion of potassium may occur, the mechanism of which is not apparent.

During alkalosis, H^+ tends to move out of the cell in exchange for extracellular K^+. This may result in hypokalaemia. Alkalosis also increases renal K^+ excretion (*see below*).

Insulin

Insulin infusion (or the response to a glucose load) is known to increase K^+ uptake into muscle and liver cells. The mechanism is believed to involve stimulation of Na/K ATPase activity by insulin, either by increasing sodium entry into the cell or by increasing the affinity of ATP for the enzyme.

Although insulin stimulates cellular uptake of glucose, PO_4^{3-} and Mg^{2+} as well as K^+, the entry of the latter is independent of the other compounds.

Adrenaline

Although a biphasic plasma $[K^+]$ response to adrenaline infusion occurs ($\uparrow [K^+]$ followed by $\downarrow [K^+]$), the major effect is the development of a sustained hypokalaemia due to increased cellular uptake of K^+. This action is mediated by β-receptor agonists.

Renal Potassium Excretion

The rate of potassium excretion by the kidney is influenced by three major factors, namely aldosterone, distal renal tubular flow rates and acid–base status.

Aldosterone

The mechanisms of aldosterone action appear to be twofold:
1. Stimulation of Na/K ATPase in the peritubular membrane of renal distal tubular cells, thereby causing increased intracellular K^+ levels
2. Increased permeability of the luminal membrane of renal tubular cells to K^+, thereby allowing greater rates of passive secretion into the lumen

The consequent overall effect of aldosterone is to promote the excretion of K^+, and to some extent H^+, in a loose exchange for Na^+ reabsorption.

The major controllers of aldosterone secretion are the renin–angiotensin–aldosterone axis, potassium and adrenocorticotrophic hormone (ACTH).

RENIN–ANGIOTENSIN–ALDOSTERONE AXIS. Angiotensin II, an octapeptide produced from angiotensinogen by the actions of renin and angiotensin-converting enzyme (ACE), stimulates the production of aldosterone by the zona glomerulosa of the adrenal gland. Recent drug developments have allowed manipulation of this axis, e.g. captopril is an inhibitor of ACE, whereas saralasin inhibits the action of angiotensin II on the adrenal gland.

The control of plasma renin activity is described on p. 240.

POTASSIUM. Small changes in plasma $[K^+]$ have a marked direct effect on aldosterone release, i.e. increased plasma $[K^+]$ causes increased aldosterone secretion, and vice versa. Plasma potassium levels greater than $8.5\,\text{mmol/l}$, however, inhibit hormone secretion.

ACTH. ACTH stimulates aldosterone secretion. The mechanism is probably of secondary importance, since pituitary failure does not affect aldosterone secretion to the same degree it does cortisol.

It is important to note that the control of aldosterone secretion by these effectors is modified by the total body concentration of sodium, the effects being augmented by sodium depletion.

Distal Renal Tubular Flow

Increased distal renal tubular flow rates result in increased clearance of potassium by a 'washout' effect. The ability to maintain the cell–lumen gradient is unaffected by high flow rates. Hence, in situations of increased tubular flow rates, e.g. osmotic diuresis, significant kaliuresis will occur. The nephron segment involved is proximal to the site of action of ADH, and thus an increased tubular flow rate does not necessarily result in a water diuresis.

Acid–Base Status

Intracellular levels of potassium are increased in alkalosis due to increased potassium entry into the cell as a result of decreased intracellular $[H^+]$ (i.e. H^+ leaves the cell in exchange for K^+). Consequently, in the renal tubular cell, an increased K^+ gradient develops between the cell and the luminal fluid, which will results in increased kaliuresis. Metabolic alkalosis is therefore a potent cause of potassium depletion and hypokalaemia.

In acute acidosis, H^+ enters the cell in exchange for K^+. As a result, the transcellular gradient for K^+ is lessened, thereby resulting in decreased renal excretion of potassium. As previously indicated, chronic acidosis, by an un-explained mechanism, results in a kaliuresis.

Hyperkalaemia

Hyperkalaemia is defined as a plasma potassium level greater than 4·5 mmol/l or a serum level greater than 5·0 mmol/l.

Consequences

Vague muscle weakness, initially in the lower limbs, is usually the first sign of hyperkalaemia. Flaccid paralysis may develop and spread to involve the entire musculature, with an associated paraesthesia. There appears no direct relation between the degree of muscle weakness and the plasma potassium level.

A major clinical feature of hyperkalaemia is cardiac arrhythmia. ECG changes may be related to the level of hyperkalaemia in a general way:

6–7 mmol/l: tall, peaked T waves
8–10 mmol/l: aberrant QRS complexes
11 mmol/l: fusion of QRS and T waves
10–12 mmol/l: ventricular fibrillation

The other features of hyperkalaemia are non-specific, such as malaise, nausea and vomiting.

Causes
As with all disorders of electrolytes, hyperkalaemia may result from defects in input, redistribution or output. These are comprehensively listed in *Table* 3.2.

Table 3.2. Causes of hyperkalaemia

Collection/Factitious	*Output*
Tourniquet/exercise	Renal failure: acute, chronic
Thrombocytosis	K^+-sparing diuretics
Leucocytosis	spironolactone
Haemolysis	triamterene
EDTA contamination	amiloride
Delayed separation of red cells	Hypoaldosteronism
Intake	Addison's disease
Oral/i.v. supplementation	hyporeninism (SHH)
K^+-containing drugs	heparin infusions
Blood transfusion	↓ tubular response
Redistribution	congenital adrenal hyperplasia
Tissue damage	K^+ transport defects
burns	Indomethacin therapy
trauma	
rhabdomyolysis	
tumour necrosis	
Hypoinsulinism: diabetes mellitus	
Drugs	
digitalis	
succinyl choline	
arginine HCl	
Hyperkalaemic periodic paralysis	
Hyperosmolality	

Factitious Hyperkalaemia
Potassium concentrations in serum are approximately 0·5 mmol/l higher than in plasma, due to release of K^+ from platelets during the clotting process. Elevated white cell or platelet numbers often result in an increased plasma $[K^+]$. This can be overcome to some degree by rapid separation of the plasma from cellular components of blood.

Haemolysis, which may result in severe hyperkalaemia, is usually the result of poor specimen collection or handling. Exercising of the forearm muscles following application of a tourniquet may also result in hyperkalaemia, as will a delay in separation of plasma from cells. The latter effect may often be detected by determining the time of collection (often not stated), or examination of other analytes such as glucose (↓), phosphate (↑) and lactate dehydrogenase (↑).

Because of the frequency of these avoidable errors, a high plasma [K$^+$] result which will markedly change management should always be verified by a second blood sample.

Intake

Infusion of potassium-rich fluids, including transfusions of whole blood, may cause an increase in plasma [K$^+$], although with the present transfusion techniques, hyperkalaemia as a result of a massive transfusion is uncommon. It should be remembered that infusions of potassium salts result in an immediate increase in urinary potassium excretion, even in severely depleted states. This is the result of failure of intracellular equilibration within the circulation time.

Adaptation of renal tubular, gastrointestinal and muscle cells to potassium loading develops if there is a high intake over a period of 2–3 days. Thus hyperkalaemia, due to oral supplements, usually does not occur unless renal function is compromised. Intravenous potassium supplementation, however, if given rapidly over a short period, may lead to hyperkalaemia. Infusions of potassium should therefore be restricted to less than 20 mmol/h, although in extenuating circumstances, 40 mmol/h has been used for short periods along with ECG monitoring.

A number of antibiotics, particularly penicillin derivatives, exist as potassium salts. Patients with compromised renal function, if given these drugs, may develop overt hyperkalaemia. Examples include Cilicaine (potassium phenoxymethylpenicillin) and Optipen (potassium phenethicillin).

Tissue Redistribution

Due to the presence of the high intracellular [K$^+$] (approximately 140 mmol/l), any shift of the ion to the extracellular space may cause hyperkalaemia. This effect may be seen in a number of situations:

Tissue Damage

Destruction of body tissues may cause release of sufficient intracellular potassium to result in hyperkalaemia. This is commonly seen in trauma, burns and rhabdomyolysis. With the introduction of potent cytotoxic agents, hyperkalaemia (as well as hyperphosphataemia and hyperuricaemia) has become a common complication of tumour therapy. This is particularly obvious in those tumours of haematological origin which often have a dramatic response to therapy.

Acidosis

With the previously noted exception of lactic acidosis, acute acidosis generally results in hyperkalaemia due to H$^+$–K$^+$ exchange across the cell membrane. In chronic acidoses, however, hyperkalaemia is not as prominent, since Na/K ATPase adaptation has time to develop.

Digitalis

This group of drugs, including ouabain, inhibit Na/K ATPase activity, therefore inhibiting intracellular K$^+$ uptake, and may result in hyperkalaemia.

Succinylcholine
A muscle relaxant used in anaesthesia, 'scoline' causes a depolarizing blockade of the neuromuscular junction, which is believed to allow release of potassium from muscle.

Hyperkalaemic Periodic Paralysis
This rare autosomal dominant disorder is heralded by the acute onset of muscle weakness which spontaneously resolves over a few hours. The disorder is often associated with exertion, cold or potassium infusions. Treatment involves stimulation of cellular uptake of potassium with Salbutamol, and increasing renal clearance with thiazide diuretics. The cause of the disorder is unknown.

Output
Since potassium homeostasis is mainly dependent on renal excretion, renal insufficiency predisposes to hyperkalaemia. In these cases, adaptive changes, mediated by aldosterone, allow increased excretion of potassium via the gut (increasing from 10% of intake to 30–40%). The individual surviving nephrons of the failing kidney respond by increasing the fractional excretion of potassium (FE_{K+}). In the normal adult, FE_{K+} is of the order of 10–15%. In renal insufficiency, FE_{K+} may approach 200–300% (p. 179).

Renal Failure
In chronic renal failure, hyperkalaemia is only prevalent at glomerular filtration rates less than approximately 20 ml/min. At rates greater than this, although plasma K^+ levels may be normal, potassium tolerance is reduced.

Other factors involved in the development of hyperkalaemia of renal failure include chronic metabolic acidosis, and failure to limit potassium intake. Since potassium excretion is markedly affected by reduced tubular flow rates, dehydration is a potent cause of hyperkalaemia in these patients.

In acute renal failure, hyperkalaemia is found frequently, with levels of 7·0 mmol/l or greater in more than 50% of cases. Major causes of the hyperkalaemia include:
1.   Increased tissue breakdown (release of K^+ from cells)
2.   Metabolic acidosis (cellular H^+–K^+ exchange)
3.   Decreased distal tubular flow ($\downarrow$ GFR)
4.   Limited adaptation to high plasma [K^+] due to rapid onset of the disorder

It is important to note that hypokalaemia may occasionally occur in acute renal failure, for example, in patients who have developed chronic hypokalaemia due to the use of diuretics or laxatives. Hypovolaemia may also develop in these patients and lead to renal insufficiency or failure.

Potassium-sparing Diuretics
The specific aldosterone antagonist, spironolactone, causes a mild natriuresis, with decreased excretion of K^+ and H^+ (p. 259). Agents such as triamterene and

amiloride act independently of aldosterone, possibly by blockade of sodium pores in the luminal membrane of the distal renal tubular cells.

A number of diuretic formulations include both a thiazide and a potassium-sparing diuretic in an attempt to overcome the kaliuretic effect of the former. These combinations have the potential to cause hyperkalaemia and it is recommended that they are not used in patients with renal or hepatic disorders. They should also be used with caution in the elderly, where the GFR is invariably reduced due to age-related 'nephron drop-out'. Oral potassium supplements should not be prescribed with these types of diuretics.

Mineralocorticoid Deficiency

In mineralocorticoid deficiency (e.g. Addison's disease), uncontrolled natriuresis with decreased clearance of K^+ and H^+ occurs. The consequent findings of hyponatraemia, and hyperkalaemic acidosis, are typical of this condition (*see* Chapter 10).

It should be remembered, however, that in adrenal failure secondary to pituitary failure, the renin–angiotensin–aldosterone axis remains functional, and hence natriuresis and hyperkalaemia rarely occur in this situation.

SYNDROME OF HYPORENINISM HYPOALDOSTERONISM (SHH, TYPE 4 RTA). Recent publications have indicated the frequent finding of hyperkalaemia associated with mild to moderately impaired renal function (plasma creatinine $<0.2\,\text{mmol/l}$). The syndrome is seen in the elderly, frequently in association with diabetes mellitus, and is often associated with a moderate metabolic acidosis.

Although most of these patients have been shown to be hyporeninaemic, the aetiology of the disorder is not clear. Although failure of renin secretion is involved, there is also evidence to suggest a decreased physiological response to renin. There may also be a decreased renal tubular response to aldosterone, resulting from damage to the nephron.

INDOMETHACIN. There have been several reports in the literature of hyperkalaemia associated with indomethacin therapy. At present, the pathogenesis is uncertain, but it is thought that the cause is due to inhibition of prostaglandin synthesis and a consequent suppression of renin secretion.

Diagnosis/Evaluation

Because of the frequency of factitious hyperkalaemia, the unexpected finding of an increased plasma $[K^+]$ requires an immediate urgent repeat sample and analysis to verify the abnormality.

A review of other analytes present in the electrolyte profile will eliminate common causes of hyperkalaemia, e.g. renal failure, diabetic ketoacidosis.

An appropriate drug history will reveal hyperkalaemia resulting from increased input (oral potassium supplements), or from potassium-sparing diuretic therapy.

Once common causes of hyperkalaemia have been eliminated, urinary measurement of $[K^+]$ may give some indication of other causes. It is often elevated in disorders of potassium redistribution, and inappropriately low in disorders of aldosterone action.

A suggested approach to the evaluation and diagnosis of hyperkalaemia is shown in *Fig.* 3.2.

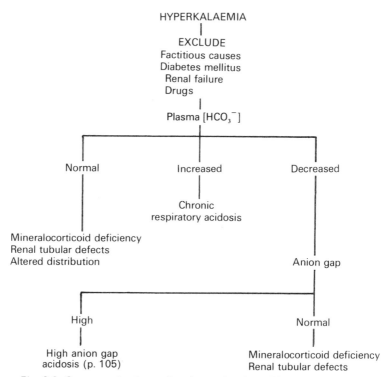

Fig. 3.2. Suggested scheme for the evaluation of hyperkalaemia.

Treatment

In situations of modest elevation of plasma potassium (e.g. up to 5·5 mmol/l), restriction of potassium intake, with increased sodium and fluid intake, is usually sufficient to reverse the trend.

Where levels exceed 6·5 mmol/l, or there is ECG evidence of bizarre QRS complexes, conduction block or ventricular arrhythmia, then a medical emergency exists, and rapid therapy is required, as outlined below.

Calcium Gluconate

Ten to twenty ml of 10% calcium gluconate are given i.v. over 2–3 min in an attempt to antagonize the cardiotoxic effects of potassium. The effect is only transitory, and must be followed with more permanent therapy.

Sodium Bicarbonate

Sodium bicarbonate, 100–200 mmol (8·4% sodium bicarbonate contains 100 mmol/100 ml) are given by i.v. infusion over 30 min in an attempt to shift potassium intracellularly. Although the effect may last for a few hours, the K^+ slowly leaks out of the cells as the alkalosis abates. Note two major precautions with bicarbonate therapy:

1. Do not infuse bicarbonate in the same line as calcium salts, or a spectacular precipitate of calcium carbonate develops, and
2. Recall that 100 mmol of bicarbonate has 100 mmol of associated sodium which may cause water retention and possible oedema

Glucose–Insulin

One hundred millilitres of 50% glucose and 50 units of soluble insulin are infused via an i.v. line. The insulin directly causes cellular K^+ uptake, whilst the glucose protects against hypoglycaemia. This effect lasts for several hours.

Resonium A (Sodium Polystyrene Sulphonate)

This cation exchange resin, when taken orally, exchanges Na^+ for K^+ in the gut, causing diffusion of potassium from the mucosa. Since the resin tends to form intestinal concretions, it is often given as an enema. The usual dose is 30 g twice daily, along with a strict reduction in potassium intake. A disadvantage of resonium A is the non-selective cation binding that occurs, so that the absorption characteristics of some drugs, such as digoxin and phenytoin, may be affected.

Haemodialysis

In the context of acute renal failure, haemodialysis is usually the treatment of choice. In this situation, renal physicians should be consulted as early as possible, so that correction of a number of analytes can be carried out with reasonable caution and greater control.

Case Examples

Incorrect Sampling (EDTA Contamination)

Routine examination of a 38-year-old executive for insurance purposes revealed a bizarre electrolyte pattern. A repeat specimen of blood revealed normal parameters (second set of results). Subsequently, it was found that the original sample had been 'topped up' with blood from an EDTA tube.

Time (h)		1000	1400	
Plasma	Na	141	142 mmol/l	(137–145)
	K	10·3	3·8 mmol/l	(3·1–4·2)
	Cl	94	96 mmol/l	(98–106)
	HCO$_3$	28	27 mmol/l	(22–32)
	Urea	5·5	5·3 mmol/l	(3·0–8·0)
	Creat	0·09	0·09 mmol/l	(0·05–0·12)
	Ca	0·56	2·14 mmol/l	(2·20–2·55)
	Alb	46	44 g/l	(39–48)
	AP	20	78 u/l	(30–110)

Comment

The effects of contamination of the first sample with potassium EDTA (ethylene diamine tetra-acetate), used as an anticlotting agent for haematological examination, are:

1.   Increased potassium level as a direct result of K^+ contamination
2.   Chelation of calcium (and magnesium) by EDTA, thereby affecting laboratory analysis of calcium-using chelating methods. To overcome this effect, calcium may be analysed using atomic absorption spectrometry techniques
3.   Inhibition of alkaline phosphatase (AP) activity, which requires magnesium as a cofactor. This effect is variable, depending upon the amount of magnesium added to the enzyme substrate prior to analysis

Insulin Deficiency

A 36-year-old male, a known insulin-dependent diabetic, attended the local hospital following a viral illness. Home monitoring had shown increasing glycosuria. The patient complained of polyuria, nausea and vomiting. Clinical examination revealed moderate dehydration, rapid respirations and acetone on his breath. Initial electrolyte parameters revealed:

Plasma			
	Na	113 mmol/l	(137–145)
	K	7·8 mmol/l	(3·1–4·2)
	Cl	80 mmol/l	(98–106)
	HCO_3	5 mmol/l	(22–32)
	Urea	18·5 mmol/l	(3·0–8·0)
	Creat	0·48 mmol/l	(0·05–0·12)
	Glu	45·6 mmol/l	(3·8–5·8)
	AG	36 mEq/l	(10–18)
	BOHB	18·3 mmol/l	(0·02–0·2)
	AcAc	4·2 mmol/l	(0·01–0·15)

(BOHB: β-hydroxybutyrate
AcAc: acetoacetate)

Rapid infusion of normal saline and insulin, with appropriate potassium replacement, allowed restoration of electrolytes to within normal limits in 48 h, with marked improvement in the patient's clinical status.

Comment

The case illustrates the common initial findings in diabetic ketoacidosis. Hyponatraemia is due to:

1.   Extracellular water shift due to the osmotic effect of glucose
2.   Loss in vomitus (but replacement of water loss by drinking low salt fluid)
3.   Obligatory loss of cation due to renal clearance of ketones (as Na^+ ketone$^-$)
4.   Factitious hyponatraemia (p. 36) due to increased plasma lipids

The hyperkalaemia is secondary to the release of K^+ from cells as a result of insulinopaenia, and severe metabolic acidosis. Investigations have shown that these patients, even though hyperkalaemic, are severely potassium depleted, often in negative balances of some 500–750 mmol of K^+.

The inappropriately high creatinine level (compared to the urea) is the result of interference with the assay of creatinine. Most laboratories analyse creatinine using an alkaline picrate reagent by the so-called Jaffé reaction. Unless special precautions are taken, this method is affected by the presence of aceto-acetate (AcAc), giving a falsely high value.

The very high levels of β-hydroxybutyrate (BOHB) and AcAc are a consistent finding in diabetic ketoacidosis. The ratio of BOHB : AcAc is a guide to the severity of the acidosis, by reflecting the mitochondrial redox potential (Chapter 9). In this case, the BOHB : AcAc ratio suggests severe intracellular acidosis.

Renal Failure

A 60-year-old lady was admitted for terminal care following a massive right-sided cerebrovascular accident 8 days previously. On examination, she was found to be unconscious, markedly dehydrated and had Kussmaul respiration. Plasma and urine examination revealed:

Plasma	Na	137 mmol/l	(137–145)
	K	8·7 mmol/l	(3·1–4·2)
	Cl	103 mmol/l	(98–106)
	HCO_3	8 mmol/l	(22–32)
	Urea	78·9 mmol/l	(3·0–8·0)
	Creat	0·65 mmol/l	(0·05–0·12)
	Osmol	376 mmol/kg	(285–297)
Urine	Na	69 mmol/l	
	K	22 mmol/l	
	Creat	5·8 mmol/l	
	Osmol	467 mmol/kg	

Despite attempts to correct the acute renal failure, the patient died 12 h after admission.

Comment

The parameters show the typical findings of acute renal failure (in this case as a result of hypovolaemia), with a marked uraemic acidosis.

The hyperkalaemia is mainly the result of increased H^+–K^+ exchange in an attempt to buffer (intracellularly) the excess H^+.

Defective renal tubular function is indicated by the inappropriately low urinary osmolality. The FE_{Na}· was 5·6% which indicates renal sodium wasting (p. 187).

Addison's Disease

An 18-year-old girl with four previous admissions for vague symptoms of abdominal discomfort, nausea and occasional vomiting attacks returned to the Accident and Emergency Department with similar complaints. Examination revealed no abnormality apart from mild dehydration. The initial electrolyte values are shown (dated 7/11). I.v. saline was instituted, to which the patient responded within 24 h, with complete normalization of the electrolyte parameters. Therapy was ceased and discharge planned a few days later, when the patient had a hypotensive crisis, at which time the second set of electrolytes was obtained (dated 12/11).

A short Synacthen test revealed no responsive rise in the plasma cortisol. Hydrocortisone therapy was instituted with a rapid clinical response, as is shown by the final set of electrolytes:

Date		7/11	12/11	15/11	
Plasma	Na	132	118	131 mmol/l	(137–145)
	K	4·6	6·2	3·8 mmol/l	(3·1–4·2)
	Cl	100	86	103 mmol/l	(98–106)
	HCO$_3$	25	19	26 mmol/l	(22–32)
	Urea	6·6	9·5	3·7 mmol/l	(3·0–8·0)
	Creat	0·07	0·09	0·05 mmol/l	(0·05–0·12)

Comment

This case illustrates the typical plasma electrolyte pattern of Addison's disease (Chapter 10). In this case, saline therapy disguised the disorder by replacement of the pathological loss of Na$^+$ in the urine. The increased renal tubular flow rates caused by the i.v. therapy induced kaliuresis and thus normalized the plasma [K$^+$].

Further studies on this patient revealed the aetiology of the disease to be idiopathic (autoimmune), and yet no evidence of the characteristic pigmentation was found. Approximately 20% of cases of Addison's disease do not show pigmentation.

It should also be remembered that, in adrenal failure, clinical symptoms appear much earlier than the biochemical changes (in this case, approximately 2 months). The sudden collapse in this patient was the result of a respiratory infection.

Hypokalaemia
Hypokalaemia is defined as a plasma potassium concentration of less than 3·0 mmol/l or a serum level less than 3·5 mmol/l.

Consequences
The non-specific signs and symptoms of hypokalaemia include anorexia and nausea. Polyuria (and polydipsia) may result from the effect of hypokalaemia on the distal renal tubular cell (nephrogenic diabetes insipidus of hypokalaemia). The development of a flaccid paralysis affecting particularly the proximal musculature may also occur if the potassium depletion is severe.

Causes

Hypokalaemia, unlike hyperkalaemia, is rarely the result of improper specimen collection; contamination by i.v. fluids (i.e. blood taken from a 'drip' arm) being the exception.

Disorders characterized by a low plasma $[K^+]$ can be defined under disordered intake, redistribution and output. The common disorders resulting in hypokalaemia are listed in *Table* 3.3.

Table 3.3. Causes of hypokalaemia

Intake	Renal
i.v. therapy	mineralocorticoid excess
Redistribution	primary hyperaldosteronism
Insulin therapy	ectopic ACTH syndrome
Alkalosis	hyperreninism
Catecholamines	Bartter's syndrome
Megaloblastic anaemia therapy (B_{12})	Liddle's syndrome
Familial periodic paralysis	diuretic therapy
Salbutamol therapy	renal tubular acidosis (Types 1 and 2)
Output	hypomagnesaemia
Gastrointestinal	acute leukaemia
vomiting	antibiotics
diarrhoea	carbenicillin
villous adenoma of colon	amphotericin B
ureterosigmoidostomy	gentamicin
Skin	
sweat	
burns	

Intake

Dietary causes of hypokalaemia are rare because of the wide distribution of potassium in both meat and vegetables. Hospitalized patients, however, on fasting regimes with i.v. infusions lacking potassium supplements, frequently become hypokalaemic. In these cases, the lack of potassium intake, as well as the increased distal tubular flow (i.v. infusion) causing kaliuresis, can result in marked hypokalaemia. This is often referred to as 'surgical hypokalaemia'.

Tissue Redistribution

As previously indicated, any shift of potassium intracellularly will result in hypokalaemia.

Insulin

Insulin infusion, or an increase in plasma insulin as a response to a glucose load, may result in intracellular K^+ shift. One of the major complications of treatment of diabetic ketoacidosis, for this reason, is hypokalaemia. In those patients, who are initially found to be hypokalaemic, large potassium supplements are required, since insulin therapy may worsen the situation, as may i.v. bicarbonate therapy.

Metabolic Alkalosis

Metabolic alkalosis, due to any cause, results in an intracellular shift of K^+ in exchange for H^+. In the distal renal tubular cell, the resulting increased intracellular K^+ will result in excessive K^+ loss in the urine. This loss will be aggravated if there is also hyperaldosteronism (e.g. secondary to hypovolaemia).

Vitamin B_{12} Therapy

The initial treatment of pernicious anaemia with vitamin B_{12} results in increased red cell production. This may be associated with hypokalaemia as extracellular potassium is taken up by the developing red cells.

Salbutamol

This drug, used in the treatment of asthma and the prevention of premature labour, is a β_2-sympathomimetic agent, which increases cellular K^+ uptake.

Hypokalaemic Familial Periodic Paralysis

Hypokalaemic familial periodic paralysis is a rare autosomal dominant condition affecting a predominance of males. The disorder is characterized by attacks of flaccid paralysis lasting 6–24 h with an associated marked hypokalaemia. Since urinary potassium levels do not indicate a renal cause, a transcellular shift of potassium is suspected. Following the attack, the plasma potassium level spontaneously returns to normal. Attacks may be precipitated by mineralocorticoids, glucose-insulin infusions or ACTH. The aetiology is thought to be due to a non-aldosterone mineralocorticoid. Although potassium supplements may alleviate the attacks, hyperkalaemia may occur on recovery. Acetazolamide therapy has been described as useful in this disorder. The drug produces a metabolic acidosis, and therefore inhibits the intracellular uptake of potassium.

Barium Poisoning

Several sporadic episodes of hypokalaemia, secondary to barium poisoning, have been recorded in the literature. The clinical findings of diarrhoea, vomiting, hypertension and flaccid paralysis have responded to potassium infusion. The aetiology of the hypokalaemia is not completely explained by the disordered gastrointestinal function, as low plasma $[K^+]$ has been reported in the absence of these symptoms. It is assumed that a transcellular shift of potassium occurs.

Output

Gastrointestinal

VOMITING. Vomiting, or nasogastric suction, with consequent loss of intestinal or gastric secretions, will cause a negative K^+ balance. The alkalosis, secondary to gastric acid loss, will potentiate the hypokalaemia, as will the secondary hyperaldosteronism due to the hypovolaemia of fluid depletion.

DIARRHOEA. Prolonged diarrhoea from any cause may result in faecal loss of potassium, as a result of:
1.   Loss of faecal water which may contain up to 100 mmol/l potassium
2.   Loss of colonic mucosal cells (shed in diarrhoea), which have high intracellular potassium levels
3.   Secondary hyperaldosteronism as a result of fluid depletion

LAXATIVE ABUSE. Laxative abuse may result in hypokalaemia by mechanisms similar to those described for diarrhoea. Since these patients are often reticent to admit their laxative abuse, an unexplained hypokalaemia should always be investigated by utilizing urinary and faecal K^+ measurements. In chronic abuse, the urine potassium may be elevated due to a pseudo-Bartter syndrome (p. 69).

VILLOUS ADENOMA. In a small percentage of patients with this tumour of the colon or rectum, there is an excessive loss of potassium in the faeces. The reason for the potassium loss is uncertain, but probably involves mechanisms similar to those of diarrhoea.

Skin

SWEAT. During severe exercise or hot climatic conditions, fluid losses via the skin may amount to several litres per day. Apart from the loss of potassium in sweat (approx. 10–20 mmol/l), the resultant fluid loss may result in hypovolaemia and secondary hyperaldosteronism, which increases renal potassium loss.

BURNS. The destruction of tissues by burns causes an initial increase in plasma $[K^+]$. Following this phase, however, fluid loss from the burnt site invokes a secondary hyperaldosteronism with resultant kaliuresis.

Diuretics

Diuretic therapy (e.g. thiazides, frusemide) is the commonest cause of hypokalaemia, even though only a small percentage of patients on diuretics develop this complication.

The inhibition of proximal Na^+ reabsorption by diuretics results in increased water delivery to the distal tubule. This increased flow rate causes kaliuresis. Secondary hyperaldosteronism, due to volume depletion, and the presence of a mild metabolic alkalosis, potentiates the kaliuresis.

The effects of diuretics on potassium status appear related to the clinical condition for which the drug is prescribed. In general, less than 5% of the patients on diuretic therapy develop hypokalaemia.

In hypertensive patients without oedema, although hypokalaemia has been recorded, there is little evidence to suggest any depletion of total body potassium. Consequently, potassium supplementation is unnecessary in these cases if there is adequate food (i.e. K^+ intake). In oedematous patients on diuretic therapy, total body potassium depletion has been shown to occur, although hypokalaemia may not be present. This depletion may be due, in part, to an associated secondary hyperaldosteronism.

Oedematous patients with poor dietary intake ('tea and toast'), and patients on cardiac glycosides, should have potassium monitoring and replacement as required. Potassium supplementation is generally required during therapy with the potent 'loop-acting' diuretics (e.g. frusemide, ethacrynic acid).

Mineralocorticoid Excess
Hyperaldosteronism, whether primary or secondary, will result in increased Na^+ reabsorption and increased K^+ excretion by the distal tubular cells of the kidney. This often results in hypokalaemia. Mineralocorticoid excess states are discussed in greater detail in Chapter 10.

PRIMARY HYPERALDOSTERONISM (CONN'S SYNDROME). In primary hyper-aldosteronism, the excessive circulating aldosterone causes increased renal tubular Na^+ reabsorption and increased K^+ and H^+ excretion. This results in increased kaliuresis and eventually potassium depletion and hypokalaemia.

A common screening procedure for detection of this syndrome involves measurement of urinary potassium levels, which are often elevated above 40 mmol/l even in the presence of severe hypokalaemia.

ECTOPIC ACTH SYNDROME. Syndromes associated with production of ACTH from extra-pituitary sites are most frequently associated with carcinomas of the lung (particularly oat cell), thymus and pancreas. They have also been described in bronchial carcinoid, phaeochromocytoma and ovarian arrhenoblastoma. Skin pigmentation, commonly described in this condition, may not always be seen even in the presence of extremely high levels of ACTH. This is due to the rapidly progressive nature of the disease, where the patient usually succumbs to the malignancy before the hyperpigmentation and classic features of Cushing's syndrome appear. The excessive mineralocorticoid activity may reflect the excessive amounts of circulating cortisol (which has some mineralocorticoid activity) or increased production of aldosterone precursors (e.g. 11-deoxy-corticosterone).

CUSHING'S SYNDROME. The cause of hypokalaemia in Cushing's syndrome is thought to be the result of the moderate mineralocorticoid activity of cortisol itself, although other steroids may also contribute.

LIQUORICE INGESTION. Chronic liquorice ingestion (and swallowed chewing tobacco) result in a pseudo-hyperaldosteronism-like state. The active ingredient, glycyrrhizinic acid, is a potent mineralocorticoid found in the natural liquorice extract. Most commercial liquorice flavouring is now artificial, although the natural product still persists in some confectionery.

RENIN-PRODUCING TUMOURS. The Robertson–Kihara syndrome, resulting from ectopic production of renin, is usually associated with haemangio-pericytomas, although renal-cell carcinoma has also been implicated.

SECONDARY HYPERALDOSTERONISM. Hyper-reninaemic states, which will stimulate aldosterone secretion, may be associated with 'malignant' hypertension and renal artery stenosis. The hypertensive state also promotes increased GFR, and hence increased distal tubular flow. Approximately 20% of these patients have hypokalaemia.

ADRENOGENITAL SYNDROMES. The adrenogenital syndromes are a group of congenital disorders resulting from complete or partial enzymatic blockade of steroid synthesis pathways. Of these syndromes, two are frequently associated with hypokalaemia, namely 11-β-hydroxylase and 17-α-hydroxylase deficiencies.

BARTTER'S SYNDROME. Patients with this disorder have a marked hypo-kalaemic alkalosis, due to renal potassium wasting. Unlike primary hyper-aldosteronism, these patients are usually normotensive, and there is an association with mental retardation. Urine-concentrating ability is impaired and juxta-glomerular hyperplasia is a consistent finding.

The aetiology of the severe renal potassium wasting has still not been conclusively established. The defect may in fact be a renal inability to conserve K^+. Initial studies suggested a decreased vascular responsiveness to angiotensin II, and it was assumed the increased plasma renin activity was a reactive mechanism to maintain blood pressure, and to increase plasma aldosterone concentrations.

Studies with the prostaglandin synthetase inhibitor, indomethacin, have shown the ability of this drug to correct the hypokalaemic alkalosis and hyper-reninism. It is now postulated that high levels of prostaglandin E secreted by the renal tubules causes increased renin production, and hence increased circulating levels of angiotensin and aldosterone. Prostaglandin E has also been shown to inhibit locally the action of ADH and therefore cause a renal concentrating defect.

LIDDLE'S SYNDROME. A familial defect first reported in 1963, this syndrome is associated with hypertension and hypokalaemic alkalosis. Plasma aldosterone measurements have been found to be low, and the hypokalaemia was unaffected by spironolactone. Triamterene was, however, found to be effective in correcting the kaliuresis, and the suggestion has been made that the defect results from a primary defect in Na^+/K^+ transport. The defect has since been shown to occur in other tissues, including red blood cells.

Renal Tubular Acidosis (RTA)

TYPE 1 (DISTAL) RTA (p. 195). In this disorder, there is a defect in excretion of hydrogen ions in the distal tubule. This results in:
1. Retention of hydrogen ions and hence metabolic acidosis
2. Inappropriately high urinary pH
3. Negligible urinary titratable acidity and ammonium secretion
4. Decreased sodium reabsorption resulting in increased natriuresis
5. Kaliuresis as a result of failure of H^+ competition with K^+ for excretion, and increased distal tubular flow rates due to decreased Na^+ reabsorption

TYPE 2 (PROXIMAL) RTA (p. 196). The defect in this disorder is the inability of the proximal tubule to secrete H^+ which enables reabsorption of HCO_3^-. The massive amount of HCO_3^- swamps the limited distal bicarbonate reabsorption mechanism, so that heavy bicarbonaturia (15–20% of filtered load) occurs. The increased distal tubular flow rate induces kaliuresis and potassium depletion.

A similar hypokalaemic acidosis is seen in patients treated with carbonic anhydrase inhibitors (e.g. acetazolamide), which are still used in the treatment of glaucoma.

Hypomagnesaemia
Several case reports now exist regarding patients presenting with hypokalaemia, alkalosis, hypomagnesaemia and dermatitis. Potassium replacement alone did not correct the abnormality. Response was noted, however, if the hypomagnesaemia was corrected first. The aetiology of the hypokalaemia is believed to be due to a defect in Na/K ATPase activity, which is magnesium dependent.

Leukaemia
In acute leukaemia, secretion of lysozyme in the urine has been suggested as the cause of the hypokalaemia seen in some cases. Lysozyme acts like an unabsorbable anion, causing increased distal tubular flow rates. There is evidence, however, to suggest that the hypokalaemia may result from a tubular defect due to the malignancy.

Antibiotics
Several antibiotics cause hypokalaemia by two different renal mechanisms. The nephrotoxicity of amphotericin B causes alteration in the membrane permeability of the distal tubule to K^+. Other antibiotics, such as carbenicillin, act as unabsorbable anions, which require a cation for excretion. They are excreted as the sodium salt, thereby increasing distal tubular flow and hence potassium excretion.

Diagnosis/Evaluation
The elucidation of the aetiology of hypokalaemia is best approached by initially excluding drugs or inappropriate i.v. therapy, since these are the most frequent causes.

An associated metabolic acidosis suggests several possibilities, listed in *Fig. 3.3*, which can be separated by further specific investigations.

If the above manoeuvres prove unrewarding, estimation of urinary potassium will often aid in locating the site of potassium loss, i.e. renal or extrarenal. In situations of inappropriately high urinary $[K^+]$, the use of urinary $[Cl^-]$ (p. 99), and other tests, such as plasma renin activity, aldosterone and other steroid estimations (p. 244) will determine the cause of the disorder.

Treatment

Potassium Supplements
Initially, oral potassium chloride tablets were found to be related to a high incidence of peptic ulceration. Since the development of slow release tablets (Slow-K, Span-K), the incidence of major gastrointestinal side-effects has decreased, but minor complaints are still common.

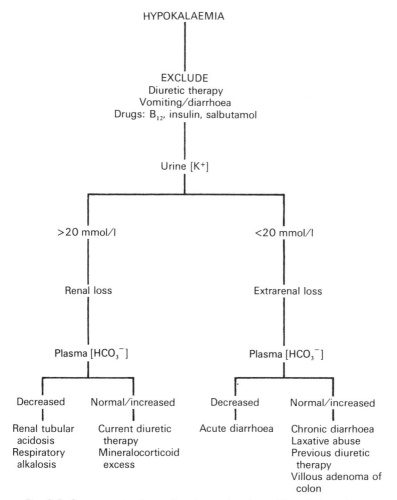

Fig. 3.3. Suggested scheme for the evaluation of hypokalaemia.

The most important factors with respect to potassium supplementation involve the actual amounts to be prescribed:

1. It should be recalled that plasma potassium represents less than 2% of the total body potassium, with more than 85% of the analyte situated intracellularly

2. Institution of potassium therapy will immediately increase the urinary excretion of potassium, particularly with i.v. therapy, because of failure of equilibration with the intracellular space

3. The usual daily intake of potassium is approximately 100 mmol. One 600-mg tablet of potassium chloride contains only 8 mmol of KCl. One gram of KCl, the usual i.v. formulation, contains 13 mmol of potassium. It should

be remembered that up to 50% of the K^+ dose may be lost immediately in the urine

Consequently, in the absence of renal failure, greater potassium supplementation may be required than is expected. It has been suggested that a patient with a plasma $[K^+]$ of 2·0 mmol/l, in the absence of transcellular shifts, has a deficit of some 500–750 mmol of potassium.

Patients with mild hypokalaemia (plasma $[K^+]$ greater than 2·5 mmol/l), requiring potassium supplementation, can usually be treated adequately by oral therapy, preferably with the slow release tablet. In the case of inability to swallow these rather large capsules, various sachets and dissolvable tablets are available, but these often contain other salts as well. Potassium bicarbonate tablets are also available (e.g. Potavescent). These are useful in the treatment of acidotic hypokalaemic disorders, such as renal tubular acidosis.

When patients have significant hypokalaemia (plasma $[K^+]$ less than 2·0 mmol/l), it is advisable to use an i.v. route for replacement therapy. To allow sufficient equilibration with the intracellular space, no more than 20 mmol/h should be given, unless in extreme emergency. The usual dosages employed are 2–4 g of KCl infused over 12 h in 500 ml of either 0·9% saline or 5% dextrose (i.e. 20–40 mmol potassium over 12 h). The plasma $[K^+]$ should be monitored at least daily, but in cases of diminished renal function, a closer monitor should be kept.

There are several case reports of cardiac arrhythmias occurring (due to hyperkalaemia) following failure to mix adequately potassium salts added to infusion bottles. This may result in infusion of high concentrations of K^+ over short periods. This problem is easily overcome by ensuring adequate mixing of the contents of infusion bottles at the time of addition of any supplement.

Case Examples

Drugs: Diuretics

A 60-year-old man complained of swelling of the ankles and increasing shortness of breath on exercise. Physical examination revealed slightly elevated blood pressure and mild signs of congestive cardiac failure. Diuretic therapy (using 80 mg frusemide) and oral potassium (16 mmol/d) was initiated following the collection of blood samples for routine electrolytes (dated 22/11).

When seen at outpatient follow-up a fortnight later, the patient complained of increasing weakness, and a second blood sample was taken for electrolyte analysis (dated 6/12). The results are shown:

Date		22/11	6/12	
Plasma	Na	139	147 mmol/l	(132–144)
	K	3·8	2·5 mmol/l	(3·1–4·8)
	Cl	104	101 mmol/l	(93–108)
	HCO$_3$	26	35 mmol/l	(21–32)
	Urea	5·9	10·0 mmol/l	(3·0–8·0)
	Creat	0·11	0·11 mmol/l	(0·06–0·12)

Comment
Diuretic therapy, the commonest cause of hypokalaemia, shows the typical pattern indicated above. A hypokalaemic alkalosis with a mild increase in urea level should always raise the suspicion of diuretic therapy.

As indicated previously, diuretics decrease renal tubular sodium reabsorption, thereby increasing distal renal tubular flow rates. This promotes excess kaliuresis. When diuretic-induced hypovolaemia occurs, there is increased proximal tubular sodium and bicarbonate reabsorption (p. 91). This, along with increased renal HCO_3^- generation due to K^+ depletion (p. 112) results in metabolic alkalosis.

Drugs: Salbutamol therapy
A 22-year-old female presented to hospital in premature labour. Suppression of labour was instituted using salbutamol infusion. The results shown below were taken before commencement of the infusion, and 4 h later:

Time (h)		1400	1800	
Plasma	Na	141	141 mmol/l	(132–144)
	K	3·8	2·8 mmol/l	(3·1–4·8)
	Cl	108	107 mmol/l	(93–108)
	HCO_3	23	18 mmol/l	(21–32)
	Urea	3·0	3·8 mmol/l	(3·0–8·0)
	Creat	0·07	0·08 mmol/l	(0·06–0·12)

Comment
The effect of the β_2-sympathomimetic, salbutamol, is to promote uptake of K^+ by the cell, in exchange for H^+. The results normalized following cessation of therapy the following day.

Drugs: Laxative abuse
A 39-year-old female presented to her local doctor complaining of malaise and weakness. Physical examination revealed generalized wasting, but nothing specific.

Initial plasma electrolytes revealed a marked hypokalaemia even though the plasma was reported as haemolysed. Repeat blood and urine samples were requested with the following results:

Plasma	Na	139 mmol/l	(137–145)
	K	2·3 mmol/l	(3·1–4·2)
	Cl	90 mmol/l	(98–106)
	HCO_3	37 mmol/l	(22–32)
	Urea	3·6 mmol/l	(3·0–8·0)
	Creat	0·07 mmol/l	(0·05–0·12)
Urine	Na	12 mmol/l	
	K	12 mmol/l	
	Cl	15 mmol/l	
	Creat	4·1 mmol/l	

Comment

Both the plasma and urine samples showed characteristic colour changes on changing pH. Further studies on the urine revealed the presence of phenolphthalein, a component of some laxatives.

The renal conservation of potassium (urinary $[K^+]$ <20 mmol/l) in the presence of persistent hypokalaemia indicates loss of the ion from a site other than the kidney, thereby suggesting examination of the gastrointestinal tract. Note that in persistent laxative abuse, a pseudo-Bartter-like syndrome may develop, in which case, urine potassium levels may be increased.

Primary Hyperaldosteronism

A 35-year-old man presented to his local doctor complaining of persistent headaches and blurring of vision. Examination revealed supine BP of 170/110, grade II retinopathy and cardiomegaly. Plasma and urine electrolytes were as indicated:

Plasma	Na	144 mmol/l	(137–145)
	K	2·7 mmol/l	(3·1–4·2)
	Cl	101 mmol/l	(98–106)
	HCO_3	34 mmol/l	(22–32)
	Urea	5·6 mmol/l	(3·0–8·0)
	Creat	0·09 mmol/l	(0·05–0·12)
Urine	Na	54 mmol/l	
	K	45 mmol/l	
	Cl	89 mmol/l	
	Creat	9·7 mmol/l	

Recumbent plasma aldosterone measurements were found to be markedly elevated, and selective venous angiography revealed very high levels of the hormone near the left adrenal vein. Computerized axial tomographic (CAT) scanning revealed the presence of a 2-cm lesion in the left adrenal gland which was found to be an adenoma at surgery.

Comment

The case illustrates the characteristic hypokalaemic alkalosis of primary hyperaldosteronism. The initial screening urinary $[K^+]$ of greater than 40 mmol/l, in the presence of a low plasma $[K^+]$, is a positive indication of renal potassium wasting.

The use of high definition CAT scanning in the location of small tumours in the abdominal cavity is well shown in this case. Previously, involved biochemical testing was required for the diagnosis of the cause of this disorder (p. 246).

Drugs: Vitamin B_{12} therapy

A 65-year-old lady presented to her local doctor complaining of weakness, shortness of breath and palpitations. Examination revealed mild congestive cardiac failure with marked pallor. Haematological parameters revealed a megaloblastic anaemia. Biochemical screening revealed a mild hyperbilirubinaemia, with marked elevation of plasma lactate dehydrogenase. The electrolyte values shown are those obtained prior to therapy, and 2 days after commencement of vitamin B_{12} therapy:

Date		15/10	27/10	
Plasma	Na	137	140 mmol/l	(137–145)
	K	4·0	3·0 mmol/l	(3·1–4·2)
	Cl	101	103 mmol/l	(98–106)
	HCO_3	26	26 mmol/l	(22–32)
	Urea	3·8	4·5 mmol/l	(3·0–8·0)
	Creat	0·06	0·08 mmol/l	(0·05–0·12)

Comment

Several reports have alluded to hypokalaemia following increased red cell production secondary to B_{12} replacement therapy. Some authors have suggested that the rare sudden death following therapy may in fact be secondary to the sudden decrease in the plasma $[K^+]$. For this reason potassium supplementation is recommended prior to initiation of therapy for megaloblastic anaemia.

Further Reading

DeFronzo R. A., Bia M. and Smith D. (1982) Clinical disorders of hyperkalaemia. *Ann. Rev. Med.* **33**, 521–554.

Kunau R. T. and Stein J. H. (1977) Disorders of hypo- and hyperkalaemia. *Clin. Nephrol.* **7**, 173–190.

Sterns R. H., Cox M., Feig P. U. and Singer I. (1981) Internal potassium balance and the control of plasma potassium concentration. *Medicine* **60**, 339–354.

4

Chloride–anion gap

Chloride Homeostasis

Distribution
Total body ~ 2000 mmol
Plasma ~ 100 mmol/l
Interstitial fluid ~ 110 mmol/l
Intracellular fluid ~ 2 mmol/l

Intake
100–200 mmol/day—mainly as NaCl.

Output
Sweat ~ 5–10 mmol/day
Faeces ~ 5–10 mmol/day
Urine ~ 100–200 mmol/day

Renal Excretion
Closely related to Na excretion.
Glomerular filtration: $\sim 14\,000$–18 000 mmol/day.
Proximal tubule: passive reabsorption following on active reabsorption of Na^+.
Ascending limb of loop of Henle: thought to be active reabsorption of Cl^- followed by passive reabsorption of Na^+ and K^+, but the exact mechanism remains controversial.
Distal nephron: both active and passive Cl^- reabsorption.

Control of Renal Excretion
Unclear, but it is closely related to control of Na excretion, i.e.

$\uparrow$ Blood volume $\longrightarrow$ $\downarrow$ Cl^- reabsorption (with Na^+)
$\downarrow$ Blood volume $\longrightarrow$ $\uparrow$ Cl^- reabsorption (with Na^+)

Under normal circumstances the excretion of urinary Cl^- tends to parallel that of Na^+. The exception to this occurs when large amounts of complex, poorly reabsorbable anions appear in the urine (e.g. SO_4^{2-}, PO_4^{2-}, ketones), i.e. poorly

76

reabsorbable anions (balanced by Na^+) are excreted in the urine, taking the Na^+ with them. This may result in moderate sodium depletion (and hypovolaemia), which is a potent stimulus to renal tubular Na^+ reabsorption. Under these circumstances most, or all, of the Na^+ not balanced by the complex anions (i.e. NaCl) will be reabsorbed along with Cl^- in the proximal renal tubule. Thus in this situation the urine, which contains significant quantities of Na^+ (excreted as Na^+. (complex ion)$^-$), will be low in Cl^- (e.g. vomiting, p. 114).

Plasma Chloride Disturbances

The plasma chloride concentration is closely related to the plasma $[Na^+]$ on the one hand, and the plasma $[HCO_3{}^-]$ on the other, i.e.

↑ Plasma $[Na^+]$—usually associated with ↑ $[Cl^-]$ except in the case of a high anion gap

↓ Plasma $[Na^+]$—invariably associated with ↓ $[Cl^-]$
↑ Plasma $[HCO_3{}^-]$—invariably associated with ↓ $[Cl^-]$
↓ Plasma $[HCO_3{}^-]$—associated with ↑ $[Cl^-]$ if the anion gap is normal.

Hyperchloraemia

Consequences

Clinical and biochemical manifestations are those of the primary disorder; hyperchloraemia *per se* appears to have no deleterious effects on the body.

Causes

Hypernatraemia (p. 24)
Normal anion gap metabolic acidosis (p. 105)
Respiratory alkalosis (p. 122)

Diagnosis/Evaluation

The major diagnostic use of estimating the plasma chloride concentration is to aid the recognition of the two types of metabolic acidosis, i.e. normal and high anion gap acidosis (p. 105).

Hypochloraemia

Consequences

Consequences are those of the primary disease and not of the hypo-chloraemia *per se*.

Causes
Hyponatraemia (p. 35)
Metabolic alkalosis (p. 113)
Respiratory acidosis (p. 119)

Diagnosis/Evaluation

In the absence of hyponatraemia a low plasma $[Cl^-]$ indicates the presence of an increased plasma bicarbonate level, which itself is usually due to the primary process, i.e. respiratory acidosis or metabolic alkalosis.

Anion Gap

Definition

The plasma anion gap (AG) is an estimation of the total unmeasured plasma anions present which, in association with Cl^- and HCO_3^-, balance the plasma cations, Na^+ and K^+. It is usually calculated from the plasma electrolyte values using the following formula:

$$AG\,mEq/l = ([Na^+]\,mmol/l + [K^+]\,mmol/l)$$
$$- ([Cl^-]\,mmol/l + [HCO_3^-]\,mmol/l).$$

N.B. Some formulae do not include the plasma $[K^+]$ in the calculation.

The above formula actually calculates the difference between the unmeasured anions (Ua) and the unmeasured cations (Uc) of the plasma, i.e. in plasma, which is electroneutral, the total cations (Tc) balance the total anions (Ta). Therefore

$$Tc = Ta$$

where

$$Tc = [Na^+] + [K^+] + Uc$$

and

$$Ta = [Cl^-] + [HCO_3^-] + Ua$$

therefore

$$[Cl^-] + [HCO_3^-] + Ua = [Na^+] + [K^+] + Uc$$

therefore

$$Ua - Uc = ([Na^+] + [K^+]) - ([Cl^-] + [HCO_3^-]) = AG.$$

The major plasma cations and anions are shown in *Table* 4.1.

From this table it can be appreciated that the anion gap should increase or decrease if:

1.   There are large changes in:
  a.   Plasma levels of Ca^{2+} or Mg^{2+}
  b.   Plasma levels of protein, SO_4^{2-}, PO_4^{2-}

Table 4.1. Major cations and anions found in plasma. Note that the units are mEq/l because it is the number of ionic charges (negative/positive) present that are important (e.g. $1.0\,Ca^{2+}$ mmol/l $= 2.0$ mEq/l)

Cations (mEq/l)		Anions (mEq/l)	
Na^+	~ 140	Cl^-	~ 100
K^+	~ 4	HCO_3^-	~ 25
Ca^{2+}*	~ 2	Protein⁻*	~ 15
Mg^{2+}*	~ 2	PO_4^{2-}*	~ 2
		SO_4^{2-}*	~ 1
		Organic acids*	~ 5
Total	~ 148	Total	~ 148

* Denotes unmeasured ionic charges.

2.   Foreign cations are introduced in large quantities, e.g. lithium
3.   Foreign anions are introduced, e.g. drugs
4.   There is an increase in organic anions, e.g. lactate, ketones

An important point to note about an anion gap estimation is that it is subject to considerable error because it is calculated from four different estimations (Na^+, K^+, Cl^- and HCO_3^-), each of which has an inherent analytical error. If the analytical error of each of these analytes is 1 mmol/l, then the error of the calculated anion gap is

$$\sqrt{1^2 + 1^2 + 1^2 + 1^2}\ mEq/l = 2\ mEq/l$$

Allowance should be made for this error when using the anion gap as a diagnostic tool.

Increased Anion Gap

Causes

Increased Unmeasured Anions
1. Decreased excretion of anions normally present
    Renal failure: acute/chronic
2. Increased production of anion
    Keto-acidosis (p. 223)
    Lactic acidosis (p. 109)
    Ingestions
        Salicylate (p. 127)
        Ethanol/methanol
        Paraldehyde
        Ethylene glycol

3. Exogenous anions
   Drugs
      Salicylate
      Carbenicillin
      Penicillin
   Haemodialysis
      Acetate

Decreased Unmeasured Cations
Hypermagnesaemia, hypercalcaemia (unlikely cause)

Laboratory Error

Diagnosis/Evaluation
High anion gaps are almost invariably associated with a metabolic acidosis. The two commonest causes, renal failure and diabetic ketoacidosis, are readily diagnosed by an inspection of other biochemical parameters, i.e. plasma creatinine, plasma glucose, qualitative tests for urine/plasma ketones.

If the aetiology is obscure it is advisable, first of all, to check the plasma electrolyte values using a fresh blood sample. Further investigations will depend on the clinical picture and the assays available. Special attention should be given to the possibility of intoxications, particularly with salicylates, ethanol and methanol.

Laboratory Tests
The following tests, if available, are helpful in elucidating the aetiology.

Ketones
Ketosis (diabetes mellitus, alcohol)

Lactic Acid
Lactic acidosis (p. 109)

Blood Gases
a. Respiratory alkalosis—salicylate toxicity
b. Low Po_2 (<40 mmHg)—lactic acidosis

Toxicology
Salicylates, alcohol

Urinalysis
Oxalate—increased in ethylene glycol toxicity

Case Examples

Metabolic Acidosis: Lactic acidosis
The following results are those of a 60-year-old male with a long history of chronic obstructive lung disease who presented at casualty with acute respiratory arrest.

Plasma	Na	136 mmol/l	(132–144)
	K	4·0 mmol/l	(3·2–4·8)
	Cl	85 mmol/l	(98–108)
	HCO_3	23 mmol/l	(23–33)
	Urea	12·5 mmol/l	(3·0–8·0)
	Creat	0·22 mmol/l	(0·06–0·12)
	AG	32 mEq/l	(7–17)
Blood	pH	7·14	(7·35–7·45)
	H^+	72 nmol/l	(35–45)
	P_{CO_2}	72 mmHg	(35–45)
	P_{O_2}	45 mmHg	(80–110)
	$AHCO_3$	24 mmol/l	(24–32)

The plasma lactate concentration, in a blood sample taken half an hour after the above sample, was 12 mmol/l (reference value: <2 mmol/l). ($AHCO_3$ refers to the blood bicarbonate concentration calculated from the pH and P_{CO_2}, p. 86.)

Comment
This patient, with an obstructive lung disease of long standing would, under normal circumstances, be expected to have a high P_{CO_2} (respiratory acidosis) and a high plasma bicarbonate level (compensation). The normal to low plasma bicarbonate shown above can be due either to laboratory error or to an associated metabolic acidosis.

A laboratory error, yielding a falsely low bicarbonate, is unlikely as the bicarbonate levels measured by two different analytical methods are in close agreement (23 and 24 mmol/l). The sodium and chloride values could also be incorrect, and therefore should be re-checked on a new blood sample.

The increased anion gap and the hyperlactataemia, coupled with the low P_{O_2}, suggest a lactic acidosis due to anoxia, i.e. an originally high bicarbonate concentration, due to compensation of the chronic respiratory acidosis, has been decreased by the lactic acidosis caused by the acute anoxia of the acute respiratory arrest.

This case demonstrates the usefulness of the anion gap in the evaluation of some acid–base disorders, particularly mixed metabolic alkalosis and metabolic acidosis. This condition may present with a normal plasma bicarbonate concentration, and unless the plasma chloride is measured and the anion gap calculated the condition may be misdiagnosed.

Laboratory/Clerical Error
The following laboratory results were taken, over the telephone, by a ward clerk for a patient awaiting surgery for a carcinoma of the breast. The patient was on digoxin and thiazide therapy for congestive cardiac failure, but otherwise appeared

well and in good health on admission.

Plasma	Na	141 mmol/l	(132–144)
	K	2·7 mmol/l	(3·2–4·8)
	Cl	99 mmol/l	(98–108)
	HCO$_3$	22 mmol/l	(23–33)
	Urea	4·8 mmol/l	(3·0–8·0)
	Creat	0·074 mmol/l	(0·06–0·12)
	AG	23 mEq/l	(7–17)

Comment

On inspection these results seem curious in that although hypokalaemia is compatible with diuretic therapy, the mild metabolic acidosis and high anion gap appears incongruous for this patient, i.e. hypokalaemia is more often associated with an alkalosis (↑ plasma [HCO$_3$$^-$]) or a hyperchloraemic metabolic acidosis (p. 105) than with a high anion gap acidosis. A laboratory check on this patient's results revealed that the bicarbonate value was in fact 32 mmol/l and an error had occurred in transcription.

Decreased Anion Gap

Causes

Decreased Unmeasured Anions
Hypoalbuminaemia

Increased Unmeasured Cations
IgG myeloma

Overestimation of Chloride
Bromism
Laboratory error

Underestimation of Sodium
Severe hypernatraemia
Hyperviscosity (e.g. myeloma)
Laboratory error

Diagnosis/Evaluation

In comparison with increased levels, low anion gaps are relatively uncommon. However, their occurrence should be viewed with suspicion because:

1.   They may be associated with otherwise unapparent disease states:
   a.   Bromism—bromide ions interfere with the colorimetric estimation of chloride, giving falsely high values.
   a.   Myeloma—IgG may have positive charges (cationic) and also plasma hyperviscosity may cause underestimation of sodium.

2.   They may indicate an analytical error, e.g. chloride too high, bicarbonate too high, sodium too low.

Case Example

Multiple Myeloma
A female aged 75 years presented with severe bone pain and a crush fracture of the thoracic vertebra 8. She was diagnosed as having an advanced IgG myeloma.

Plasma	Na	134 mmol/l	(132–144)
	K	3·7 mmol/l	(3·2–4·8)
	Cl	108 mmol/l	(98–108)
	HCO_3	28 mmol/l	(23–33)
	Urea	4·8 mmol/l	(3·0–8·0)
	Anion gap	2 mEq/l	(7–17)
	Total protein	120 g/l	(62–82)
	Albumin	27 g/l	(36–52)

Comment
The possible causes of the small anion gap are threefold:
1. Presence of protein cations—IgG protein
2. Decreased unmeasured anion—hypoalbuminaemia
3. Underestimation of plasma sodium concentration.
(Most modern instruments for electrolyte analyses sample an aliquot of plasma by suction into a probe. Highly viscous plasma, which can occur in myeloma, may result in the aliquot containing less plasma water than it should and therefore a falsely low plasma sodium level.)

Further Reading
Emmett M. and Narins R. G. (1977) Clinical use of the anion gap. *Medicine* **56**, 38–54.

5

Acid–base

Units

The SI system of units requires that the partial pressure of a gas (P_{CO_2}, P_{O_2}) be reported in kilopascals (kPa). To convert the traditional units, millimetres of mercury (mmHg), to kPa multiply by 0·133. The reverse conversion is obtained by multiplying kPa by 7·5. Throughout this chapter traditional units are used because (a) the greater part of the published work on acid–base metabolism originates in the USA, which has not yet converted to SI units, and (b) in many laboratories where SI units are accepted the traditional units are still in use.

Definitions

Acid

A substance that dissociates in water to produce hydrogen ions (H^+). A strong acid almost completely dissociates, e.g. hydrochloric acid

$$HCl \longrightarrow H^+ + Cl^-.$$

A weak acid shows poor dissociation, e.g. acetic acid:

$$CH_3COOH \rightleftharpoons CH_3COO^- + H^+.$$

Acidaemia

A raised blood concentration of H^+ (>45 nmol/l) or a low pH ($<7·35$).

Acidosis

A primary process that generates excessive H^+. Depending on the relevant buffering and compensatory processes it may, or may not, result in acidaemia.

Alkali

A substance that dissociates in water to form hydroxyl ions (OH^-), e.g. sodium hydroxide:

$$NaOH \longrightarrow Na^+ + OH^-.$$

Alkalaemia
A low blood concentration of H^+ ($<35\,nmol/l$) or a high pH ($>7\cdot45$).

Alkalosis
A primary process that produces excessive hydroxyl ions (OH^-). It does not always result in alkalaemia (e.g. compensation).

Base
A substance that can accept H^+. A weak base barely combines with H^+ (e.g. Cl^-). A strong base has a high affinity for H^+ (e.g. CH_3COO^-).

Conjugate Base
The conjugate base of an acid is its dissociated anionic product, e.g. carbonic acid:

$$H_2CO_3 \rightleftharpoons H^+ + HCO_3^-.$$

The conjugate base of H_2CO_3 is bicarbonate (HCO_3^-).

Buffer
A mixture of a weak acid and its conjugate base which attenuates a change in $[H^+]$ when a strong acid or base is added to it. It acts by the formation of a weaker acid or base, e.g. carbonic acid + bicarbonate

a.   Buffer + strong acid (H^+):

$$H^+ + HCO_3^- \longrightarrow H_2CO_3 \text{ (weak acid).}$$

b.   Buffer + strong base (OH^-):

$$OH^- + H_2CO_3 \longrightarrow H_2O + HCO_3^- \text{ (weak base).}$$

Blood Buffer Systems
The three most important blood buffer systems are: (a) bicarbonate system—HCO_3^-/H_2CO_3, (b) phosphate system—$HPO_4^{2-}/H_2PO_4^-$, (c) proteins—protein$^-$/protein$^+$.

pH
A measure of the hydrogen ion concentration $[H^+]$ defined as the logarithm of the reciprocal of the $[H^+]$.

$$pH = \log 1/[H^+] = -\log[H^+].$$

pH of a Buffer System
This may be calculated from the Henderson–Hasselbalch equation which relates the pH to the concentration of buffer acid and base.

$$pH = pK + \log[\text{base}]/[\text{acid}].$$

K is the overall dissociation equilibrium constant.

For the bicarbonate buffer system pK $= 6\cdot1$. Therefore for the bicarbonate system:

$$pH = 6\cdot1 + \log\frac{[HCO_3{}^-]}{[H_2CO_3]}.$$

From this equation it can be seen that the pH of a buffer system is directly related to the ratio of base to acid.

$$pH \propto \frac{[HCO_3{}^-]}{[H_2CO_3]}.$$

In a solution, e.g. plasma, the $[H_2CO_3]$ is directly related to the P_{CO_2} (partial pressure of CO_2) of the system. The solubility constant of CO_2 is $0\cdot03$ and thus:

$$P_{CO_2}\,(mmHg) \times 0\cdot03 = [H_2CO_3]\,mmol/l$$

therefore

$$pH \propto \frac{[HCO_3{}^-]}{P_{CO_2}}.$$

The $[H^+]$ of the bicarbonate system can be calculated from the following formula:

$$[H^+] = \frac{24 \times P_{CO_2}\,(mmHg)}{[HCO_3{}^-]\,mmol/l}\,nmol/l.$$

This formula has been calculated for the bicarbonate buffer system utilizing the law of mass action and the solubility constant of CO_2.

Respiratory Component
This term defines the blood P_{CO_2} level as it is ultimately controlled by respiration. Respiratory acidosis is defined as a high P_{CO_2} ($>45\,mmHg$); respiratory alkalosis as a low P_{CO_2} ($<35\,mmHg$).

Metabolic Component
This term describes the plasma $[HCO_3{}^-]$ as this part of the bicarbonate buffer system reflects the non-respiratory component of acid–base homeostasis. A metabolic alkalosis is defined as a high $[HCO_3{}^-]$ ($>33\,mmol/l$), and a metabolic acidosi as a low $[HCO_3{}^-]$ ($<23\,mmol/l$).

Compensation
From the Henderson–Hasselbalch equation it can be seen that as long as the ratio of $[HCO_3{}^-]$ to $[H_2CO_3]$ remains constant (approximately $20:1$) the pH will remain at $7\cdot40$ (mean normal plasma pH), i.e.

$$pH = 6\cdot1 + \log\frac{[HCO_3{}^-]}{[H_2CO_3]}$$

$$pH = 6\cdot1 + 1\cdot3 = 7\cdot40$$

therefore if

$$\log\frac{[\text{HCO}_3^-]}{[\text{H}_2\text{CO}_3]} = 1\cdot3 \text{ then the pH} = 7\cdot40$$

(antilog of $1\cdot3 = 20$).

Therefore if the $[\text{HCO}_3^-] : [\text{H}_2\text{CO}_3] = 20 : 1$ then the pH will be $7\cdot40$.

If a primary disorder, e.g. diabetic keto-acidosis, lowers the $[\text{HCO}_3^-]$ then the pH could be returned to $7\cdot40$ by lowering the $[\text{H}_2\text{CO}_3]$ (or $P\text{CO}_2$), i.e.

$$\text{pH (N)} \propto \frac{[\text{HCO}_3^-](\downarrow)}{P\text{CO}_2(\downarrow)}.$$

This process is called compensation, i.e. return of the pH back towards 'normal' (pH of $7\cdot40$). Metabolic disorders evoke a compensatory respiratory change ($\downarrow [\text{HCO}_3^-] \longrightarrow \downarrow \text{CO}_2$, etc.) and respiratory disorders causes a metabolic change ($\uparrow P\text{CO}_2 \longrightarrow \uparrow [\text{HCO}_3^-]$, etc.). These compensatory processes return the pH *towards* normal, and only rarely to normal.

Normal Acid–Base Homeostasis

Intermediary metabolism results in the continuous production of non-volatile acids which must be excreted by the kidney and, although pulmonary function plays an important role in the maintenance of body fluid hydrogen ion concentration, only the kidney can regulate H^+ balance.

The acid–base status, and body fluid $[\text{H}^+]$, reflects the metabolism of hydrogen ion on the one hand and that of carbon dioxide on the other.

H^+ Metabolism

Hydrogen ions, produced during intermediary metabolism, are secreted by the cells into the extracellular fluid where they are buffered. During this process the extracellular $[\text{HCO}_3^-]$ is lowered (bicarbonate consumption). This $[\text{HCO}_3^-]$ is eventually restored to its original level by the kidneys during the process of H^+ excretion. Thus, it is convenient to consider H^+ metabolism from three aspects:
1. H^+ production
2. Extracellular H^+ buffering
3. Renal H^+ excretion

H^+ Production

The daily turnover of hydrogen ion in a normal adult is around 150 mol. Of this amount the net gain is approximately 15–20 mol ($\sim 10\%$). The major portion of the 150 mmol of H^+ is re-utilized in metabolic processes.

More than 90% of the H^+ produced is the result of hydrolysis of ATP, respiratory chain reactions and the reduction of nicotinamide nucleotides, i.e.
1. $\text{ATP}^{4-} + \text{H}_2\text{O} \longrightarrow \text{ADP}^{3-} + \text{HPO}_4^{2-} + \text{H}^+$

2. $2Fe^{3+}$ (cytochrome) $+ 2H \longrightarrow 2Fe^{2+} + 2H^+$
3. $NAD^+(NADP^+) + 2H.R \longrightarrow NADH (NADPH) + H^+ + R$

Under normal circumstances these three reactions do not result in a net gain in H^+ because the generated H^+ is usually removed by the reverse reactions, i.e. when ATP is resynthesized, and when the reduced cytochromes and nicotinamide nucleotides are reoxidized.

The other major source of H^+ is the respiratory production of $CO_2(CO_2 + H_2O \longrightarrow H_2CO_3 \longrightarrow H^+ + HCO_3^-)$. This reaction results in the net gain of the 15–20 mol of H^+ mentioned above but, as will be shown later, these are normally removed by the lungs.

Another source of H^+ production is the formation of non-volatile acids. These acids which accumulate at the rate of 40–80 mmol/d will result in a net gain in H^+ unless they are excreted by the kidneys.

Non-volatile Acid (H^+) Production
The majority of the organic acids formed during metabolism of fat, protein and carbohydrate are almost completely burned to carbon dioxide and water, and hydrogen ions normally do not accumulate. Nevertheless, there is a daily production of some 40–80 mmol of H^+ (0·5–1·0 mmol/kg) resulting from:
1. Oxidation of sulphhydryl groups (—SH) of cystine and methionine $\longrightarrow H_2SO_4$
2. Hydrolysis of phosphoesters $\longrightarrow H_3PO_4$
3. Incomplete oxidation of carbohydrate and fat $\longrightarrow$ lactic acid, ketoacids

Extracellular Buffering
After secretion from the cells of origin the hydrogen ions are buffered by the extracellular buffering systems (bicarbonate, phosphate, protein). Of these buffers the carbonic acid/bicarbonate system is the most important because of the high turnover of carbon dioxide; the capacity of the lungs to vary the extracellular P_{CO_2}; and the capacity of the kidney to regulate the plasma bicarbonate level.

The addition of acid (H^+A^-) to this system results in a fall in the bicarbonate level—'consumption' of bicarbonate (A^- represents acid anion, e.g. SO_4^{2-}), i.e.

$$H^+A^- + NaHCO_3 \longrightarrow Na^+A^- + H_2CO_3$$

which results in:
1. $\downarrow$ [$NaHCO_3$]—consumption of bicarbonate
2. $\uparrow$ [Na^+A^-]—increase in acid anions
3. $\uparrow$ [H_2CO_3] ($\uparrow P_{CO_2}$)—accumulation of carbonic acid

The amount of HCO_3^- consumed is equal to the amount of H^+ added to the buffer system and will also be equal to the increase in acid anion concentration [A^-]. This low [HCO_3^-] and increased P_{CO_2} will result in a fall in pH of the buffer system, i.e.

$$pH(\downarrow) \propto \frac{[HCO_3^-](\downarrow)}{P_{CO_2}(\uparrow)}.$$

Therefore the venous blood returning to the lungs from the cells where the above reactions occur will have:
1. ↓ $[HCO_3^-]$
2. ↑ P_{CO_2}
3. ↓ pH

In the lungs much of the blood CO_2 is removed by respiration which results eventually in arterial blood with:
1. ↓ $[HCO_3^-]$
2. ↓ P_{CO_2}
3. ∼normal pH

This arterial blood is then delivered to the kidneys where H^+ is excreted and HCO_3^- generated. Consequently the renal venous blood will have an increased $[HCO_3^-]$ which replaces the HCO_3^- removed by the addition of H^+ at the cell level.

Renal H^+ Excretion and HCO_3^- Reabsorption

The kidney's role in acid–base homeostasis is threefold:
1. Excretion of H^+ and regeneration of HCO_3^-
2. Excretion of acid anions
3. Reabsorption of filtered HCO_3^-

Excretion of H^+ and Regeneration of HCO_3^-

In the distal nephron, mainly the collecting ducts, H^+ is secreted into the tubular fluid and eventually excreted in the urine. During this process bicarbonate ions, equivalent to the amount of H^+ excreted, are generated and pass back into the blood. Hydrogen ion excretion by the kidney involves three separated but closely related mechanisms (*Fig. 5.1*).
1. Formation of H^+ in tubular cells
2. Secretion of H^+ into tubular lumen
3. Excretion of H^+ in the urine

FORMATION OF H^+. In the tubular cell, due to the presence of carbonic anhydrase, carbon dioxide and water combine to produce H^+ and HCO_3^-. It is believed by some investigators that the chemical reaction is: $CO_2 + OH^-$ (+carbonic anhydrase) $\longrightarrow HCO_3^-$, rather than $CO_2 + H_2O$ (+carbonic anhydrase) $\longrightarrow H^+ + HCO_3^-$. Whichever reaction is correct the net result is the same, i.e. formation of H^+ and HCO_3^-.

SECRETION OF H^+. Intracellular H^+ is secreted into the tubular fluid across the cell membrane in exchange for Na^+. This reabsorbed Na^+ is then returned to the blood accompanied by the cell-generated HCO_3^-. The amount of HCO_3^- generated by the distal nephron is equivalent to that bicarbonate consumed when the non-volatile acids were originally added to the buffer system.

EXCRETION OF H^+. The amount of H^+ the distal nephron has to excrete is of the order of 40–80 mmol/d, i.e. the amount produced by metabolism (0·5–1·0 mmol/kg/d). However, the kidney is unable to decrease the urine pH to below 4·4 ([H^+] of 40 μmol/l), i.e. it is not able to produce a cell to tubular lumen

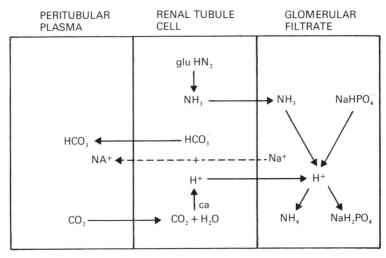

Fig. 5.1. Excretion of H+, and HCO_3^- regeneration, by the distal nephron. ca, Carbonic anhydrase.

H^+ concentration gradient greater than $1:1000$ (assuming an intracellular $[H^+]$ of 40 nmol/l and a urine $[H^+]$ of 40 μmol/l). Therefore to excrete 40 mmol of H^+ daily the kidney would either have to lower the urine pH to around 1·4 ($[H^+]$ of 40 mmol/l) or pass around 1000 litres of urine with a pH of 4·4 ($[H^+]$ of 40 μmol/l). Both of these are obviously impossible. However, the problem is overcome by the presence of urinary buffers, mainly phosphate (Na_2HPO_4/NaH_2PO_4) and ammonia (NH_3/NH_4^+), which bind the secreted H^+ and thus prevent a high $[H^+]$ gradient occurring (*Fig.* 5.1).

The phosphate buffer (Na_2HPO_4), which is limited by the amount filtered at the glomerulus, accounts for the excretion of 20–40 mmol of H^+ daily. This is measured in the urine as titratable acidity (TA). The H^+ not removed by the phosphate is bound by urinary ammonia (NH_3) to form ammonium ions (NH_4^+) and then excreted (normally around 30–50 mmol/d). This ammonia is produced in the tubular cells from amino acids, mainly glutamine, and diffuses across the cell membrane into the tubular lumen where it binds H^+. The ammonia production rate of the cell, unlike renal phosphate excretion, can be increased some tenfold, and is responsible for the excretion of the massive amounts of H^+ which may be produced in disorders such as diabetic ketoacidosis.

There are other substances in the urine that may accept H^+, e.g. urate and creatinine, but they do not play a significant role in acid–base homeostasis.

Excretion of Acid Anion

The acid anions produced during metabolism (SO_4^{2-}, PO_4^{2-}, etc.) are filtered by the glomeruli and, provided the GFR is adequate, cleared from the plasma. If renal function is impaired these anions may be retained and result in a high anion gap (p. 78).

Reabsorption of Filtered Bicarbonate
Each day some 4000 mmol of HCO_3^- are filtered by the glomeruli and if the plasma level is to be maintained this amount has to be returned to the blood. This is accomplished by renal tubular reabsorption (around 80–90% in the proximal tubule and the remainder in the distal nephron). This process, like the mechanism of H^+ excretion in the distal nephron, involves tubular secretion of H^+ coupled with reabsorption of Na^+ (*Fig.* 5.2).

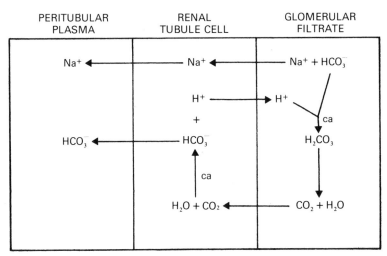

Fig. 5.2. Bicarbonate reabsorption in the proximal renal tubule. ca, Carbonic anhydrase.

In the proximal tubular cells hydrogen and bicarbonate ions are produced under the influence of carbonic anhydrase. The H^+ is then secreted into the tubular lumen in exchange for Na^+ and then combines with the filtered HCO_3^- to form carbonic acid, and then CO_2 and water. This reaction is catalysed by carbonic anhydrase located in the cell brush borders. The tubular-generated CO_2 diffuses back into the cell and re-enters the H^+/HCO_3^- production process. The cell-generated HCO_3^- and the reabsorbed Na^+ are secreted back into the bloodstream.

An important concept to appreciate with regard to renal H^+ manipulation is that some 4–4·5 thousand mmol are secreted by the tubules daily but only about 1–2% (40–80 mmol) is actually excreted in the urine, i.e. around 98–99% of the secreted H^+ is involved in HCO_3^- reabsorption.

Under normal circumstances little or no bicarbonate is excreted in the urine. However, if the plasma level rises sufficiently (to a threshold level of 26–28 mmol/l) the amount filtered by the glomeruli will exceed the tubular reabsorptive capacity and bicarbonate will appear in the urine. The rate of reabsorption, and the renal threshold, is influenced by a number of factors which include plasma P_{CO_2}, plasma volume and plasma $[K^+]$.

Increased reabsorption occurs if there is:
1.   ↑ Plasma $P\text{CO}_2$
2.   ↓ Plasma volume
3.   Hypokalaemia

Carbon Dioxide Metabolism

The carbon dioxide produced during metabolism of carbohydrate, fat and protein is carried by the blood to the lungs where it is excreted. Disturbances in CO_2 metabolism which may result in respiratory acid–base disorders are due to alterations in the pulmonary excretion rate and not to variations in production, or bufferings, of carbonic acid.

Carbon Dioxide Production

In the adult the complete oxidation of fat, carbohydrate and protein produces 15 000–20 000 mmol of CO_2 daily. This CO_2 diffuses out of cells to the blood where it enters into a number of reactions with the eventual formation of carbonic acid, bicarbonate and carbamino compounds.

Carbon Dioxide Transport

The major portion (>90%) of the CO_2 entering the blood diffuses into the red cells, a small fraction remaining in the plasma in the dissolved state.

In the red cells (*Fig.* 5.3) carbonic anhydrase catalyses the hydration of CO_2 to form carbonic acid which then dissociates into H^+ and HCO_3^-. The liberated H^+ is buffered by haemoglobin (reduced haemoglobin is a potent buffer), whilst most of the generated HCO_3^- diffuses across the cell wall to enter the plasma in exchange for Cl^- (chloride shift). A small fraction of the red cell CO_2 combines with the nitrogen groups on haemoglobin to form carbamino compounds.

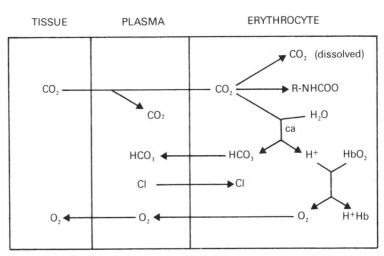

Fig. 5.3. Carbon dioxide transport in the blood: reactions which occur in the red cells at the tissue level. ca, Carbonic anhydrase.

The driving force behind these reactions is the P_{CO_2}. An increase, or decrease, in the P_{CO_2} level will result in a rise, or fall, in the blood levels of HCO_3^- as well as that of carbamino compounds. In the lung alveoli the low P_{CO_2} level will cause diffusion of CO_2 down its chemical gradient and a reversal of the above chemical reactions.

Carbon Dioxide Excretion

In the lung the low P_{CO_2}, and reduced buffering power of oxyhaemoglobin (release of H^+), results in CO_2 excretion.

In the red cells (*Fig.* 5.4) the H^+ released from oxygenated haemoglobin combines with HCO_3^- to form carbonic acid and then CO_2 which is excreted into the alveoli. As the red cell concentration of HCO_3^- falls more diffuses in from the plasma (in exchange for red cell Cl^-). The carbamino compounds also release CO_2 in response to the low P_{CO_2}.

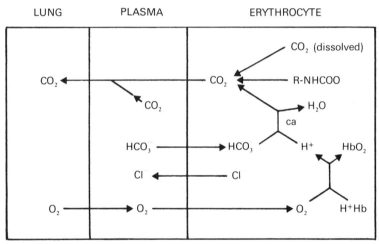

Fig. 5.4. Excretion of carbon dioxide by the lungs: reactions which occur in the red cells at the lung level. ca, Carbonic anhydrase.

The degree of pulmonary CO_2 excretion depends on the respiratory rate and the extent of the pulmonary gas exchange area. Factors influencing the respiratory rate, other than voluntary control, are pH ($\uparrow$ with $\downarrow$ pH), P_{CO_2} ($\uparrow$ with $\uparrow$ P_{CO_2}), and blood oxygen content (hypoxia stimulates respiration).

Disturbances of Acid–Base Metabolism

The primary disturbances in disordered acid–base metabolism involves changes in the blood levels of P_{CO_2} (respiratory component) or $[HCO_3]$ (metabolic component). These conditions referred to as acidosis or alkalosis result, in the first instance, in acidaemia ($\downarrow$ pH, $\uparrow$ [H$^+$]) or alkalaemia ($\uparrow$ pH, $\downarrow$ [H$^+$]). However, if the initial disorder is continuous the compensatory process will return the pH towards normal.

An important concept regarding compensation is that in simple disorders the pH is returned towards normal, and not completely to normal (pH of 7·40). If an acid–base disturbance results in a pH of around 7·40 a mixed disorder (alkalosis and acidosis) should be suspected. The exceptions to this rule are (a) chronic respiratory alkalosis which may attain full compensation (pH to $\sim$7·40) after a period of 1–2 weeks, and (b) minor degrees of chronic respiratory acidosis ($P_{CO_2} < 60$ mmHg) which may present in the fully compensated form.

Simple Metabolic Acidosis

Metabolic acidosis results from any process that reduces the plasma [HCO$_3$]. It may be primary, or secondary to a lowered P_{CO_2} (respiratory alkalosis). In the primary disorder the lowered [HCO$_3$$^-$] results in an acidaemia ($\downarrow$ pH, $\uparrow$ [H$^+$]) which stimulates respiration and this lowers the blood P_{CO_2}. This compensatory process (respiratory alkalosis) returns the pH towards normal, but not completely to normal. The limit to which the P_{CO_2} can fall in severe metabolic acidosis is around 10 mmHg. Maximum compensation occurs within 12–24 h of the initial disturbance and the level of P_{CO_2} reached, for a given [HCO$_3$$^-$], may be calculated from the following equation:

$$P_{CO_2} \text{ (mmHg)} = 1\cdot5 \times [\text{HCO}_3] + 8 \pm 2.$$

This, and the following compensation equations, may be found in the review by Narins R.G. and Emmett M. (1980).

Simple Metabolic Alkalosis

Metabolic alkalosis results from any process which increases the plasma [HCO$_3$$^-$]. This may be secondary to an increased blood P_{CO_2} (respiratory acidosis), or a primary disorder. In the latter the increased [HCO$_3$$^-$] and the ensuing lowered [H$^+$] suppresses respiration and increases the blood P_{CO_2} level. This compensation (respiratory acidosis) reaches its maximum in 12–24 h with an upper limit of 55–60 mmHg. Unlike metabolic acidosis, the level of compensatory change in P_{CO_2} is unpredictable. Nevertheless, the following formula is helpful in estimating the P_{CO_2} for a given [HCO$_3$$^-$] in metabolic alkalosis:

$$P_{CO_2} \text{ (mmHg)} = 0\cdot9 \times [\text{HCO}_3{}^-] + 9.$$

Simple Respiratory Acidosis

Any process that raises the blood P_{CO_2} level, whether it be primary, or secondary to metabolic alkalosis, results in a respiratory acidosis. The primary disorder, due to compromised pulmonary gas exchange, may present as an acute or chronic disturbance.

In the acute disorder the retention of CO_2 results in a 2–4 mmol/l increase in the plasma [HCO$_3$$^-$] within 10 min of the original disturbance. The increase in

CO_2 pushes the reaction, $CO_2 + H_2O \rightleftharpoons H_2CO_3 \rightleftharpoons H^+ + HCO_3^-$ to the right and the excess H^+ are buffered by the non-bicarbonate buffer systems. This increase in $[HCO_3^-]$ rarely produces a plasma level greater than 28–30 mmol/l.

In chronic respiratory acidosis the increased P_{CO_2} and $[H^+]$ stimulates distal nephron H^+ excretion and HCO_3^- generation. This compensatory process produces a maximum level of plasma $[HCO_3^-]$ in 2–4 days, the level reached being less than 45 mmol/l (limit of compensation). This level may be estimated from the following equation:

$$\text{Plasma } [HCO_3^-] \text{ mmol/l} = 0\cdot36 \times P_{CO_2} \text{ mmHg} + 10.$$

Simple Respiratory Alkalosis

Respiratory alkalosis results from processes that decrease the blood P_{CO_2} level, either as a primary lesion, or secondary to metabolic acidosis. The primary disorder, due to increased pulmonary gas exchange, may be acute or chronic.

Acute respiratory alkalosis is attended by a fall in plasma $[HCO_3^-]$ of about 2–4 mmol/l which produces a plasma level of around 18–20 mmol/l. In this disorder the lowered blood P_{CO_2} forces the equation, $CO_2 + H_2O \rightleftharpoons H_2CO_3 \rightleftharpoons H^+ + HCO_3^-$, to the left. The fall in $[H^+]$ is buffered by the non-bicarbonate buffer systems (phosphate, protein).

In the chronic situation the lowered P_{CO_2} decreases distal nephron H^+ excretion, resulting in decreased renal regeneration of HCO_3^-, whilst in the proximal renal tubules it suppresses HCO_3^- reabsorption. These two processes of compensation produce a lowered plasma $[HCO_3^-]$ which reaches a plateau in 2–4 days. The limit of compensation is a plasma $[HCO_3^-]$ of around 12–15 mmol/l.

A feature of the respiratory alkalosis compensatory mechanism is that it may proceed to completion (pH of $\sim$7·40) if the primary disorder lasts for 1–2 weeks.

Mixed Acid–Base Disorders

In clinical practice it is not unusual to find more than one primary acid–base disorder in the same patient. In these cases a knowledge of the compensatory processes discussed above, and listed in *Table 5.1*, is helpful in determining the nature of the disturbances.

Metabolic and Respiratory Acidosis

In this double disorder there is an increased P_{CO_2} (respiratory acidosis) associated with a decreased plasma $[HCO_3^-]$ (metabolic acidosis). The pH will be low and out of proportion to that expected from the levels of P_{CO_2} or $[HCO_3^-]$, if either were the primary process. Occasionally this type of acidosis presents with a low $[HCO_3^-]$ (metabolic acidosis) and a normal P_{CO_2} level (35–45 mmHg). This situation constitutes a relative respiratory acidosis, i.e. if the disorder was a pure metabolic acidosis a low compensatory P_{CO_2} ($<$35 mmHg) would be expected.

Metabolic and Respiratory Alkalosis

This disorder is associated with a low P_{CO_2}, a high plasma $[HCO_3{}^-]$ and a high pH. The disorder may be mild with the P_{CO_2} in the 'normal range' (35–45 mmHg). In this case there is a relative respiratory alkalosis, i.e. if the disorder was a simple metabolic alkalosis a high P_{CO_2} (>45 mmHg) would be expected.

Respiratory Acidosis and Metabolic Alkalosis

In this mixed disorder there is a high P_{CO_2} associated with a high $[HCO_3{}^-]$ and a pH level near, or within, the normal range. This condition differs from compensated respiratory acidosis, and compensated metabolic alkalosis, in that it has a normal or near-normal pH. In the latter two conditions the pH is either low ($<7·35$ in respiratory acidosis) or high ($>7·45$ in metabolic alkalosis) because neither of these conditions will compensate completely. The other feature of this mixed condition is that both the P_{CO_2} and the $[HCO_3{}^-]$ are usually outside of the range expected in compensation of simple disorders (*see Table* 5.1).

Table 5.1. Simple acid–base disturbances; characteristics of compensation

Disorder	Primary lesion	Compensation	Compensation limits
Metabolic acidosis	$\downarrow [HCO_3{}^-]$	$\downarrow P_{CO_2}$	Limit: $P_{CO_2} \sim 10$ mmHg Expected P_{CO_2} mmHg: $1·5 \times [HCO_3{}^-] + 8 \pm 2$
Metabolic alkalosis	$\uparrow [HCO_3{}^-]$	$\uparrow P_{CO_2}$	Limit: P_{CO_2} 55–60 mmHg Expected P_{CO_2} mmHg: $0·9 \times [HCO_3{}^-] + 9$
Respiratory acidosis			
Acute	$\uparrow P_{CO_2}$	$\uparrow [HCO_3{}^-]$	Limit: $[HCO_2{}^-] \sim 30$ mmol/l Expected $[HCO_3{}^-]$ mmol/l: $\uparrow$ by 2–4
Chronic	$\uparrow P_{CO_2}$	$\uparrow [HCO_3{}^-]$	Limit: $[HCO_3{}^-] \sim 45$ mmol/l Expected $[HCO_3{}^-]$ mmol/l: $0·36 \times P_{CO_2} + 10$
Respiratory alkalosis			
Acute	$\downarrow P_{CO_2}$	$\downarrow [HCO_3{}^-]$	Limit: $[HCO_3{}^-] \sim 18$ mmol/l Expected $[HCO_3{}^-]$ mmol/l: $\downarrow$ by 2–4
Chronic	$\downarrow P_{CO_2}$	$\downarrow [HCO_3{}^-]$	Limit: $[HCO_3{}^-] \sim 12$ mmol/l Expected; pH to $\sim 7·40$

Respiratory Alkalosis and Metabolic Acidosis

Depending on the severity of this condition the pH will be normal, or mildly deviated from normal, and associated with a low P_{CO_2} and a low $[HCO_3{}^-]$. The two conditions that may cause confusion are compensated metabolic acidosis and chronic respiratory alkalosis. In simple metabolic acidosis the P_{CO_2} will not be as low for a given $[HCO_3{}^-]$ (*see Table* 5.1) and the pH will be depressed (i.e. complete compensation does not occur). Chronic respiratory alkalosis may compensate completely but only if the disorder has been present for a period of 1–2 weeks. A 'compensated' respiratory alkalosis occurring prior to this period suggests a mixed disorder. Another clue to the diagnosis may be obtained from the anion gap value (p. 78). A high anion gap in the presence of a 'normal' pH and low levels of P_{CO_2} and $[HCO_3{}^-]$ is suggestive of a mixed disorder.

Mixed Metabolic Acidosis and Alkalosis
In this condition the P_{CO_2} and $[HCO_3]$ may be high, low or normal with a pH only moderately deviated from normal limits. It results from a metabolic alkalosis (↑ plasma $[HCO_3{}^-]$) which has a superimposed metabolic acidosis (↓ plasma $[HCO_3{}^-]$). If the metabolic acidosis is of the high anion gap variety identification of the disorder may be made on the basis of the plasma electrolyte picture, i.e. high anion gap with a normal or near-normal plasma $[HCO_3{}^-]$. In the case of a normal anion gap acidosis associated with a metabolic alkalosis the condition may become apparent only after treatment of either disorder is instituted. Otherwise the disorder should be suspected from the clinical findings, e.g. concurrent vomiting and diarrhoea.

Evaluation of Acid–Base Disorders
The evaluation of a patient with a suspected acid–base disorder involves analysis of three sets of data:
1. Clinical picture
2. Plasma electrolyte results
3. Blood gas values

Clinical Picture
A careful history and physical examination may provide information that leads the clinician to suspect a certain type of disorder, e.g. metabolic acidosis in diarrhoea, diabetes mellitus and renal failure; metabolic alkalosis in vomiting and diuretic therapy; respiratory acidosis in chronic lung disease; respiratory alkalosis in pneumonia and congestive cardiac failure; mixed respiratory alkalosis and metabolic acidosis in salicylate overdose.

Plasma Electrolytes
An inspection of the plasma electrolytes, particularly bicarbonate, potassium, chloride, anion gap and creatinine levels provides considerable information about possible acid–base disturbances.

Bicarbonate
↓ $[HCO_3{}^-]$ suggests metabolic acidosis or a compensated respiratory alkalosis.

↑ $[HCO_3{}^-]$ suggests metabolic alkalosis or a compensated respiratory acidosis.

(*Figs.* 5.5 and 5.6)

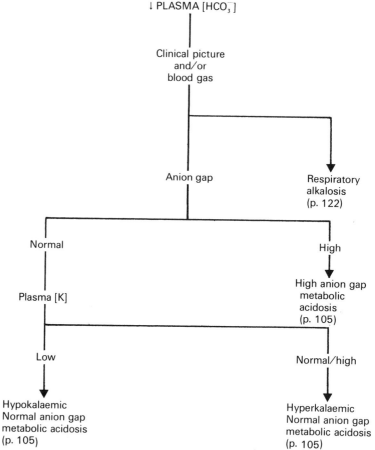

Fig. 5.5. Suggested scheme for the evaluation of a low plasma bicarbonate concentration.

Potassium

↑ [K$^+$] suggests acidosis (K$^+$ moves out of cells in exchange for H$^+$).
↓ [K$^+$] suggests alkalosis (K$^+$ moves into cells in exchange for H$^+$).

Chloride

↑ [Cl$^-$] suggests compensated respiratory alkalosis or hyperchloraemic metabolic acidosis.

↓ [Cl$^-$] suggests metabolic alkalosis or compensated respiratory acidosis.

Anion Gap (p. 78)

A high anion gap suggests a metabolic acidosis even if the plasma [HCO$_3$$^-$] is normal. This may occur in mixed metabolic acidosis and alkalosis.

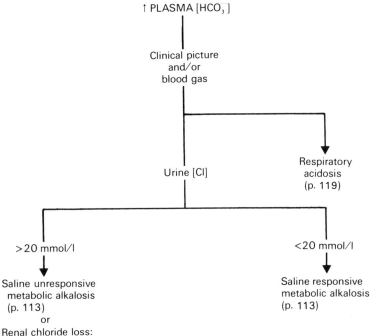

Fig. 5.6. Suggested scheme for the evaluation of a high plasma bicarbonate concentration.

Creatinine
High plasma levels suggest renal failure.

Blood Gas Values
When interpreting blood gas results consider the pH, the $[HCO_3^-]$, and the P_{CO_2} values separately and then combine the information to arrive at a diagnosis (*Figs.* 5.7, 5.8, 5.9). It is helpful to bear in mind the Henderson–Hasselbalch relationship:

$$pH \propto \frac{[HCO_3^-]}{P_{CO_2}}$$

pH may be ↑, N, or ↓

↑ = alkalaemia
N = normality, or compensation, or mixed disorder
↓ = acidaemia

$[HCO_3^-]$ may be ↑, N, or ↓.

↑ = metabolic alkalosis
↓ = metabolic acidosis

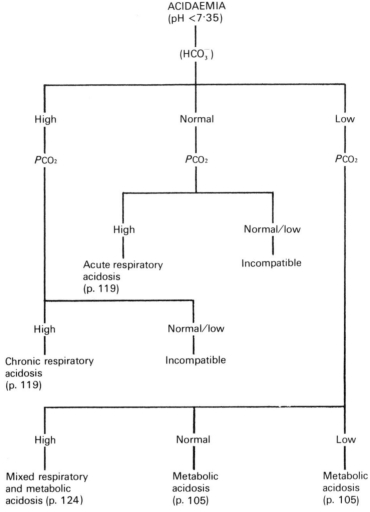

Fig. 5.7. Suggested scheme for the evaluation of acidaemia. (Reproduced with permission from Walmsley R. N. and White G. H. (1983) *A Guide to Diagnostic Clinical Chemistry.* Melbourne, Blackwell Scientific, p. 114.)

$P\text{CO}_2$ may be ↑, N, or ↓.

↑ = respiratory acidosis
↓ = respiratory alkalosis

It is also a useful exercise to check the validity of the blood gas values by calculating the $[H^+]$ from the $P\text{CO}_2$ and the $[HCO_3^-]$.

$$[H^+] = \frac{24 \times P\text{CO}_2\,(\text{mmHg})}{[HCO_3^-]\,\text{mmol/l}}\,\text{nmol/l}.$$

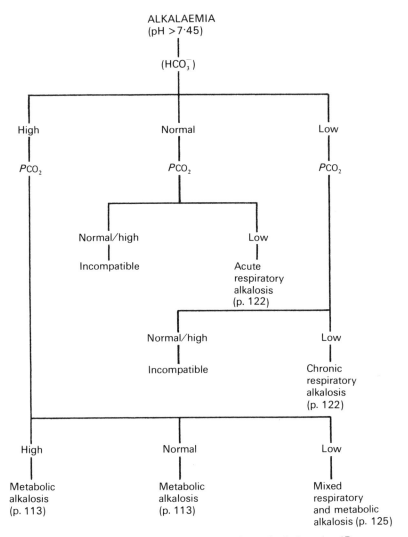

Fig. 5.8. Suggested scheme for the evaluation of alkalaemia. (Reproduced with permission from Walmsley R. N. and White G. H. (1983) *A Guide to Diagnostic Clinical Chemistry*. Melbourne, Blackwell Scientific, p. 115.)

In this regard useful values to remember are:

$$pH \text{ of } 7\cdot50 \sim 30\,nmol/l \text{ of } [H^+]$$
$$7\cdot40 \sim 40\,nmol/l \text{ of } [H^+]$$
$$7\cdot30 \sim 50\,nmol/l \text{ of } [H^+]$$
$$7\cdot20 \sim 60\,nmol/l \text{ of } [H^+]$$

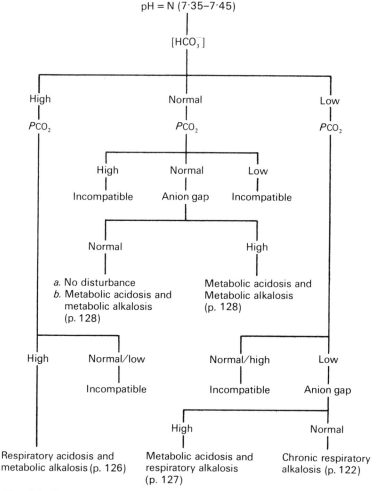

Fig. 5.9. Suggested scheme for the investigation of a patient with a suspected acid–base disorder, but with a normal pH. (Reproduced with permission from Walmsley R. N. and White G. H. (1983) *A Guide to Diagnostic Clinical Chemistry.* Melbourne, Blackwell Scientific, p. 116.)

N.B. In the following examples, and later case material, the term 'AHCO$_3$' indicates the 'actual' bicarbonate concentration which has been calculated (by the 'blood gas' instrument) from its measured pH and P_{CO_2} values, i.e. utilizing the Henderson–Hasselbalch equation. 'Plasma HCO$_3$' indicates the measured plasma bicarbonate concentration.

Example 1

pH   = 7·30   (7·35–7·45)
AHCO$_3$ = 15 mmol/l (23–33)

P_{CO_2} $= 30\,\text{mmHg}$ (35–45)

$$\text{pH}\ (\downarrow) \propto \frac{[HCO_3{}^-]\ (\downarrow)}{P_{CO_2}\ (\downarrow)}.$$

1. $[H^+] = (24 \times 30)/15 = 48\,\text{nmol/l}$ (pH 7·3 = 50 nmol/l)
2. pH $= \downarrow$ = acidaemia
3. $[HCO_3{}^-] = \downarrow$ = metabolic acidosis
4. $P_{CO_2} = \downarrow$ = respiratory alkalosis

This patient has a metabolic acidosis and a respiratory alkalosis. The pH shows an acidaemia and therefore the primary disorder is the acidosis and the respiratory alkalosis is compensatory. The primary lesion could not have been a respiratory alkalosis because 'over compensation' never occurs.

Example 2

pH $= 7·39$ (7·35–7·45)
$AHCO_3$ $= 15\,\text{mmol/l}$ (23–33)
P_{CO_2} $= 24\,\text{mmHg}$ (35–45)
Anion gap $= 25\,\text{mEq/l}$ (7–17)

$$\text{pH (N)} \propto \frac{[HCO_3{}^-](\downarrow)}{P_{CO_2}\ (\downarrow)}.$$

1. $[H^+] = (24 \times 24)/15 = 38\,\text{nmol/l}$ (pH 7·39 = 40 nmol/l)
2. pH = normal = ? normality, ? mixed disorder, ? fully compensated disorder
3 $[HCO_3{}^-] = \downarrow$ = metabolic acidosis
4. $P_{CO_2} = \downarrow$ = respiratory alkalosis

This patient has a respiratory alkalosis and a metabolic acidosis. This could represent a mixed disorder or a compensated primary disorder (respiratory alkalosis or a metabolic acidosis). Four points suggest it is a mixed disorder:

1. pH = normal ($\sim$7·40). It is unusual for primary disorders to compensate fully.
2. If the primary disorder was a metabolic acidosis the expected P_{CO_2} would be

$$1·5 \times [HCO_3{}^-] + 8 = \sim 30\,\text{mmHg}.$$

The measured P_{CO_2} of 24 mmHg is far too low for a compensated metabolic acidosis with a $[HCO_3{}^-]$ of 15 mmol/l.

3. If the primary disorder was a respiratory alkalosis complete compensation would be unlikely unless the condition was present for at least a week, and in this disorder the anion gap would be expected to be normal.
4. The high anion gap suggests a metabolic acidosis, and, as noted above, if this was the only abnormality the expected P_{CO_2} would be of the order of 30 mmHg.

These blood gas values were those of a patient who took an overdose of salicylate. This situation often results in a mixed respiratory alkalosis, and metabolic acidosis of the high anion gap variety.

Metabolic Acidosis

Metabolic acidosis results from any process that lowers the plasma bicarbonate concentration. It may be primary, or secondary to respiratory alkalosis (compensation). A low plasma $[HCO_3^-]$ is not always associated with acidaemia, e.g. compensation of respiratory alkalosis; and a metabolic acidosis can be associated with a normal or high plasma bicarbonate concentration, e.g. mixed metabolic acidosis and alkalosis.

Consequences

The effects of acidaemia *per se* are usually overwhelmed by the features of the primary disease process, e.g. renal failure, diabetes mellitus. However, some of the consequences have diagnostic and management implications and should be evaluated prior to treatment.

Potassium Metabolism

Hyperkalaemia is usually associated with acidaemia (movement of K^+ out of cells in exchange for extracellular H^+); however, most disorders which present with metabolic acidosis and hyperkalaemia usually have deranged potassium metabolism due to causes other than the high $[H^+]$, e.g. insulin deficiency in diabetes and decreased renal excretion in renal failure. Experimental evidence suggests that a high $[H^+]$ due to organic acids (lactic, ketoacids) does not cause K^+ to move out of cells whereas an acidosis due to HCl (e.g. NH_4Cl ingestion) will result in K^+ movement from the cells.

Some patients with metabolic acidosis can present with hypokalaemia (*Table* 5.3). This usually occurs in conditions where there is excessive loss of K^+ from the body, e.g. renal tubular acidosis.

During prolonged acidosis there is increased renal potassium excretion which may result in severe potassium depletion. This is thought to be due to increased distal tubular flow rate as a consequence of decreased proximal tubular sodium reabsorption (cause unknown).

Calcium Metabolism

Acidaemia enhances the bone mobilization of calcium, decreases its protein binding and reduces renal tubular Ca^{2+} reabsorption resulting in hypercalciuria. This can cause a negative calcium balance and consequently bone disease; the hypercalciuria may result in nephrocalcinosis and nephrolithiasis. These features are common in untreated Type 1 renal tubular acidosis.

Myocardial Function

Acidaemia impairs myocardial contraction and can result in cardiac failure, especially if the pH falls below 7·00 ($[H^+]$ of 100 nmol/l).

Compensation

As stated above the acidaemia of metabolic acidosis stimulates respiration and the consequent hypocapnia (respiratory alkalosis) returns the pH towards, but not to, normal.

Causes

In order to understand the pathophysiology of metabolic acidosis and to classify it along diagnostic lines it is helpful to arrange the causes into two groups: pathophysiological (*Table* 5.2) and diagnostic (*Table* 5.3).

Table 5.2. Classification of metabolic acidosis according to pathophysiology

---

Increased acid production
  Ketosis: diabetes mellitus, starvation, ethanol
  Lactic acidosis: (*Table* 5.4)
  Toxins: salicylate, ethylene glycol, methanol, paraldehyde
  Therapy: NH_4Cl, lysine and arginine HCl

Decreased acid excretion
  Renal failure: acute, chronic
  Renal tubular acidosis: Type 1, Type 4

Loss of bicarbonate
  Diarrhoea
  Renal tubular acidosis Type 2
  Diversion of urine to gut: ureterosigmoidostomy, vesico-colic fistula, ileal bladder

---

Table 5.3. Diagnostic classification of metabolic acidosis

High anion gap
  Renal failure
  Ketoacidosis
  Lactic acidosis (*Table* 5.4)
  Toxins: methanol, salicylate, ethylene glycol, paraldehyde

Normal anion gap (hyperchloraemic)
  Hyperkalaemia
    Early uraemia acidosis
    Obstructive nephropathy
    Therapy with NH_4Cl, lysine and arginine HCl
    Hypoaldosteronism (Type 4 renal tubular acidosis)
  Hypokalaemia
    Diarrhoea
    Renal tubular acidosis (Types 1 and 2)
    Carbonic anhydrase inhibitors (acetazolamide)
    Post-hypocapnia
    Diversion of urine into gut: vesico-colic fistula, ureterosigmoidostomy, ileal bladder

---

The basic biochemical lesion in simple metabolic acidosis is a decreased plasma level of bicarbonate which may come about by:

1. Addition of H^+ (↑ production, ↓ excretion) to the buffer system.

$$H^+ + NaHCO_3 \longrightarrow Na^+ + H_2CO_3 \longrightarrow CO_2 + H_2O.$$

2.   Loss of HCO_3^- from the extracellular fluid:
  a.   Diarrhoea (small bowel secretions contain HCO_3^-)
  b.   Renal tubular loss ($\downarrow$ proximal reabsorption in Type 2 renal tubular acidosis)

Diagnosis/Evaluation
  After a thorough clinical examination of the patient, which may provide clues about a possible acid–base disorder, the plasma electrolytes should be evaluated. In many patients this can provide sufficient information for diagnosis and management. In others, especially the very ill or if there is the possibility of a mixed disorder, arterial blood gases may be required.

Plasma Electrolytes
Particular attention should be given to the $[HCO_3^-]$, the anion gap and the potassium concentration.

Bicarbonate
A low plasma $[HCO_3^-]$ suggests either a primary metabolic acidosis or a compensated respiratory alkalosis (*see Fig.* 5.5). A normal, or even a high, level does not exclude metabolic acidosis (*see* Mixed metabolic acidosis and alkalosis, p. 128).

Anion Gap
The normal plasma anion gap ($[Na^+]mmol/l + [K^+]mmol/l - [Cl^-]mmol/l - [HCO_3^-] mmol/l$) is of the order of 7–17 mEq/l. A high level, except in rare circumstances (p. 78), indicates a metabolic acidosis. For diagnostic purposes metabolic acidosis can be classified into high and normal anion gap types (*see Table* 5.3).

Potassium
An inspection of the plasma potassium level is an important part of the evaluation of patients with metabolic acidosis because of the possibility of life-threatening hyperkalaemia. It is also helpful in the evaluation of the normal anion gap acidoses (*see Table* 5.3).

Blood Gas Values
If arterial blood gas results are available particular attention should be given to:
1.   The degree of acidaemia (pH)
2.   The possibility of a mixed disorder
3.   The blood Po_2 level

Acidaemia
The decision whether or not to employ alkali therapy (e.g. bicarbonate) rests on the degree of acidaemia. Most clinicians would seriously consider intervention if the patient's pH is less than 7·20 ($[H^+]$ of around 60 nmol/l).

Mixed Disorders

The possibility of a mixed disorder should always be borne in mind, especially if the pH is very low, e.g. <6·9 (combined respiratory and metabolic acidosis), or near normal, e.g. ~7·40 (combined respiratory alkalosis and metabolic acidosis).

Blood Po$_2$

The level of Po$_2$ gives some indication of the patient's oxygen status, e.g. anaerobic glycolysis and increased lactic acid production probably does not occur at Po$_2$ levels greater than 40 mmHg.

Principles of Management

Therapy of metabolic acidosis is aimed at increasing the extracellular bicarbonate concentration. This may be accomplished by treating the initial disease or, in severe cases, alkali therapy.

The decision to institute bicarbonate therapy depends on: (*a*) the type of disorder, e.g. Type 1 RTA will require oral bicarbonate therapy but patients with diabetic ketoacidosis may be able to generate sufficient bicarbonate from the circulating ketones after insulin is administered; (*b*) the severity of the acidaemia (many clinicians consider a pH of 7·20 to be the point of intervention for bicarbonate therapy).

Parenteral Bicarbonate Therapy

Indication

pH less than 7·00–7·20.

Aim

To increase the pH to 7·20–7·30 or the [HCO$_3$⁻] to 15–20 mmol/l.

Amount

A rough estimation of the amount required can be calculated from the plasma bicarbonate level and the patient's weight. Assume the bicarbonate 'space' to be ~50% of the body weight and calculate the amount of bicarbonate required to raise the level to 15–20 mmol/l.

E.g. 70-kg patient with a [HCO$_3$⁻] of 10 mmol/l.
To raise the [HCO$_3$⁻] to 15 mmol/l approximately 175 (0·5 × 70 × 5) mmol will be required. However, in practice the patient is 'titrated' by infusing bicarbonate and regularly checking the plasma level.

Complications

1.   Sodium overload—Each mmol of bicarbonate is balanced by 1 mmol of sodium and the infusion of large quantities may result in sodium (and water) overload. Particular care in this regard must be exercised in patients with renal impairment.

2. Hypokalaemia—Infusion of HCO_3^- and the subsequent rise in pH increases the passage of K^+ into cells. This cellular movement is an important consideration in potassium-depleted conditions (e.g. renal tubular acidosis) where severe hypokalaemia consequent to HCO_3^- therapy can result in respiratory paralysis. If hypokalaemia is present it is important to commence potassium repletion before giving parenteral bicarbonate therapy.

3. Tetany—Alkalaemia enhances the binding of Ca^{2+} to protein which can result in a low plasma $[Ca^{2+}]$ and tetany. The patients most at risk are those with renal failure.

4. Alkalosis: 'Overshoot' alkalosis can occur in patients who have large quantities of circulating organic acids.

E.g. in diabetic ketoacidosis insulin therapy increases cell uptake and conversion of ketone bodies to bicarbonate. The ketone bodies are taken up by the cells in the acid form ($H^+KETONE^-$), the H^+ coming from the extracellular CO_2 and water. This process generates bicarbonate, i.e.

1. $CO_2 + H_2O \longrightarrow H_2CO_3$
2. $Na^+.KETONE^- + H_2CO_3 \longrightarrow Na^+.HCO_3^- + H^+.KETONE^-$
3. $H^+.KETONE^-$ removed by cell uptake

Case Examples

Lactic Acidosis

A 71-year-old female was admitted to hospital with peripheral circulatory collapse due to cardiogenic shock (myocardial infarction). On examination she was cyanotic, had a pulse rate of 140, and a systolic blood pressure of 95 mmHg. The results below are those of blood samples taken prior to resuscitation.

Plasma	Na	141 mmol/l	(142–144)
	K	5·3 mmol/l	(3·2–4·8)
	Cl	102 mmol/l	(98–108)
	HCO_3	12 mmol/l	(23–33)
	Creat	0·15 mmol/l	(0·06–0·12)
	Anion gap	32 mEq/l	(7–17)
	Lactate	16·3 mmol/l	(<2)
Blood	pH	7·15	(7·35–7·45)
	H^+	70 nmol/l	(35–45)
	P_{CO_2}	26 mmHg	(35–45)
	P_{CO_2}	32 mmHg	(80–110)
	$AHCO_3$	9 mmol/l	(24/32)

Comment

The plasma analyte values indicate that the patient has a high anion gap metabolic acidosis which is due to accumulation of lactic acid. This has resulted from tissue hypoxia (circulatory collapse, and P_{O_2} 32 mmHg).

An inspection of the blood gas results shows:

1. A calculated $[H^+]$ (from P_{CO_2} and $[HCO_3^-]$, p. 86) of 69 nmol/l which correlates with the measured value of 70 nmol/l.

2. The estimated level of P_{CO_2} (compensation) for a metabolic acidosis with a plasma $[HCO_3^-]$ of 9 mmol/l is 21.5 ± 2 mmHg (*see Table* 5.1) which is close to, but lower than, the measured value. This infers, not a concurrent respiratory acidosis, but a respiratory response which has not yet reached a plateau, i.e. the maximum compensation may not be evident for 12–24 h.

Lactic acidosis is defined as a metabolic acidosis with an acidaemia (pH < 7.35) and a plasma lactate level greater than 7 mmol/l (reference range < 2 mmol/l). The causes can be divided into two groups: (1) those with overt tissue hypoxia (Type A), and (2) those where tissue hypoxia is not apparent (Type B)—*Table* 5.4.

Table 5.4. Causes of lactic acidosis

Type A—tissue hypoxia apparent
  Severe hypoxia
  Severe anaemia
  Shock/haemorrhage/hypotension
  Congestive cardiac failure

Type B—tissue hypoxia not apparent
  Acquired disease: diabetes mellitus, liver failure, seizures, tumours
  Drugs/toxins: biguanides, ethanol, methanol
  Congenital disorders: deficiency of: glucose-6-phosphatase, fructose-1,6-diphosphatase

Lactic acidosis should be suspected if there is a severe acidaemia associated with a high plasma anion gap and a suggestive clinical story (hypoxia, drugs, etc.). A plasma lactate estimation is not necessary for diagnosis providing other causes of a high anion gap acidosis (*see Table* 5.3) are excluded.

Diarrhoea and Metabolic Acidosis

The results below are those of a 76-year-old male who presented with a 5-day history of severe diarrhoea. He was later diagnosed as having the carcinoid syndrome (5-hydroxyindole acetic acid of 650 µmol/day—reference range < 60).

Plasma	Na	140 mmol/l	(132–144)
	K	2.8 mmol/l	(3.2–4.8)
	Cl	116 mmol/l	(98–108)
	HCO$_3$	15 mmol/l	(23–33)
	Creat	0.16 mmol/l	(0.06–0.12)
	Anion gap	12 mEq/l	(7–17)
Blood	pH	7.33	(7.35–7.45)
	H$^+$	47 nmol/l	(35–45)
	P_{CO_2}	31 mmHg	(35–45)
	P_{O_2}	86 mmHg	(80–110)
	AHCO$_3$	16 mmol/l	(24–32)

Comment

The calculated [H^+] of 46 nmol/l (from P_{CO_2} and [HCO_3^-]) checks with the measured value of 47 nmol/l, and the estimated (compensatory) P_{CO_2} of 32 ± 2 mmHg (*see Table* 5.1) correlates with the measured value of 31 mmHg.

This patient has a normal anion gap (hyperchloraemic) metabolic acidosis associated with hypokalaemia (*see Table* 5.3). In diarrhoea there is loss of sodium bicarbonate, potassium and water from the gut which results in metabolic acidosis, hypokalaemia and hypovolaemia. The hypovolaemia stimulates renal sodium reabsorption (as NaCl) and retention of ingested, or infused, NaCl which effects a hyperchloraemia (Na^+ lost in the diarrhoea fluid as $NaHCO_3$ is replaced by NaCl).

An important point to note in metabolic acidosis due to diarrhoea is that new bicarbonate can only be generated by the kidney (excretion of H^+ as NaH_2PO_4 and NH_4Cl). This process takes some days to maximize (dependent on ability of the kidney to increase production of NH_3) and intravenous bicarbonate therapy may be necessary. Potassium should be replaced with the bicarbonate because the increased [HCO_3^-] will force extracellular K^+ into the cells and aggravate the hypokalaemia.

Early Uraemia Acidosis

A 35-year-old female presented with a long history of vague symptoms of depression, anxiety and headaches which were self-treated with analgesics. She was given a diagnosis of analgesic nephropathy.

Plasma	Na	139 mmol/l	(132–144)
	K	6·1 mmol/l	(3·2–4·8)
	Cl	113 mmol/l	(98–108)
	HCO_3	17 mmol/l	(23–33)
	Creat	0·28 mmol/l	(0·06–0·12)
	Anion gap	15 mEq/l	(7–17)
Blood	pH	7·31	(7·35–7·45)
	H^+	49 nmol/l	(35–45)
	P_{CO_2}	34 mmHg	(35–45)
	P_{O_2}	95 mmHg	(80–110)
	$AHCO_3$	16 mmol/l	(24–32)

Comment

The calculated [H^+] of 51 nmol/l, and calculated compensatory P_{CO_2} of 32 ± 2 mmHg, correlates with the measured values and indicates a simple compensated metabolic acidosis.

The differential diagnosis of hyperkalaemic, hyperchloraemic metabolic acidosis is listed in *Table* 5.3. The commonest cause is early uraemic acidosis, the diagnosis of which is usually evident from the history and an inspection of the plasma electrolyte values. The next commonest cause is Type 4 renal tubular acidosis (hypoaldosteronism, p. 199 which shows a similar biochemical picture, i.e. hyperkalaemia and hyperchloraemic metabolic acidosis with mild to moderately impaired renal function (↑ plasma [creatinine]).

Patients with analgesic nephropathy have, early in the disease, distal nephron dysfunction (H^+ and K^+ retention) associated with a moderate decrease in GFR (retain the ability to excrete acid anions). The renal loss of Na^+ ($\downarrow$ distal nephron Na^+–H^+ exchange) results in hypovolaemia which increases the proximal nephron reabsorption of NaCl, and encourages retention of ingested NaCl. Thus the decrease in plasma [HCO_3^-] ($\downarrow$ distal nephron generation) is accompanied by an increase in [Cl^-] which may result in hyperchloraemia.

Metabolic Alkalosis
Any process that raises the plasma bicarbonate level is considered to be metabolic alkalosis. This may occur as a primary process, or be secondary to respiratory acidosis. It need not necessarily be associated with alkalaemia or a raised plasma bicarbonate concentration, e.g. mixed metabolic acidosis and alkalosis.

Under normal circumstances the body's respiratory system compensates for the alkalaemia of a high plasma bicarbonate level by decreasing respiration and increasing the Pco_2. This compensation process returns the H^+ concentration towards normal but, like most other acid–base compensatory processes, rarely to normal.

Consequences
The major effect of alkalaemia is enhanced protein binding of Ca^{2+} with consequent increased neuromuscular activity. This becomes apparent in severe alkalaemia when positive Chvostek and Trousseau signs, twitching and tetany may occur.

Other metabolic effects include:
1. Hypokalaemia—passage of K^+ into cells (exchange for H^+) and increased renal K^+ excretion
2. Increased renal calcium reabsorption
3. Enhanced glycolysis resulting in increased lactic acid production and a small increase (1–2 mEq/l) in the plasma anion gap
4. Cellular uptake of phosphate resulting occasionally in mild hypophosphataemia

The alkalaemia of metabolic alkalosis suppresses respiration with a consequent increased blood Pco_2 (hypercapnia) and return of the pH towards normal (compensation). This compensatory response is limited by the concurrent decrease in oxygenation which is a potent stimulus for increased respiration. Thus, unlike metabolic acidosis, there is not a well-defined relationship between the blood [HCO_3^-] and the blood Pco_2. The limit of compensation is a blood Pco_2 of around 55–60 mmHg. Several formulae have been constructed to estimate the level of Pco_2 for a given [HCO_3^-], ((1) and (2) below), but generally they have proved unreliable.

1. P_{CO_2} (mmHg) $= 0.9 \times [HCO_3^-]$ (mmol/l) $+ 15.6$
2. P_{CO_2} (mmHg) $= 0.9 \times [HCO_3^-]$ (mmol/l) $+ 9$

Causes

The primary biochemical lesion in metabolic alkalosis is a raised plasma bicarbonate concentration, the level of which depends on the rate of generation of new bicarbonate on the one hand, and the rate of renal excretion on the other. In order to produce a sustained plasma level at least two mechanisms have to be brought into play: (1) generation of new bicarbonate, and (2) maintenance of the high plasma bicarbonate concentration.

Generation of Bicarbonate

The production of HCO_3^-, over and above basal levels, may occur in the following situations:

1. Increased exogenous alkali
  a. Ingestion and i.v. infusion of bicarbonate
  b. Infusion of substances metabolized by cells to bicarbonate (lactate, citrate, acetate)
2. Increased endogenous alkali
  a. Gastrointestinal—loss of H^+ in vomitus, chloride diarrhoea
  b. Renal—increased renal excretion of H^+: potassium depletion, aldosteronism, hypercapnia

Maintenance of Increased Plasma $[HCO_3^-]$

The generation, or ingestion, of 'new' bicarbonate usually does not result in hyperbicarbonataemia unless there is a mechanism to maintain the plasma level, e.g. a normal adult has to ingest some 100–120 g (> 1000 mmol) of sodium bicarbonate daily before there is a significant rise in the plasma level. This is due to the efficiency of the kidney in excreting bicarbonate loads.

Increased renal HCO_3^- reabsorption, and maintenance of a high plasma level, may occur in:

1. Hypovolaemia
2. Potassium depletion
3. Hyperaldosteronism
4. Hypercapnia

Potassium depletion and hyperaldosteronism are closely related, and the associated increased renal HCO_3^- generation, and reabsorption, probably requires that both be present. Either in isolation appear not to be able to maintain a high plasma bicarbonate level. The suggested sequence of events is: ↑ aldosterone ⟶ ↑ renal K^+ excretion ⟶ K^+ depletion ⟶ ↑ renal NH_3 production and excretion ⟶ ↑ renal H^+ excretion and ↑ bicarbonate generation (provided aldosterone is present in excess to encourage tubular Na^+–H^+ exchange).

Depending on the mechanism of hyperbicarbonataemia maintenance, the metabolic alkaloses can be divided into two groups:

1. Those associated with hypovolaemia which will respond to volume expansion with saline by lowering the plasma $[HCO_3^-]$—'saline responsive', i.e.

    ↑ Plasma   volume   (saline   infusion) $\longrightarrow$ ↓ renal HCO_3^- reabsorption $\longrightarrow$ loss of excess bicarbonate in the urine.

2. Those with normovolaemia, or hypervolaemia, who do not respond to saline infusions—'saline unresponsive'—i.e. those with aldosterone excess and potassium depletion.

    Tables 5.5 and 5.6 list the causes of metabolic alkalosis according to pathophysiology, and the response to saline.

Table 5.5. Classification of metabolic alkalosis based on pathophysiology

---

Loss of H^+
  Gastrointestinal
    Stomach: vomiting, gastric aspiration
    Bowel: chloride diarrhoea
  Renal
    Mineralocorticoid excess (p. 243)
    Potassium deficiency (p. 65)

Exogenous alkali load
  Bicarbonate: oral, intravenous
  Antacid therapy: magnesium carbonate
  Organic acid salts: lactate, acetate, citrate

Post-hypercapnia

Contraction alkalosis

Table 5.6. Classification of metabolic alkalosis according to response to saline load

---

Saline responsive
  Gastrointestinal: vomiting, gastric suction, chloride diarrhoea
  Renal: diuretic therapy
      post-hypercapnia
  Exogenous alkali bicarbonate,
    antacids,
    organic acid salts (lactate citrate, acetate)
  Contraction alkalosis

Saline unresponsive
  Mineralocorticoid excess
    Primary aldosteronism, ectopic ACTH syndrome
    Enzyme defects: 11- and 17-hydroxylase
    Bartter's syndrome
    Liddle's syndrome
    Liquorice ingestion
    Carbenoxolone therapy
  Severe potassium depletion

Diagnosis/Evaluation

In the majority of patients with metabolic alkalosis the cause is readily established from the clinical picture. In those cases with obscure aetiology special consideration should be given to the possibility of surreptitious vomiting and diuretic administration, especially if severe to moderate hypokalaemia is present. Further information may be obtained from the urinary chloride concentration (*see Fig.* 5.6). The saline-responsive group (*see Table* 5.5) has a low concentration (<20 mmol/l) and the unresponsive group has a level greater than 20 mmol/l.

A high anion gap associated with a metabolic alkalosis suggests a concurrent metabolic acidosis. Although alkalaemia is associated with increased lactate production this does not raise the plasma anion gap more than 2–3 mEq/l.

If blood gas results are available the $P\text{co}_2$ value should be checked for the possibility of an associated respiratory disorder. A low level (<35 mmHg) suggests a concurrent respiratory alkalosis, whilst a level greater than 60 mmHg indicates a possible underlying respiratory acidosis.

Principles of Management

The management of metabolic alkalosis depends on the cause and severity. In all cases the general principle is to reduce the alkalaemia by lowering the plasma bicarbonate level. This involves attention to the causes of generation and maintenance of the increased plasma bicarbonate.

In the volume-contracted or saline-responsive group the generating mechanism (vomiting, diuretics, etc.) should be returned to normal, the hypovolaemia resolved (intravenous saline if necessary), and any potassium deficit corrected. In mineralocorticoid excess the treatment depends on the aetiology but if it is of the endogenous type spironolactone administration will alleviate the problem until definitive treatment can be carried out.

Drastic measures aimed at lowering the bicarbonate level such as acid (HCl) administration, haemodialysis and carbonic anhydrase therapy are rarely necessary.

Case Examples

Vomiting

A 6-month-old infant was admitted to hospital with a 5-day history of projectile vomiting (pyloric stenosis). His admission acid–base parameters, and those 10 h later after intravenous normal saline infusion, with potassium supplements, are shown below.

Date		13/02	14/02	
Time (h)		2200	0800	
Plasma	Na	131	134 mmol/l	(132–144)
	K	2·1	3·6 mmol/l	(3·2–4·8)
	Cl	66	94 mmol/l	(98–108)
	HCO₃	>40	34 mmol/l	(23–33)
	Creat	0·05	0·04 mmol/l	(0·06–0·12)

Urine	Na	22	—mmol/l	
	K	28	—mmol/l	
	Cl	<10	—mmol/l	
Blood	pH	7·54	7·48	(7·35–7·45)
	H^+	29	33 nmol/l	(35–45)
	PCO_2	50	43 mmHg	(35–45)
	PO_2	51	75 mmHg	(80–110)
	$AHCO_3$	41	32 mmol/l	(24–32)

Comment

The admission blood gas and electrolyte values are typical of a patient who is vomiting from above the pylorus (gastric vomiting), e.g.

A. Loss of HCl and water (gastric juice):

HCl loss ⟶
1. Metabolic alkalosis (generation of HCO_3^-)
2. Hypochloraemia

Water loss ⟶ hypovolaemia ⟶
1. ↑ Aldosterone ⟶ ↑ renal K^+ loss
2. ↑ Renal NaCl reabsorption ⟶ ↓ urine $[Cl^-]$
3. ↑ Renal HCO_3^- reabsorption (maintenance of alkalosis)

B. The high plasma $[HCO_3^-]$ floods the renal reabsorption mechanism resulting in:
1. $NaHCO_3$ excretion ⟶ ↑ urine $[Na^+]$ (>20 mmol/l)
2. ↑ Distal nephron flow rate ⟶ ↑ renal K^+ excretion

C. The alkalaemia suppresses respiration producing:
1. ↑ PCO_2 (compensation)
2. ↓ PO_2

In metabolic alkalosis complete compensation (pH to 7·40) is rarely achieved because the decreased respiratory response to alkalaemia not only results in hypercapnia, but also in hypoxia. Both of these are potent respiratory stimulants and they eventually over-ride the alkalaemic suppression of respiration.

The metabolic alkalosis of vomiting is an example of the saline-responsive type (hypovolaemia, urine $[Cl^-]$ <20 mmol/l). This is illustrated in the above case where after appropriate saline infusion the $[HCO_3^-]$ has dropped from 41 to 32 mmol/l within a few hours.

Diuretic Therapy

The electrolyte and blood gas values shown below are those of a 76-year-old female, with congestive cardiac failure, who had been on diuretic (thiazide) therapy for 4 months.

Plasma	Na	124 mmol/l	(132–144)
	K	2·4 mmol/l	(3·2–4·8)
	Cl	76 mmol/l	(98–108)
	HCO_3	38 mmol/l	(23–33)
	Creat	0·07 mmol/l	(0·06–0·12)

Urine	Na	34 mmol/l	
	K	68 mmol/l	
	Cl	26 mmol/l	
Blood	pH	7·49	(7·35–7·45)
	H^+	32 nmol/l	(35–45)
	P_{CO_2}	47 mmHg	(35–45)
	P_{O_2}	62 mmHg	(80–110)
	$AHCO_3$	37 mmol/l	(24–32)

Comment

Hypokalaemic metabolic alkalosis is a common complication of diuretic therapy in patients treated for oedematous conditions (cardiac failure, nephrosis, cirrhosis). It is unusual in non-oedematous patients on diuretic therapy (e.g. essential hypertension). This difference may be due to increased aldosterone activity which is common in the former (secondary hyperaldosteronism), but not in the latter.

The probable sequence of events in the above patient is:

A. Diuretic therapy $\longrightarrow$ ↑ renal Na^+ loss $\longrightarrow$
1.   Hypovolaemia $\longrightarrow$ ↑ aldosterone
2.   ↑ Distal nephron flow rate
       (1)+(2) $\longrightarrow$ ↑ K^+ excretion $\longrightarrow$ hypokalaemia
B.
1.   Hypokalaemia + hyperaldosteronism $\longrightarrow$ ↑ renal HCO_3^- generation (H^+ excretion)
2.   Hypovolaemia + K^+ depletion $\longrightarrow$ ↑ proximal tubule HCO_3^- reabsorption
       (1)+(2) $\longrightarrow$ generation and maintenance of HCO_3^- $\longrightarrow$ metabolic alkalosis.

The high urine $[Cl^-]$ in this patient (>20 mmol/l) suggests saline resistance alkalosis. However, in this patient it is due to the continued action of the diuretic. If the diuretic was discontinued her urine $[Cl^-]$ would fall to low levels (<20 mmol/l).

Mineralocorticoid Excess

A male patient aged 55 years with a carcinoma of the bronchus presented with severe weakness in the upper and lower limbs and an 'Addisonian' type of pigmentation. A diagnosis of the ectopic ACTH syndrome was made on the basis of the clinical picture, the plasma electrolytes and the value of the random plasma cortisol.

Plasma	Na	144 mmol/l	(132–144)
	K	1·7 mmol/l	(3·2–4·8)
	Cl	85 mmol/l	(98–108)
	HCO_3	>40 mmol/l	(23–33)
	Creat	0·05 mmol/l	(0·06–0·12)
	Cortisol	1750 nmol/l	(160–690)
Urine	Na	71 mmol/l	
	K	22 mmol/l	
	Cl	35 mmol/l	

Blood	pH	7·53	(7·35–7·45)
	H^+	30 nmol/l	(35–45)
	P_{CO_2}	58 mmHg	(35–45)
	P_{O_2}	68 mmHg	(80–110)
	$AHCO_3$	47 mmol/l	(24–32)

Comment

In the ectopic ACTH syndrome there is excessive mineralocorticoid activity due either to the massive amounts of circulating cortisol (cortisol has weak mineralocorticoid activity) or to increased adrenal secretion of the aldosterone precursors, corticosterone and deoxycorticosterone (DOC).

In the distal nephron mineralocorticoids increase tubular cell H^+ (and K^+) secretion, and tubular fluid Na^+ reasorption which results in:
1.   ↑ K^+ excretion ⟶ hypokalaemia
2.   ↑ H^+ excretion ⟶ ↑ HCO^+ generation
3.   ↑ Na^+ reabsorption ⟶ hypervolaemia

The hypokalaemia, in turn, (*a*) increases renal tubular NH_3 secretion which then enhances renal H^+ excretion (and HCO_3^- generation), and (*b*) increases proximal renal tubular reabsorption of HCO_3^-. Thus, the metabolic alkalosis is generated and maintained by K^+ depletion and mineralocorticoid excess.

The hypervolaemia encourages renal Na^+ excretion by decreasing the reabsorption of NaCl in the proximal tubule, and the ascending limb of the loop of Henle. This brings body sodium back into balance (↑ reabsorption in the distal tubules and ↓ reabsorption in the proximal tubules), and results in excretion of dietary NaCl in the urine (urinary $[Cl^-] > 20$ mmol/l). The above patient is an example of saline-resistant metabolic alkalosis.

The blood P_{CO_2} level in this patient (58 mmHg) indicates that compensation has reached its limit (55–60 mmHg). If the P_{CO_2} was higher (>60 mmHg) a superimposed respiratory acidosis would have to be considered.

Respiratory Acidosis

Respiratory acidosis is defined as any process that increases the blood P_{CO_2} (hypercapnia). This is the result of CO_2 excretion lagging behind production, and is never due to increased CO_2 production. The increased P_{CO_2} may be the primary process, or it may be secondary to compensation of a primary metabolic alkalosis.

Consequences

Brain

Hypercapnia induces cerebral vasodilatation, and consequently the increased blood flow may result in an increased intracranial pressure. This could be responsible for the drowsiness, headache, stupor and coma which can be associated with respiratory acidosis.

Heart

Acidaemia depresses cardiac contractility but this is usually offset by the simultaneous acidaemic-induced release of adrenaline.

Potassium Metabolism

Hyperkalaemia occasionally accompanies acute respiratory acidosis (K^+ release from the cells) but it is unusual in chronic respiratory acidosis. In the kidney, acute acidaemia depresses potassium excretion, but in chronic acidaemia there is increased potassium excretion (exact cause unknown) which may result in mild body depletion.

Phosphate

Acidaemia may be associated with hyperphosphataemia due to phosphate efflux from cells.

Compensation

Within 5–10 min of acute hypercapnia there is a 2–4 mmol/l increase in plasma $[HCO_3^-]$ which may raise the plasma level to 28–30 mmol/l, i.e. the equation, $CO_2 + H_2O \rightleftharpoons H_2CO_3 \rightleftharpoons H^+ + HCO_3^-$, is forced to the right and the H^+ are removed by the non-bicarbonate buffer systems. This small increment in bicarbonate is followed, in chronic hypercapnia, by a steady rise in the plasma level which reaches a plateau within 2–4 days.

This sustained rise in bicarbonate is due to the effect of the raised plasma P_{CO_2} on the renal tubules, i.e.

$\uparrow P_{CO_2} \longrightarrow \uparrow$ renal $Na^+ - H^+$ exchange $\longrightarrow \uparrow$ renal H^+ excretion (mainly as NH_4Cl) $\longrightarrow \uparrow HCO_3^-$ generation $\longrightarrow$ $\uparrow$ plasma $[HCO_3^-]$.

This plasma bicarbonate response is fairly consistent for a given level of P_{CO_2} and may be roughly calculated from the following formula:

$$\text{Plasma } [HCO_3^-] \text{ mmol/l} = 0.36 \times P_{CO_2} \text{ mmHg} + 10.$$

The limit of compensation is a plasma bicarbonate level of around 45 mmol/l.

As the plasma bicarbonate rises there is a fall in the plasma chloride concentration. This is due to increased renal Cl^- excretion in association with increased urinary NH_3 excretion (as NH_4Cl).

Causes

Hypercapnia is due to pulmonary alveolar hypoventilation which may be a consequence of intrathoracic disease, central depression of respiration, or neuromuscular and chest wall disorders (*Table* 5.7).

Diagnosis/Evaluation

The clinical examination and inspection of plasma electrolyte values cannot be relied upon for the assessment of alveolar ventilation. Arterial blood gas

Table 5.7. Causes of respiratory acidosis

Central depression
  Trauma/cerebrovascular accident
  Infections of nervous system
  Intracranial neoplasms
  Drug overdose (hypnotics, narcotics)

Neuromuscular
  Poliomyelitis
  Guillain–Barré syndrome
  Multiple sclerosis
  Myopathy

Thoracic disease
  Restrictive defects
    hydrothorax
    pneumothorax
    flail chest
  Obstructive disease
    foreign body
    bronchitis
    asthma
    emphysema (chronic obstructive lung disease)
    severe pulmonary oedema

---

estimations are necessary if hypoventilation is suspected. Patients with respiratory acidosis are not immune to mixed acid–base disorders and a careful examination of the degree of acidaemia and blood bicarbonate levels should be made.

pH

Compensation of respiratory acidosis returns the pH towards normal but rarely to normal. Thus a near-normal pH suggests an underlying metabolic alkalosis. However, minor degrees of chronic hypercapnia (P_{CO_2} < 60 mmHg) may exhibit near-complete compensation (pH ~ 7·40).

[HCO$_3^-$]

The combination of metabolic alkalosis and respiratory acidosis is relatively common as a result of vomiting or diuretic therapy in patients with chronic obstructive lung disease. A bicarbonate concentration greater than 45 mmol/l or greater than the calculated compensatory response suggests this mixed disorder.

If, in addition to hypercapnia, there is tissue hypoxia there may be a metabolic acidosis superimposed on the respiratory disorder (anaerobic glycolysis produces lactic acid). In these circumstances the [HCO$_3^-$] may be low (< 25 mmol/l), but the diagnosis is usually evident from the blood gas results ($\downarrow$ P_{O_2}, and $\uparrow$ anion gap). On the other hand the [HCO$_3^-$] can be raised, but less than expected for the level of P_{CO_2}. In this case there can be confusion with a compensatory response that has not proceeded to completion. An estimation of the plasma anion gap may be helpful in these cases (a high anion gap usually indicates metabolic acidosis).

Principles of Management

Treatment is aimed at lowering the P_{CO_2} by relieving the initiating lesion. An important point to bear in mind is that following correction of the precipitating factors the plasma $[HCO_3^-]$ will take some 12–24 h to return to normal. Thus severe alkalaemia (post-hypercapnic metabolic alkalosis) may develop if the P_{CO_2} is lowered quickly, e.g. by mechanical ventilation.

Case Examples

Acute Respiratory Acidosis

A male of 18 years presented with acute asthma and bronchitis. His initial treatment included bronchodilatation therapy and oxygen. The admission blood gas values and those 90 min later are shown below.

Date		11/12	11/12	
Time	(h)	0315	0445	
Blood	pH	7·29	7·38	(7·35–7·45)
	H^+	51	42 nmol/l	(35–45)
	P_{CO_2}	63	47 mmHg	(35–45)
	P_{O_2}	48	118 mmHg	(80–110)
	$AHCO_3$	29	27 mmol/l	(24–32)

Comment

The blood gas picture in acute respiratory acidosis presents with hypercapnia, acidaemia and a plasma bicarbonate level in the upper half of the reference range but less than 30 mmol/l. The actual rise in bicarbonate is of the order of 0·1 mmol/l for each 1 mmHg rise in P_{CO_2} or around 2–4 mmol/l.

In the above case of acute hypoventilation the calculated rise in $[HCO_3^-]$ of around 2 mmol/l is in agreement with his measured values, i.e. if it is assumed that the second set of results are 'normal' for this patient.

Chronic Respiratory Acidosis

A 64-year-old male with chronic obstructive lung disease had a respiratory arrest whilst in hospital. The three blood gas results below show the patient's acid–base status prior to respiratory arrest, immediately after the arrest during oxygen therapy, and after cessation of oxygen therapy.

Date		28/05	29/05	29/05	
Time	(h)	2130	0045	0150	
Blood	pH	7·27	7·15	7·21	(7·35–7·45)
	H^+	54	70	62 nmol/l	(35–45)
	P_{CO_2}	83	115	91 mmHg	(35–45)
	P_{O_2}	55	122	55 mmHg	(80–110)
	$AHCO_3$	38	40	37 mmol/l	(24–32)

Comment

The compensatory rise in plasma bicarbonate in chronic respiratory acidosis, provided it is of at least 2 days' duration, is of the order of 0·35 mmol/l for each

1 mmHg rise in the $P\text{CO}_2$. A rough calculation of the final $[\text{HCO}_3{}^-]$ level can be made using the formula on p. 118. In the above case the compensatory plasma $[\text{HCO}_3{}^-]$, for a $P\text{CO}_2$ of 83 mmHg, should be around 40 mmol/l which is near the measured level of 38 mmol/l.

The second set of values shows the effect of an acute respiratory acidosis superimposed on the chronic form, i.e. an acute increase in the $P\text{CO}_2$ resulting in an acute increase of 2 mmol/l in the plasma bicarbonate and an increase of 16 nmol/l in the $[\text{H}^+]$. This increase is dissipated as the $P\text{CO}_2$ returns towards its original level (third set of results).

Respiratory Alkalosis
Respiratory alkalosis (hypocapnia) occurs when CO_2 excretion rate exceeds production rate. The only process resulting in this disorder is pulmonary hyperventilation.

Consequences
The main clinical features of respiratory alkalosis are those of alkalaemia, i.e. increased protein binding of Ca^{2+} with increased neuromuscular activity (tetany, etc.). The occasional central nervous system effects of light headedness and nausea may be related to hypocapnic cerebral vasoconstriction.

Occasionally, depending on the severity and duration of the alkalosis, there can be slight to mild disturbances of potassium, glucose and phosphate metabolism.

Potassium
Initially there can be a slight decrease in plasma $[\text{K}^+]$ (entry into cells, increased renal excretion) but this does not usually result in hypokalaemia.

Glucose
Alkalaemia enhances glycolysis and increases lactate production. This lactate increase may result in a 2–3 mEq/l increase in the anion gap.

Phosphate
Hypophosphataemia, due to alkalaemic-induced phosphate entry into cells, often occurs, and may be marked if the alkalaemia is prolonged.

Compensation
In the acute phase of hypocapnia there is a fall of some 2–4 mmol/l in the plasma $[\text{HCO}_3{}^-]$, i.e. the equation, $\text{CO}_2 + \text{H}_2\text{O} \rightleftharpoons \text{H}_2\text{CO}_3 \rightleftharpoons \text{H}^+ + \text{HCO}_3{}^-$, is forced to the left and the decrease in $[\text{H}^+]$ is buffered by the non-bicarbonate systems. This fall rarely produces a plasma $[\text{HCO}_3{}^-]$ below 18 mmol/l.

In the chronic phase there is a further fall in $[\text{HCO}_3{}^-]$ due to renal tubular H^+ retention ($\downarrow$ $\text{HCO}_3{}^-$ generation), and reduced proximal renal tubular $\text{HCO}_3{}^-$

reabsorption. The plasma level reaches a plateau in 2–4 days at around 12–15 mmol/l (limit of compensation).

As the plasma $[HCO_3^-]$ falls the plasma $[Cl^-]$ rises due to increased tubular reabsorption of NaCl, i.e. $\downarrow$ P_{CO_2} $\longrightarrow$ $\downarrow$ renal Na^+–H^+ exchange $\longrightarrow$ $\uparrow$ renal Na^+ loss (as $NaHCO_3$) $\longrightarrow$ hypovolaemia $\longrightarrow$ $\uparrow$ proximal renal tubule Na^+ reabsorption (as NaCl). Thus, Na^+ is lost in the urine as $NaHCO_3$, and is replaced in the plasma by NaCl.

Causes

As stated above the cause of respiratory alkalosis is hyperventilation. This may be due to central or pulmonary mechanisms (*Table* 5.8).

Table 5.8. Causes of respiratory alkalosis

Central
　　Anxiety/hysteria
　　Pregnancy
　　Hypoxaemia
　　Hepatic encephalopathy
　　Gram-negative septicaemia
　　Salicylate overdose
　　Cranial pathology: infection, tumour, injury

Pulmonary
　　Pulmonary embolism
　　Congestive cardiac failure
　　Asthma
　　Pneumonia

Mechanical Ventilation

Diagnosis/Evaluation

The plasma electrolyte pattern of respiratory alkalosis (hypobicarbonataemia and hyperchloraemia) resembles that of hyperchloraemic metabolic acidosis. In some cases blood gas estimations may be required to distinguish between the two.

Hypocapnia may be primary (acute, chronic), or secondary to metabolic acidosis. In the latter disorder there is an acidaemia and only if the P_{CO_2} is below the metabolic acidosis compensation limit (~ 10 mmHg) can a separate element of respiratory alkalosis be evoked.

In chronic primary respiratory alkalosis complete compensation can occur, and there can be difficulty in distinguishing the blood gas picture of this disorder from that of a mixed respiratory alkalosis and metabolic acidosis (*see below*). However, the clinical picture should provide sufficient clues for a diagnosis to be made.

Principles of Management

Treatment is directed at normalizing the blood P_{CO_2} by removing the cause, and in most cases no other therapy is required. However, there have been reports of severe alkalaemia occurring in respiratory alkalosis, and these can be associated with cardiac arrhythmias. In these cases controlled mechanical ventilation (after respiratory paralysis) has been successful. Other therapeutic measures that have been used in these situations are acetazolamide, NH_4Cl and HCl administration with the object of decreasing the alkalaemia by lowering the plasma $[HCO_3^-]$.

Case Examples

Acute Respiratory Alkalosis

A 49-year-old female with a long history of asthma presented in acute distress with severe shortness of breath and paraesthesia in both hands and around the mouth.

Blood	pH	7·61	(7·35–7·45)
	H^+	24 nmol/l	(35–45)
	P_{CO_2}	19 mmHg	(35–45)
	P_{O_2}	70 mmHg	(80–110)
	$AHCO_3$	20 mmol/l	(24–32)

Comment

In acute respiratory alkalosis the fall in plasma $[HCO_3^-]$ is of the order of 0·2 mmol/l for each 1-mmHg fall in P_{CO_2}. This occurs within 10 min of the onset of hyperventilation and usually results in a plasma bicarbonate concentration which is often below the lower limit of the reference range, but generally greater than 18 mmol/l.

The blood gas picture associated with acute asthma is variable, and may present as respiratory alkalosis or respiratory acidosis.

Chronic Respiratory Alkalosis

A male of 72 years with congestive cardiac failure presented with bilateral ankle oedema and increasing shortness of breath over the previous 3 days.

Plasma	Na	135 mmol/l	(132–144)
	K	3·4 mmol/l	(3·2–4·8)
	Cl	110 mmol/l	(98–108)
	HCO_3	16 mmol/l	(23–33)
	Creat	0·19 mmol/l	(0·06–0·12)
Blood	pH	7·47	(7·35–7·45)
	H^+	34 nmol/l	(35–45)
	P_{CO_2}	25 mmHg	(35–45)
	P_{O_2}	62 mmHg	(80–110)
	$AHCO_3$	17 mmol/l	(24–32)

Comment

The persistent hyperventilation associated with congestive cardiac failure is due partly to hypoxia ($\downarrow P_{O_2}$) and partly to pulmonary reflex mechanisms. Within hours of the initial acute fall in plasma [HCO_3^-] the level declines further, and over a period of 2–4 days, reaches a steady state. The lowest level reached in the most severe cases is around 12–15 mmol/l.

This fall in bicarbonate, which is of the order of 0·5 mmol/l for each mmHg fall in P_{CO_2}, is due to increased renal excretion, and decreased renal generation of HCO_3^-. This plasma bicarbonate decrease is accompanied by an increased plasma [Cl^-] which is due to renal Cl^- retention, i.e.

$$\downarrow CO_2 \longrightarrow \downarrow \text{renal tubular Na}^+\text{-H}^+ \text{ exchange} \longrightarrow .$$

1.   (a) ↓ Tubule HCO_3^- generation
        (b) ↓ Proximal tubule HCO_3^- reabsorption
        (a) + (b) ⟶ ↓ plasma [HCO_3^-]
2.   Renal Na^+ loss (as $NaHCO_3$) ⟶ Na^+ depletion ⟶ hypovolaemia ⟶ ↑ proximal tubular Na^+ reabsorption (as $NaCl$ ⟶ hyperchloraemia.

Chronic respiratory alkalosis is the only simple acid–base disorder, other than mild respiratory acidosis, which can show complete compensation (pH to ~7·40). This compensation usually takes up to 1–2 weeks to develop.

Mixed Acid–Base Disorders

A mixed acid–base disorder is the occurrence of two or more primary acid–base disturbances in the same patient. Although their presence may be suspected from the clinical picture the definitive diagnosis depends on examination, and correct interpretation, of the blood gas values. In this context a knowledge of the nature and magnitude of the compensatory mechanisms of simple (primary) acid–base disorders is essential (*see Table* 5.1).

Respiratory and Metabolic Acidosis

Causes
This combination commonly occurs when there is respiratory depression (respiratory acidosis) associated with severe hypoxia (anaerobic glycolysis ⟶ ↓ lactate production).
1.   Cardiopulmonary arrest
2.   Drug overdose (sedatives, narcotics)
3.   Severe obstructive pulmonary disease
4.   Severe pulmonary oedema

Diagnosis
The hallmark of this disorder is:
1.   Very low pH—acidaemia
2.   Low plasma [HCO_3^-]—metabolic acidosis

3.   Normal to high P_{CO_2}—respiratory acidosis, i.e.

$$\text{pH} (\downarrow \downarrow) \propto \frac{[HCO_3^-] (\downarrow) \text{ (metabolic acidosis)}}{P_{CO_2} (\uparrow) \text{ (respiratory acidosis)}}.$$

Case Example
A 70-year-old male with cardiopulmonary collapse.

Blood	pH	6·85	(7·35–7·45)
	H^+	141 nmol/l	(35–45)
	P_{CO_2}	77 mmHg	(35–45)
	P_{O_2}	21 mmHg	(80–110)
	$AHCO_3$	13 mmol/l	(24–32)

Plasma anion gap: 27 mEq/l (7–17)

Comment
In this case the severe hypoxia (respiratory and circulatory collapse) results in anaerobic glycolysis and excessive lactic acid production (increased anion gap). The diagnosis is straightforward as both the respiratory and metabolic components indicate a primary acidosis.

Respiratory and Metabolic Alkalosis

Causes
This disorder is usually the result of two different processes:
1.   Diuretic therapy (metabolic alkalosis) in hepatic failure (respiratory alkalosis)
2.   Mechanical ventilation (respiratory alkalosis) in patients with nasogastric suction (metabolic alkalosis)
3.   Pneumonia (respiratory alkalosis) and vomiting (metabolic alkalosis)

Diagnosis
This disorder usually shows a low P_{CO_2} and a normal to increased plasma $[HCO_3^-]$, i.e.

$$\text{pH}(\uparrow \uparrow) \propto \frac{[HCO_3^-] (N \longrightarrow \uparrow) \text{ (metabolic alkalosis)}}{P_{CO_2} (\downarrow) \text{ (respiratory alkalosis)}}.$$

This disturbance differs from simple respiratory alkalosis in that the plasma bicarbonate concentration is inappropriately high, i.e. the simple disorder is associated with a low, or low normal, plasma level.

Case Example
Female of 60 years with right lower lobe pneumonia and vomiting.

Blood	pH	7·58	(7·35–7·45)
	H^+	26 nmol/l	(35–45)
	P_{CO_2}	32 mmHg	(35–45)
	P_{O_2}	62 mmHg	(80–110)
	$AHCO_3$	30 mmol/l	(24–32)

Comment

If this patient had a simple respiratory alkalosis (pneumonia) the expected bicarbonate level would be low, and usually less than 25 mmol/l, due to compensation. In the above case, although the bicarbonate concentration is within the 'normal' range, it is inappropriately high due to vomiting (metabolic alkalosis).

Respiratory Acidosis and Metabolic Alkalosis

Causes

These two disorders can occur together in a number of situations, but are commonest in patients with chronic obstructive lung disease (respiratory acidosis), who are receiving diuretic therapy (metabolic alkalosis).

Diagnosis

The features are:
1. Normal, or near-normal, pH ($\sim 7\cdot 40$) but it may be $\uparrow$, N, or $\downarrow$
2. Raised P_{CO_2}
3. Raised plasma [HCO_3], i.e.

$$pH\ (\sim N) \propto \frac{[HCO_3{}^-]\ (\uparrow)\ (\text{metabolic alkalosis})}{P_{CO_2}\ (\uparrow)\ (\text{respiratory acidosis})}.$$

The above pH equation could represent a compensated respiratory acidosis or a compensated metabolic alkalosis. The diagnosis of a mixed disorder is suspected on the basis of inappropriate compensatory responses, i.e.
1. pH: simple disorders tend not to completely compensate (pH is rarely returned to normal).
2. [$HCO_3{}^-$]: in compensated respiratory acidosis plasma levels above 45 mmol/l rarely occur, if at all.
3. P_{CO_2}: compensation of a metabolic alkalosis usually does not result in a P_{CO_2} above 60 mmHg.

Case Example

A male aged 83 years with a long history of chronic obstructive lung disease and left ventricular failure which was treated with thiazide diuretic therapy.

Blood			
	pH	7·42	(7·35–7·45)
	H^+	38 nmol/l	(35–45)
	P_{CO_2}	75 mmHg	(35–45)
	P_{O_2}	61 mmHg	(80–110)
	$AHCO_3$	48 mmol/l	(24–32)

Comment

In this patient three factors suggest a mixed disorder:
1. pH: normal
2. P_{CO_2}: >60 mmHg which is too high for a compensated metabolic alkalosis
3. [$HCO_3{}^-$]: >45 mmol/l which is too high for a compensated respiratory acidosis

Respiratory Alkalosis and Metabolic Acidosis

Causes
This disorder may occur in:
1. Salicylate overdose
2. Pulmonary embolism
3. Septic shock

Diagnosis
Characteristic features are:
1. pH: normal ($\sim$7·40) or near normal but may be ↑ or ↓ depending on severity of each disorder
2. P_{CO_2}: decreased
3. Plasma [HCO_3^-]: decreased, i.e.

$$\text{pH } (\sim N) \propto \frac{[HCO_3^-]\ (\downarrow)\ \text{(metabolic acidosis)}}{P_{CO_2}\ (\downarrow)\ \text{(respiratory alkalosis)}}.$$

The above features suggest either a compensated respiratory alkalosis or a compensated metabolic acidosis. The diagnosis of a mixed disorder is based on:
1. pH: normal, or near normal, which is unusual for compensation of a simple disorder
2. P_{CO_2}: usually below range of compensation for the level of [HCO_3^-], i.e. compensation of metabolic acidosis
3. [HCO_3^-]: inappropriately low for compensation of acute respiratory alkalosis, i.e. usually >18 mmol/l if compensation of acute respiratory alkalosis

Case Example
A female patient who presented with a salicylate overdose.

Blood	pH	7·48	(7·35–7·45)
	H^+	33 nmol/l	(35–45)
	P_{CO_2}	19 mmHg	(35–45)
	P_{O_2}	96 mmHg	(80–110)
	$AHCO_3$	14 mmol/l	(24–32)

Plasma anion gap: 22 mEq/l (7–17)

Comment
This patient has a mild alkalaemia and *prima facie* appears to have a well-compensated respiratory alkalosis. However, two points suggest that there is also an underlying primary metabolic acidosis:
1. Compensation of an acute respiratory alkalosis rarely results in a blood [HCO_3^-] less than 18 mmol/l. Chronic respiratory alkalosis may result in complete compensation but only after 1–2 weeks.
2. Patient has a high anion gap. Although alkalosis *per se* may result in an increased anion gap (mild increase in lactic acid due to increased glycolysis

in response to alkalaemia), the increment is usually less than 2–3 mEq/l. The above anion gap suggests the presence of a metabolic acidosis.

Severe salicylate toxicity, in many cases, presents with a respiratory alkalosis (stimulation of the respiratory centre) and a high anion gap metabolic acidosis (increased production of organic acids due to alteration of intermediary metabolism by the salicylates).

Metabolic Acidosis and Alkalosis

Causes
This mixed disorder may develop in two situations:
1. Long-standing metabolic acidosis (e.g. renal failure) with a superimposed acute metabolic alkalosis (e.g. vomiting).
2. Long-standing metabolic alkalosis (e.g. diuretic therapy) and superimposed acute metabolic acidosis (e.g. diabetic ketoacidosis).

Diagnosis
The P_{CO_2} and $[HCO_3^-]$, depending on the intensity of the individual disturbances, may be high, normal or low. The pH may be normal or moderately displaced from normal.

The disorder should be suspected if:
1. The plasma $[HCO_3^-]$ does not reflect the clinical picture, e.g. normal, or near-normal, concentration in diabetic ketoacidosis, or in chronic renal failure.
2. A high anion gap is present.

Case Example
A 59-year-old female, who had been on thiazide diuretic therapy for cardiac failure, presented in a semicomatosed state. Her urine was found to contain glucose and ketone bodies, and she was given a diagnosis of diabetic ketoacidosis.

Plasma	Na	119 mmol/l	(132–144)
	K	2·7 mmol/l	(3·2–4·8)
	Cl	71 mmol/l	(98–108)
	HCO_3	18 mmol/l	(23–33)
	Creat	0·32 mmol/l	(0·06–0·12)
	Anion gap	33 mEq/l	(7–17)
	Glucose	88 mmol/l	(3·5–5·5)
Blood	pH	7·35	(7·35–7·45)
	H^+	45 nmol/l	(35–45)
	P_{CO_2}	32 mmHg	(35–45)
	P_{O_2}	88 mmHg	(80–110)
	$AHCO_3$	17 mmol/l	(24–32)

Comment
The clue to this patient's mixed acid–base disturbance lies in the very high anion gap associated with a moderate decrease in the plasma $[HCO_3^-]$. A patient with

diabetic ketoacidosis and an anion gap of 33 mEq/l would be expected to have a much lower plasma [HCO_3^-], i.e. if we assume her normal anion gap was at the upper limit of normal (17 mEq/l), then the anion gap increment is 16 mEq/l (33–17). If this increase were due to the addition of ketoacid (16 mmol/l of hydrogen ion) then her plasma [HCO_3^-] would decrease by about 16 mmol/l. Thus her original bicarbonate concentration would have to be about 33 mmol/l or greater (metabolic alkalosis).

This patient's metabolic alkalosis was most likely due to diuretic therapy and potassium depletion but vomiting could not be ruled out.

Triple Acid–Base Disturbance

This uncommon condition occurs when a respiratory acid–base disorder (alkalosis or acidosis) is associated with the above type of mixed metabolic acidosis and alkalosis.

Further Reading

Arruda J. A. L. and Kurtzman N. A. (1977) Metabolic acidosis and alkalosis. *Clin. Nephrol.* **7**, 201–205.

Emmett M. E. and Narins R. G. (1977) Clinical use of the anion gap. *Medicine* **56**, 38–54.

Fulop M. E. and Hoberman H. D. (1975) Alcoholic ketosis. *Diabetes* **24**, 785–790.

Kriesberg R. A. (1976) Diabetic ketoacidosis: new concepts and trends in pathogenesis and treatment. *Ann. Intern. Med.* **84**, 633–638.

McCurdy D. K. (1972) Mixed metabolic and respiratory acid–base disturbances: diagnosis and treatment. *Chest* (Suppl.) **62**, 35S–44S.

Martinez-Maldonado M. and Schanez-Montserrat M. (1977) Respiratory acidosis and alkalosis. *Clin. Nephrol.* **7**, 191–200.

Narins R. G. and Emmett M. (1980) Simple and mixed acid–base disorders: a practical approach. *Medicine* **59**, 161–187.

Park R. and Arieff A. I. (1980) Lactic acidosis. *Adv. Intern. Med.* **25**, 33–68.

6

Calcium—Phosphate—Magnesium

CALCIUM

Homeostasis

Input

On the average daily intake of 10–20 mmol of calcium, approximately 35–40% is absorbed in the duodenum and small intestine. The amount absorbed may vary from 10 to 90% depending on calcium requirements. Gut absorption is controlled mainly by vitamin D, but it also depends on age, being increased in children and decreased in the elderly.

Absorption of calcium occurs from the gut by both passive and active mechanisms. The passive component requires 10 times the average oral intake to satisfy normal body requirements so that active absorption, requiring vitamin D, is necessary if normal calcium homeostasis is to be maintained.

In addition to absorption, secretion of calcium occurs into the gut as part of the obligatory intestinal secretions. In overall terms, some 5–7 mmol excess of calcium is absorbed (*Fig.* 6.1). Apart from the major effect of vitamin D, other factors also have some effect on calcium absorption in the gut:

1. Increased absorption:
   Acidity
   High protein intake
   High NaCl intake
   High lactose intake
2. Decreased absorption:
   Calcium binders (e.g. PO_4, oxalate)
   Alkali
   Fatty acids
   High Mg^{2+} intake

Distribution

Of the approximately 35 000 mmol of calcium in the adult, the major portion is found in the skeleton, as shown by percentage distribution in the various

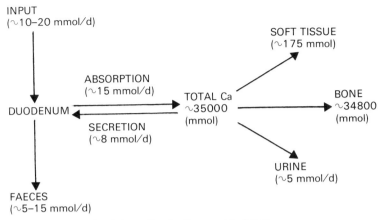

Fig. 6.1. Normal calcium distribution and balance.

tissues:

Bone	~99%
Teeth	~0·5%
Soft tissue	~0·5%
Plasma	~0·02%

The composition of bone is such that 60–70% is in the form of mineral and 30% as a protein matrix. The calcium present in bone is mainly in the form of hydroxyapatite, a crystalline structure containing mainly calcium and phosphate, with varying amounts of hydroxide and carbonate. Approximately 1% of bone calcium is available for rapid exchange with the extraskeletal calcium.

The remaining 30% of bone structure is a protein matrix, mainly collagen. This protein contains large amounts of hydroxyproline and hydroxylysine, which may be mobilized and excreted in the urine in increased amounts if there is increased turnover of bone matrix (e.g. primary hyperparathyroidism).

The plasma composition of calcium is as indicated:

Ionized	48%
Protein bound	46% (albumin 80%, globulins 20%)
Calcium phosphate	1·5%
Calcium citrate	1·5%
Calcium complexes	3% (including HCO_3)

Approximately 50% of the total plasma calcium is bound to circulating albumin, and alterations in the plasma level of this protein will affect the plasma concentration of both the bound, and the total, calcium. The concentration of free plasma calcium (often referred to as the 'ionized calcium') is maintained within narrow limits by the action of parathyroid hormone (PTH). A fall, or rise, in plasma albumin concentration of 10 g/l is usually associated with a fall, or rise, in the total plasma calcium of about 0·25 mmol/l. Use of this formulation provides a 'corrected' calcium level.

The intracellular distribution of calcium has important consequences because of the influence of this ion on neural and muscle activity. Recent discoveries of a cell regulator, calmodulin, suggests that this molecule regulates the intracellular activity of calcium as a second messenger. Normally cytosolic calcium levels are of the order of $0.1\,\mu mol/l$ (i.e. one-tenthousandth that of plasma), whereas intramitochondrial levels ($0.1-10\,mmol/l$) are similar to plasma levels. A number of mechanisms which regulate the intracellular concentration, and distribution, of calcium have been described, but are beyond the scope of this text.

Output
Calcium is lost from the body via two major sites:
1.   Gastrointestinal secretions (*see above*).
2.   Renal excretion.
The renal handling of calcium involves reabsorption of some 98% of the Ca^{2+} presented to the renal tubules by glomerular filtration. The mechanisms involve:

1. Na^+-linked reabsorption in the proximal tubule (approx. 60% of Ca^{2+} reabsorbed). The significance of this mechanism becomes apparent in situations where there is avid sodium reabsorption, such as occurs in thiazide diuretic therapy. In this case calcium reabsorption is also increased, and may result in hypercalcaemia.

2. Action of a number of hormones and vitamins, including PTH, calcitonin, and vitamin D (*see below*).

Controlling Hormones
Although total plasma calcium levels may vary considerably, as a result of changes in plasma albumin levels, the concentration of plasma 'free' calcium is maintained within relatively tight limits by two hormones and a vitamin, i.e. parathyroid hormone (PTH), calcitonin and metabolites of vitamin D.

Parathyroid Hormone (PTH)
This hormone, which is an 84 amino acid peptide, is produced as a 'pre-pro' and 'pro-hormone' prior to release from the chief cells of the parathyroid glands. The hormone is metabolized, mainly in the liver, to form a 34 amino acid NH_2-terminal peptide, which is biologically active. The remaining COOH-terminal fragment has no biological activity, but has a sustained plasma half-life. The plasma half-life of the intact hormone is of the order of 20 min. The major actions of PTH, mediated via cyclic-AMP, include:
1.   Increases bone resorption
2.   Increases renal Ca^{2+} (and Mg^{2+}) reabsorption
3.   Decreases renal H^+ secretion—this action, mainly in the proximal tubule, may result in a mild hyperchloraemic acidosis in primary hyperparathyroidism
4.   Increases 1,25-dihydroxycholecalciferol (1,25-DHCC) production
5.   Increases urine hydroxyproline excretion
6.   Decreases renal HCO_3^- reabsorption

7.   Decreases renal sodium reabsorption
8.   Decreases renal phosphate reabsorption
9.   Modulates activity of renal 1-α-hydroxylase
10.   Increases urinary c-AMP excretion
   The classic biochemical features of excessive PTH action activity are:
1.   Hypercalcaemia—↑ bone resorption, ↑ renal Ca^{2+} reabsorption, ↑ gut absorption (↑ 1,25-DHCC)
2.   Hypophosphataemia—↑ renal excretion
3.   ↑ Plasma alkaline phosphatase activity—↑ osteoblastic activity.
   These actions are summarized in *Fig.* 6.2.

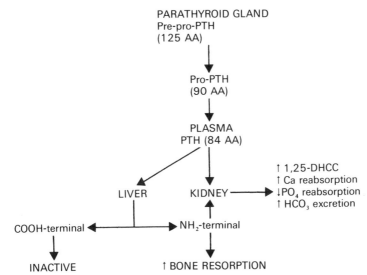

Fig. 6.2. Parathyroid hormone metabolism and actions. 1,25-DHCC: 1,25-dihydroxycholecalciferol.

Calcitonin

Secreted by the parafollicular or 'C-cells' of the thyroid gland, this 32 amino acid peptide hormone, which appears to be mainly metabolized in the kidney, has a plasma half-life of the order of 18 min. Although calcitonin has significant calcium-controlling actions in a number of species, its action in man appears to be significant only in those situations of increased calcium turnover, e.g. in children, Paget's disease and malignant hypercalcaemia.
   The major actions of the hormone, mediated by cyclic-AMP, are:
1.   Inhibition of osteoclastic activity
2.   Possible decreased osteoblastic activity
3.   Decreased renal reabsorption of calcium and magnesium
4.   Decreased renal reabsorption of sodium and potassium
5.   Decreased renal reabsorption of phosphate
6.   Decreased secretion of gastrin

Vitamin D

The sources of vitamin D (cholecalciferol) are twofold:

1. Dietary intake of vitamin D_3 or D_2 (ergocalciferol from plants)
2. Action of u.v. light (sunlight) on 7-dehydrocholecalciferol (present in the skin) to form vitamin D_3.

Vitamin D_3 is metabolized in the liver to 25-hydroxycholecalciferol (25-HCC). The 25-HCC is then transported in the blood, bound to an α_2-macroglobulin, to the kidney. Here, depending upon a number of factors (*see below*), the 25-HCC may be converted to the active 1,25-dihydroxycholecalciferol (1,25-DHCC) by an hydroxylase located in the renal tubules (*Fig.* 6.3).

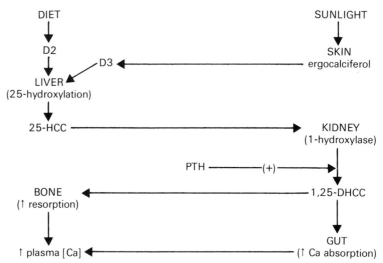

Fig. 6.3. Vitamin D metabolism and its effect on plasma calcium levels. 25-HCC: 25-hydroxycholecalciferol; 1,25-DHCC: 1,25-dihydroxycholecalciferol.

The control of 1,25-DHCC synthesis is affected by:

1. Increased:
   Increased PTH
   Decreased circulating 1,25-DHCC
   Decreased dietary calcium
   Decreased dietary PO_4
2. Decreased:
   Decreased PTH
   Renal tubular destruction
   ($\downarrow$ 1-α-hydroxylase)

The major actions of 1,25-DHCC include:

1. Increased absorption of calcium from the gut
2. Increased absorption of phosphate from the gut
3. Increased resorption of calcium from bone
4. Increased calcium reabsorption in the renal tubules

Glucocorticoids

Steroid hormones, particularly glucocorticoids, affect calcium homeostasis by a number of mechanisms, including:

1. Increased body catabolism (including osteoid)
2. Decreased osteoblastic activity
3. Decreased bone formation
4. Decreased GIT calcium absorption
5. Increased calciuresis
6. Decreased metabolic response to 1,25-DHCC

The overall effect of corticosteroids, therefore, is to inhibit gastrointestinal intake of calcium, and slightly decrease bone resorption. However, the over-riding action of PTH causes mobilization of bone calcium, and increased urinary excretion. This offsets any effect that corticosteroids may have on the plasma calcium level.

Thyroxine

This hormone, because of its general effects in increasing the body metabolic rate, increases the rate of the bone turnover, thereby mobilizing calcium stores. This can result in increased calcium excretion, and occasionally hypercalcaemia.

Glucagon

Recent findings suggest that glucagon increases plasma calcitonin levels, as well as having a direct suppressive effect on bone resorption. The overall effect is to cause a decrease in the plasma calcium level.

Growth Hormone (GH)

Acting via the intermediary somatomedins, GH causes calciuresis. The hormone also promotes an increase in the plasma phosphate concentration, as is seen in growing children (i.e. plasma phosphate levels are significantly higher than those found in adults).

Androgens

These hormones have been shown, in some cases, to increase bone growth and calcium deposition. This can result in decreased urinary calcium excretion.

Oestrogens

These hormones stimulate osteoblasts to increase bone deposition.

Analytical Methods

i-PTH

Due to the technical difficulties in the measurement of PTH, this assay has not been particularly helpful in the investigation of disorders of calcium homeostasis. Most routine assays are based on radioimmunoassay (RIA) techniques (hence i-PTH), the major difficulty being associated with the selection of antibody. The antibody, which is difficult to produce, may be directed against the whole PTH molecule, the COOH-terminal, or the NH_2-terminal portion. The better assays available are those using antibodies directed against the COOH-terminal, which is biologically inactive, and therefore may not reflect parathyroid gland activity, e.g. the COOH-terminal levels are elevated in renal insufficiency (since the major catabolic pathway involves glomerular filtration). All of the available NH_2-terminal assays, at present, have insufficient sensitivity to measure low plasma PTH levels.

Plasma Calcium

In the routine laboratory, plasma calcium levels are normally estimated by one of three techniques:
1.   Atomic absorption spectrophotometry
2.   Colorimetric techniques
3.   Ion-specific electrode.

Atomic absorption spectrophotometry (AAS) involves aspiration of a sample into a flame of sufficient temperature to atomize the calcium content. A special light source, with a wavelength known to be absorbed by calcium atoms, is then shone through the atomized sample. The resultant decrease in light energy passing through the flame is hence an estimation of the amount of element present in the sample. AAS techniques, because of the high temperatures involved, are unaffected by most of the inhibitors affecting the colorimetric methods (e.g. EDTA), and estimate the total plasma calcium present in the sample.

Most colorimetric methods involve combining the calcium ion with a complexing agent, usually cresolphthalein complexone. The major disadvantage of this method of analysis is that other complexing agents, particularly EDTA, inhibit the binding of calcium to the cresolphthalein complexone, thereby causing falsely low values.

Ion-specific electrodes rely on the specific characteristics of specially prepared 'membranes' to allow the passage of particular ions. This causes the generation of small electrical currents which are directly related to the concentration of the ion in the sample. This technique detects the presence of 'free' calcium ions, i.e. not bound to protein or other anions. Free calcium levels in plasma are approximately $1.04-1.17$ mmol/l. It is this fraction of the total plasma calcium which is biologically active and is closely regulated by PTH.

'Corrected' Calcium

As noted above, alterations in the plasma albumin concentration will result in changes in the plasma total calcium concentration. A helpful formula to calculate the 'corrected' plasma [Ca] in the presence of abnormalities of plasma albumin concentration is:

Corrected [Ca] mmol/l = (measured total [Ca] (mmol/l) + 0.025 (40 − [Alb]))

(where [Alb] is in g/l, and 40 g/l is the mean of the plasma albumin reference range).

Hypercalcaemia

Consequences

The clinical effects of hypercalcaemia relate to the level of the plasma calcium, usually showing little acute effect until levels of 3·0 mmol/l or greater are attained. Complaints of anorexia, nausea, vomiting, constipation, fatigue and muscle weakness are frequent. Polyuria and polydipsia often occur as a result of the increased solute load in the kidney. Mental clouding, dysphoria, and occasionally coma may also occur if the total plasma calcium level exceeds 3·5 mmol/l.

Deposition of calcium salts in the tissues may lead to conjunctival deposits (e.g. the 'red eye' of uraemia), band keratopathy, and nephrocalcinosis. If there is increased renal excretion of calcium salts, renal calculi may form.

The removal of mineral from bone, e.g. hyperparathyroidism, is often associated with bone pain, and pathological fractures (e.g. wedge fracture of the spinal vertebrae). It may also be associated with osteoclastomas.

Hypercalcaemia predisposes patients to a number of other disorders, including pancreatitis and duodenal ulcer. Associations with other diseases, including the Zollinger–Ellison syndrome and familial multiple endocrine neoplasia (FMEN), have been recorded.

Causes

Although the causes of hypercalcaemia can be discussed under the headings of input, redistribution and output, a more satisfactory approach is to describe the more frequent causes of the disorder. A list, in approximate order of decreasing frequency, is shown in *Table* 6.1.

Table 6.1. Common causes of hypercalcaemia

Factitious	*Hormonal*
Haemoconcentration	Thyrotoxicosis
Postprandial	Acromegaly
Malignancy	Hypoadrenalism
Breast, lung, myeloma	Phaeochromocytoma
Primary hyperparathyroidism	*Granulomas*
Drugs	Tuberculosis
Thiazides	Sarcoidosis
Vitamin D	*Renal failure*
Lithium	*Milk–alkali syndrome*
Vitamin A	*Immobilization*

Haemoconcentration

Frequently, a mild hypercalcaemia results from concentration of the blood by the use of a tourniquet during the blood collection procedure. Evidence suggests that this effect, due to fluid shifts into the interstitial space, may occur within 30 sec of application of the tourniquet. For this reason, blood collected for plasma calcium estimation requires the use of non-stasis techniques.

Postprandial

Ingestion of calcium causes a mild increase in the plasma calcium level as a result of rapid gut absorption. Patients should fast for 8–12 h prior to blood collection to eliminate this effect.

Malignancy

Approximately 20% of patients with malignant tumours have episodes of hypercalcaemia, particularly in the late stages of the disease process. Carcinomas of the breast, lung, kidney and prostate are frequently associated with hypercalcaemia. It may also occur in multiple myeloma, lymphoma and leukaemia.

The causes of the hypercalcaemia in malignancy are multiple, and may include:
1. Direct invasion of bone (release of Ca^{2+})
2. Tumour secretion of PTH-like material, which may not be detected by routine i-PTH assays
3. Tumour secretion of prostaglandin E ($\uparrow$ bone resorption)
4. Secretion of 'osteoclastic activating factor', particularly by myeloma tumours, which causes local bone resorption
5. Secretion of vitamin D-like sterols
6. Concurrent primary hyperparathyroidism
7. Ectopic PTH production by the tumour

Primary Hyperparathyroidism

Primary hyperparathyroidism usually results from a chief cell adenoma of the parathyroid glands. Prior to multiple biochemical screening, most of these patients suffered from massive resorption of calcium from bone, due to the excessive PTH action. This resulted in severe bone changes, and often renal disease (nephrocalcinosis, nephrolithiasis), as a consequence of the increased urinary excretion of Ca. In recent times, however, due to widespread biochemical 'screening', the disorder is often diagnosed before major clinical signs become apparent.

The biochemical findings of primary hyperparathyroidism can include:
1. Increased plasma calcium levels, usually in the range of 2·55–3·0 mmol/l
2. Decreased plasma $[PO_4]$ (direct effect of PTH on renal PO_4 excretion)
3. Tendency to hyperchloraemic acidosis due to the inhibition of renal tubular secretion of H^+ by PTH
4. Increased plasma alkaline phosphatase activity, in up to 50% of cases
5. Increased urine hydroxyproline excretion, due to increased bone resorption
6. Increased urinary Ca and PO_4 excretion
7. Increased urinary c-AMP levels
8. Increased plasma i-PTH levels

The biochemical features of primary hyperparathyroidism and hypercalcaemia of malignancy are similar and hence a number of clinical and biochemical manoeuvres have been tried to differentiate between the two disorders. However, none have proved completely successful, but in most cases the differentiation of these two disorders can usually be made on clinical grounds.

An association of primary hyperparathyroidism with other endocrine disorders has been reported, e.g. familial multiple endocrine neoplasia (FMEN), where primary hyperparathyroidism is associated with phaeochromocytoma, and medullary carcinoma of the thyroid.

Familial Hypocalciuric Hypercalcaemia
A recently recognized disease, this autosomal dominant disorder is believed to be a variant of primary hyperparathyroidism. The major feature appears to be a marked reduction in the renal excretion of calcium. Although hyperplasia of the parathyroid glands has been described in most cases, as have moderately elevated plasma levels of i-PTH, the disorder does not respond to surgical intervention.

Secondary/Tertiary Hyperparathyroidism
In renal disease, which results in prolonged renal calcium wasting, the persistent stimulus of hypocalcaemia may lead to autonomous overproduction of PTH. Consequently, a patient with severe renal disease who has been previously hypocalcaemic, and then develops hypercalcaemia, may be found to have an adenoma of the parathyroid gland. This syndrome, previously called tertiary hyperparathyroidism, is frequently seen following recovery from acute renal failure, or after renal transplantation.

Endocrine Disorders
In thyrotoxicosis, the increased metabolic activity resulting from the increased plasma thyroxine levels may be reflected in increased bone resorption and hypercalcaemia.

In acromegaly, the frequent finding of hypercalcaemia is believed to be the result of increased gut absorption of calcium, although a direct action of growth hormone on the parathyroid gland has not been excluded.

Approximately 40% of cases of adrenal insufficiency are found to be mildly hypercalcaemic. The mechanism is often ascribed to haemoconcentration, but the loss of the inhibitory action of cortisol on bone resorption may also be an important factor.

Vitamins
Ingestion of excess vitamin D, or its metabolites, may cause significantly increased gut absorption of Ca and consequent hypercalcaemia. Although 1,25-DHCC is the active metabolite, 25-HCC has approximately one-thousandth of the activity of 1,25-DHCC, but it is present in plasma at about one thousand times the concentration of 1,25-DHCC. Consequently, 25-HCC, if ingested in significant amounts, can have marked effects on Ca homeostasis.

Vitamin A overdosage has also been associated with hypercalcaemia, probably as a result of increased bone resorption.

Granulomatous Diseases
Sarcoidosis and tuberculosis both may result in hypercalcaemia. In these disorders, there appears to be an increased sensitivity to 25-HCC with increased

conversion of this precursor to 1,25-DHCC. Berylliosis, coccidioidomycosis and histoplasmosis have also been reported to produce a similar effect.

Acute Renal Failure

Acute hypercalcaemia is often noted during the polyuric phase of acute renal failure, particularly if the renal failure has been secondary to rhabdomyolysis. Mechanisms proposed include:

1.   Mobilization of soft tissue Ca deposits which occurred during the oliguric phase when plasma PO_4 levels were elevated
2.   Persistently increased PTH secretion following the initial stimulus of hypocalcaemia

Drugs

Hypercalcaemia may be associated with lithium therapy. The mechanism is believed to result from stimulation of PTH release from the parathyroid glands.

Thiazide diuretics, by decreasing the proximal renal tubular flow rates (hypovolaemia), cause increased proximal tubular reabsorption of calcium as well as that of Na^+. This results in decreased renal excretion of Ca, and may be associated with hypercalcaemia. This factor is often used to advantage in the treatment of nephrolithiasis due to calcium salts, i.e. decreasing the amount of Ca excreted. Occasionally, latent disorders which may cause hypercalcaemia are unmasked when thiazide therapy is initiated. In one reported series of investigations, more than 50% of patients who developed hypercalcaemia whilst on thiazide therapy were subsequently shown to have primary hyperparathyroidism.

Milk-alkali Syndrome

This syndrome, characterized by hypercalcaemia, alkalosis and renal dysfunction is a consequence of excessive ingestion of absorbable calcium salts, such as $CaCO_3$ (usually in doses greater than 5 g/d). As a result of the massive calcium load in the gut, passive absorption mechanisms, independent of vitamin D, become a significant source of calcium uptake. The development of the alkalosis is due to ingestion of alkali, and this in turn decreases renal calcium excretion, further aggravating the hypercalcaemia.

Although frequently mentioned as a cause of hypercalcaemia, the disorder is rarely seen nowadays, due to changing therapeutic methods in the treatment of peptic ulcers.

Immobilization

Since bone is metabolically active, prolonged immobilization will result in increased resorption as a consequence of less muscle stress on the skeleton. Hypercalciuria occurs in all patients following immobilization. In some cases, however, where there is significant bone turnover, the calcium resorbed from bone may exceed the renal clearance, and hypercalcaemia results. The hypercalcaemia of immobilization is often seen in the young, and in patients with Paget's disease.

Diagnosis/Evaluation

In the majority of patients presenting with hypercalcaemia, the aetiology is usually obvious clinically, or can be elucidated by a process of elimination. For those cases where the cause is obscure, a logical approach to evaluation is shown in *Fig.* 6.4. A major problem that can arise is the differentiation of primary hyperparathyroidism from hypercalcaemia due to an occult malignancy. Factors that may be helpful in the differentiation are indicated in *Table* 6.2.

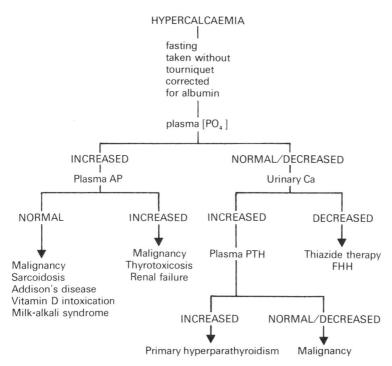

Fig. 6.4. Suggested scheme for the evaluation of hypercalcaemia. AP, alkaline phophatase; FHH, Familial hypocalciuric hypercalcaemia.

Table 6.2. Characteristics of hypercalcaemia of malignancy and primary hyperparathyroidism

	Malignancy	Primary Hyper- parathyroidism
Degree of hypercalcaemia	>3·0 mmol/l	<3·0 mmol/l
Duration	months	years
Renal calculi	rare	frequent
Plasma chloride	low, normal	normal, high
Plasma i-PTH	low, normal	high
Plasma 1,25-DHCC	low	high
Urinary Ca	>10 mmol/d	<10 mmol/d

Treatment

Although a number of techniques are available for the treatment of hypercalcaemia, the clinical situation usually indicates the therapeutic manoeuvre of choice. These regimes can be divided into acute and chronic therapies.

Acute Therapy

Phosphate Infusion

An i.v. infusion of 500 ml of 0·1 molar phosphate solution will rapidly cause a decrease in plasma [Ca]. The mechanism is believed to be the result of $Ca_3(PO_4)_2$ deposition in soft tissues. This technique has lost favour because of the strong possibility of precipitating renal failure, and should not be used in cases where the plasma $[PO_4]$ is elevated.

Saline/Frusemide Diuresis

An infusion of normal saline to expand the ECV, followed by frusemide therapy, will result in a calcium diuresis. This diuresis is due to inhibition of the function of the ascending loop of Henle by the diuretic, which will result in increased excretion of Na^+ and Ca^{2+}.

The effectiveness of this therapy relies on increasing the ECV prior to the administration of frusemide. If the patient is hypovolaemic, avid sodium reabsorption in the proximal tubule will negate the effect of frusemide which acts distally. Consequently, it is recommended that 2 litres of normal saline be infused, followed by 40 mg frusemide (i.v.), then alternating 1 litre of saline and 20 mg frusemide. Contraindications to this form of therapy are renal insufficiency and congestive cardiac failure. Significant losses of potassium and magnesium can also occur, and may require replacement therapy.

Calcitonin/Glucocorticoid

Calcitonin, which inhibits bone resorption and causes calciuresis, was initially thought to be an excellent form of therapy for hypercalcaemia. Unfortunately, some patients do not respond to this therapy, whilst other patients, after an initial response, became refractory to the treatment. The addition of prednisone to the therapeutic regime has been found to suppress the calcitonin 'escape'. This steroid also inhibits the intestinal absorption of calcium.

Cytotoxic Agents

Mithramycin, an antineoplastic agent, has been used successfully in the treatment of hypercalcaemia. The action of the drug is the result of a direct toxic effect on the bone-resorbing tissues. In doses of 25 µg/kg, a decrease in the plasma Ca level is usually apparent within 12–24 h, although maximal effect takes 2–3 days. Because of the severe toxicity of the drug (thrombocytopaenia, haemorrhage, renal impairment), this form of therapy is usually reserved for those cases resistant to other types of treatment.

Bleomycin has also been reported to have successfully suppressed elevated plasma calcium levels in cases of myeloma.

Chronic Treatment

Specific therapeutic manoeuvres aimed at the underlying cause of the hypercalcaemia are obviously the manoeuvres of choice in chronic hypercalcaemia. In some cases, however, this is not feasible, and direct suppression of plasma calcium levels are required.

For primary hyperparathyroidism in clinically symptomatic patients, surgical intervention, with cautious clinical and biochemical monitoring postoperatively (in case of hypocalcaemia), is the method of choice. In cases which are inoperable for some reason, recent reports of the use of diphosphonates (potent inhibitors of bone resorption) have indicated good responses.

Where mild hypercalcaemia is found, the use of dietary control, and the use of binding agents (e.g. oral phosphate in the form of 'buffered' phosphate) to inhibit gut uptake of calcium, are often very effective. The use of oral phosphate therapy is contraindicated in cases of renal impairment.

Corticosteroid therapy, particularly in sarcoidosis, often has an excellent effect. Steroids have also been used in the treatment of hypercalcaemia of malignancy. The long term use of steroid therapy has significant clinical side effects, however, and other treatment forms should be considered.

Case Examples

Multiple Myeloma

A 56-year-old man presented to his local doctor complaining of low back pain, unassociated with trauma. Clinical examination revealed some tenderness in the lower thoracic spine. Spinal X-rays revealed a 'crush' fracture of the twelfth thoracic vertebra. Biochemical analyses revealed:

Plasma			
	Ca	2·68 mmol/l	(2·05–2·55)
	PO_4	1·11 mmol/l	(0·6–1·2)
	Alb	31 g/l	(30–52)
	Globs	58 g/l	(22–34)
	AP	83 u/l	(30–110)

Protein electrophoresis revealed a heavy single band of IgM consistent with IgM myeloma. Cytotoxic therapy was initiated with good response, as indicated by reduction in the level of plasma γ-globulins. The patient also became normocalcaemic.

Comment

Hypercalcaemia in the adult, as previously mentioned, is most commonly the result of a malignancy. In multiple myeloma, the aetiology of the hypercalcaemia may be threefold:

1. Binding of Ca^{2+} to globulins, thereby causing an increase in total plasma Ca levels

2. Direct invasion of bone, thereby increasing release of calcium from this source

3. The release of 'osteoclastic activating factor' from the tumour. This hormone is believed to have a physiological role in the control of the bone marrow space, i.e. to allow for normal expansion of bone marrow within bone

Sarcoidosis

A 70-year-old man presented to hospital in mid-summer with complaints of increasing shortness of breath, constipation, thirst and polyuria. Clinical examination revealed tachycardia, an elevated jugular pulse and peripheral oedema. A past history of sarcoidosis, diagnosed previously by findings of interstitial lung disease, splenomegaly, and confirmed by biopsy, was noted.

Following admission, routine blood analysis revealed:

Plasma	Ca	3·35 mmol/l	(2·05–2·55)
	PO_4	0·98 mmol/l	(0·6–1·2)
	Alb	39 g/l	(30–52)
	AP	110 u/l	(30–110)

Chest X-ray revealed features of mild congestive cardiac failure, and interstitial lung disease consistent with sarcoidosis.

Further biochemical investigations revealed:

ACE	93 nmol/ml/min	(14–41)
i-PTH	5·1 u/l	(2–6)

Prednisolone therapy was initiated (as well as frusemide and digoxin for the cardiac failure), and two weeks later the following results were noted:

Plasma	Ca	2·47 mmol/l	(2·05–2·55)
	PO_4	0·82 mmol/l	(0·6–1·2)
	Alb	41 g/l	(30–52)
	AP	84 u/l	(30–110)

Steroid therapy was decreased slowly, and the patient remained normo-calcaemic. Hypercalcaemia recurred the following summer, and further steroid therapy was required.

Comment

This case illustrates the association of hypercalcaemia with sarcoidosis, possibly as a result of increased production of 1,25-DHCC by the granulation tissue. The following points are of interest:
1. The onset of hypercalcaemia in summer, when vitamin D levels are at their highest as a result of increased u.v. light
2. Rapid response to steroids, as is often the case in sarcoidosis
3. Use of frusemide to treat the mild cardiac failure in this case, rather than a thiazide, which may have made the hypercalcaemia worse ($\downarrow$ renal excretion)
4. Elevated angiotensin-converting enzyme (ACE) which is characteristic of active sarcoidosis, though not specific, for the disease

5.   The normal i-PTH level suggests that hyperparathyroidism is probably not
the cause of the increased plasma [Ca]

Familial Hypocalciuric Hypercalcaemia

A 57-year-old female was reviewed by her local practitioner for routine check-up
for employment purposes. Clinical findings were negative, but biochemical screening revealed:

Plasma	Na	140 mmol/l	(132–144)
	K	3·9 mmol/l	(3·1–5·6)
	Cl	109 mmol/l	(98–106)
	HCO$_3$	24 mmol/l	(21–32)
	Ca	3·02 mmol/l	(2·05–2·55)
	PO$_4$	0·62 mmol/l	(0·6–1·2)
	Alb	44 g/l	(30–52)
	AP	77 u/l	(30–110)

Repeat analyses revealed persistent hypercalcaemia and hyperchloraemia.
Further history revealed that her son had recently undergone parathyroid surgery
for primary hyperparathyroidism without success. Further investigations on the
above patient showed:

i-PTH	6·3 u/l	(2–6)
Urine Ca	2·5 mmol/d	(2·5–7·5)

Considering the benign course of the hypercalcaemia in this patient, the
presence of a family history, and the hypocalciuria, the case was diagnosed as
familial hypocalciuric hypercalcaemia (FHH), and no surgical intervention was
contemplated.

Comment

The syndrome of FHH has only recently been recognized. This syndrome appears
to have a benign clinical course, though occasional cases of associated pancreatitis
have been reported. The genetic expression of the disease appears to be that of an
autosomal dominant disorder.

Biochemically, there is usually hypercalcaemia, hypophosphataemia and
hyperchloraemia similar to that seen in primary hyperparathyroidism. The plasma
i-PTH, although often elevated, is not as high as that frequently found in
hyperparathyroidism. Interestingly, the plasma magnesium level is often elevated,
suggesting a defect in the homeostasis of divalent metals. Urine studies reveal low
levels of calcium excretion, which may explain the absence of renal symptoms in
these patients.

Primary Hyperparathyroidism

A 35-year-old female had a history of recurrent renal calculi, depression and
constipation. Clinical and biochemical features were consistent with hyperparathyroidism, and a parathyroid adenoma was found at operation.

Biochemical findings prior to operation, and one day following the operation are indicated:

Date		21/10	22/10	
Plasma	Ca	2·88	1·84 mmol/l	(2·05–2·55)
	PO$_4$	0·55	0·60 mmol/l	(0·6–1·2)
	Alb	42	41 g/l	(30–52)
	AP	205	195 u/l	(30–110)
	Urea	5·0	6·5 mmol/l	(3·0–8·0)

Comment

The results obtained prior to operation (21/10) are classical for primary hyperparathyroidism, i.e. the elevated PTH level causes:

1.   ↑ Bone resorption ⟶ ↑ plasma [Ca]
2.   ↑ Osteoblastic activity ⟶ ↑ plasma AP
3.   ↑ Renal PO$_4$ excretion ⟶ ↓ plasma [PO$_4$]
4.   ↑ Renal Ca reabsorption ⟶ ↑ plasma [Ca]

Prolonged exposure to hypercalcaemia results in suppression of the normal parathyroid tissue. On removal of the parathyroid adenoma, calcium continues to be deposited in the bones, and this often leads to hypocalcaemia postoperatively. Eventually, the normal parathyroid tissue will respond to the hypocalcaemia by producing PTH which then returns the plasma calcium level to normal.

With the advent of biochemical screening, patients with primary hyperparathyroidism are diagnosed earlier in the disease process. Consequently, some of the classic features of this disease, such as hypophosphataemia and elevated plasma AP activity, may not be observed on presentation.

It should also be noted that hypercalcaemia of malignancy may present with similar biochemical findings to those of primary hyperparathyroidism (i.e. ↓ plasma PO$_4$ and ↑ plasma AP levels.

Lung Carcinoma

A 58-year-old man presented to hospital with a six-month history of unproductive cough, recent haemoptysis and weight loss. He had smoked heavily since the age of eighteen. Biochemical parameters revealed:

Plasma	Ca	3·90 mmol/l	(2·05–2·55)
	PO$_4$	0·52 mmol/l	(0·6–1·2)
	Alb	36 g/l	(30–52)
	AP	240 u/l ·	(30–110)
	Urea	5·5 mmol/l	(3·0–8·0)

Sputum cytological examination and bronchoscopy revealed the presence of an oat-cell carcinoma of the lung, and chemotherapy was instituted.

Comment

An estimated 20% of patients with malignancy present, at some time during the course of their disease, with hypercalcaemia. The possible mechanisms include:

1.   Erosion of bone by secondary tumour deposits
2.   Ectopic production of PTH by the tumour

3. Production of a PTH-like material by the tumour
4. Prostaglandin production by the tumour
5. Production of osteoclastic activating factor (OAF) by some tumours, particularly myeloma
6. Coincidental hypercalcaemia from some other cause (e.g. primary hyperparathyroidism)

The biochemical features in this case are similar to those of primary hyperparathyroidism, which suggests the possibility of ectopic production of PTH or a PTH-like substance. i-PTH assay in this patient yielded a normal result, so that the suggested humoral factor was not detected by an antibody recognizing the COOH-terminal end of the normal PTH molecule.

Hypocalcaemia

Consequences

Both acute and chronic changes may occur as a result of hypocalcaemia.

Acute hypocalcaemia is heralded by tetany and paraesthesia of the extremities and circumoral areas, reflecting increased neuromuscular excitability. Muscle cramps and carpopedal spasm may also be apparent. The signs are not specific to hypocalcaemia, as they also occur in acute respiratory alkalosis and in hyperkalaemia.

Tapping the facial nerve may elicit a facial twitch (Chvostek's sign), and inflation of a sphygmomanometer cuff above the diastolic pressure on the arm for 3 min may elicit carpopedal spasm (Trousseau's sign). ECG findings include a prolonged Q–T interval and abnormality of the T-wave. Hypotension is also a frequent finding.

Chronic hypocalcaemia, usually as a result of hypoparathyroidism, may cause significant changes in the function of a number of organ systems, including:
1. Mental retardation
2. Extrapyramidal symptoms
3. Skeletal malformations, including exostoses, and premature closure of the epiphyses (particularly metacarpals 4 and 5) resulting in short stature
4. Poor formation of teeth
5. Dermatitis and hyperpigmentation

Causes

The major causes of hypocalcaemia are listed in *Table* 6.3. A number of the more important causes are discussed below.

Decreased Protein-bound Calcium

The commonest cause of hypocalcaemia is hypoalbuminaemia. Although the total plasma [Ca] is reduced, the free [Ca^{2+}] is unaltered when assayed by ion-specific electrode techniques. Correction of plasma [Ca] levels for deviations in plasma albumin levels is described under 'analytical techniques' (p. 136).

Table 6.3. Causes of hypocalcaemia

Factitious	*Acute pancreatitis*
EDTA contamination	*Hyperphosphataemia*
Hypoalbuminaemia	Renal failure
Decreased PTH activity	Phosphate supplements
Hypoparathyroidism	Leukaemia therapy
Pseudohypoparathyroidism	*'Hungry bone' syndrome*
Pseudo-idiopathic hypoparathyroidism	*Drugs*
Hypomagnesaemia	Mithramycin
Decreased vitamin D activity	Diuretics (frusemide, ethacrynic
See Table 6.4	acid)

EDTA Contamination

Ethylene diamine tetra-acetate (EDTA), an anticoagulant used in collection of blood samples for haematological examination, inhibits the clotting process by chelation of calcium, which is required for normal coagulation. Colorimetric analytical techniques (e.g. cresolphthalein complexone) also rely on the chelation of calcium, which, if already complexed to EDTA, does not react. Occasionally, very low plasma calcium levels are measured in the laboratory, which are later found to be the result of EDTA contamination. An example of the effect of EDTA contamination is shown on p. 61.

Renal Failure

Mild hypocalcaemia is seen in most cases of chronic renal failure. In acute renal failure, hypocalcaemia may be marked, the proposed mechanisms include:
1.   Decreased renal reabsorption of Ca^{2+}
2.   Phosphate retention, with consequent soft-tissue metastatic calcification
3.   Decreased intestinal uptake
4.   Decreased 1-α-hydroxylation of 25-HCC by the kidney
5.   Uraemia *per se* has also been shown to cause PTH resistance in bone resorption.

Failure of PTH Action

Decreased activity of PTH may result from a number of defects in PTH production, action or metabolism, e.g.
1.   Parathyroid disease/surgical removal
2.   Inability of the chief cells in the parathyroid tissue to modify pre-pro or pro-hormone to the active PTH molecule
3.   Inability to secrete PTH molecule
4.   Inability to cleave the PTH molecule to the active 34 amino acid molecule
5.   Failure of renal receptor interaction with circulating PTH
6.   Failure of adenylate kinase response to PTH-receptor interaction

   The commonest cause of a pathologically decreased plasma PTH level is destruction of the parathyroid glands. This may follow surgery (usually of the thyroid), irradiation of the neck, or infiltration of the glands by malignancy, or amyloid.

Idiopathic Hypoparathyroidism
Frequently, this disease is an isolated event, but may be associated with other autoimmune disorders, such as pernicious anaemia and Addison's disease.

Pseudo-idiopathic Hypoparathyroidism
This disorder is similar to idiopathic hypoparathyroidism, except that plasma levels of i-PTH have been found to be elevated, suggesting failure of metabolism of PTH to the active metabolite. As distinct from pseudohypoparathyroidism, infusion of exogenous PTH results in a normal response.

Pseudohypoparathyroidism
This disease results from the failure of the target organ to respond to PTH, as is shown by failure of elevation of nephrogenic cyclic-AMP following infusion of PTH. Clinically, the patients are short, mentally retarded, and have shortening of the 4th and 5th metacarpals. Two types of this disorder exist:
Type 1 No c-AMP response to PTH due to a defect in receptor-adenyl cyclase coupling protein
Type 2 The c-AMP response is present on testing

Pseudopseudohypoparathyroidism
This is a further variant of pseudohypoparathyroidism in which the clinical signs of pseudohypoparathyroidism are present, but no biochemical deficit is detectable.

Defective Vitamin D Metabolism
The clinical findings of rickets in childhood, or osteomalacia in adults, is usually the result of defective vitamin D metabolism. A number of possible causes are as shown in *Table* 6.4.

Table 6.4. Causes of defective vitamin D metabolism

Nutritional ↓ Intake: Rickets; Osteomalacia	*Decreased response to 1,25-DHCC* Vitamin D-resistant rickets
Malabsorption Coeliac syndrome Tropical sprue Short bowel syndrome	*Increased clearance of 1,25-DHCC* Nephrotic syndrome Drugs Dilantin Alcohol Glutethimide
Decreased 25-hydroxylation Liver disease	
Decreased 1-hydroxylation Renal disease Vitamin D-resistant rickets	

Hungry Bone Syndrome
Following parathyroidectomy, vitamin D therapy for osteomalacia, and in some osteoblastic malignancies, new bone formation rate may outstrip bone resorption and the intestinal uptake of calcium. This may result in low plasma calcium and phosphate levels, which can be associated with an increased plasma AP level.

Hypomagnesaemia
Severe hypomagnesaemia (less than 0·3 mmol/l) may suppress the secretion of PTH as well as inhibiting the action of this hormone on the various target organs.

Acute Pancreatitis
Occasionally, in severe acute pancreatitis, marked hypocalcaemia may develop. The aetiology is believed to involve:
1.   Formation of calcium soaps as a result of lipase activity within the damaged gland
2.   Release of glucagon which may stimulate calcitonin release, as well as directly suppressing bone resorption
3.   Hypoalbuminaemia
4.   Hypomagnesaemia.

Diagnosis/Evaluation
As for hypercalcaemia, the causes of hypocalcaemia are usually obvious from the clinical and biochemical features. In those cases where the aetiology is obscure, an approach to evaluation is shown in *Fig.* 6.5.

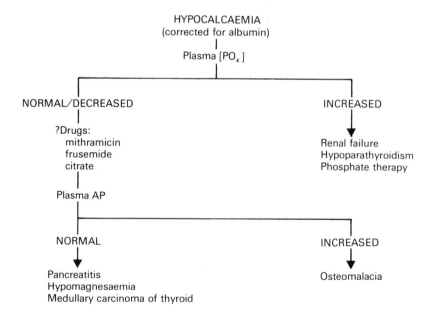

Fig. 6.5. Suggested scheme for the evaluation of hypocalcaemia.

Treatment

In the clinical situation of frank tetany, an i.v. infusion of 10–20 ml of 10% calcium gluconate (2·3 mmol/10 ml) will rapidly elevate the plasma calcium level, and alleviate the symptoms. Calcium chloride is also available for infusion, but often causes marked thrombophlebitis at the site of administration. If re-occurrence of tetany occurs, then a slow infusion of 0·35 mmol/kg of calcium gluconate over 6 h is recommended. In refractory cases, hypomagnesaemia and hyperkalaemia need to be excluded, as both these situations may cause tetanic symptoms.

In cases of chronic hypocalcaemia, as a result of hypoparathyroidism or vitamin D deficiency, treatment with oral calcium supplements is recommended. Vitamin D analogues are initiated concurrently, to increase gut absorption of the calcium. Approximately 2–4 g of elemental calcium are given daily, with variable amounts of vitamin D analogue, depending on the type (e.g. 2·5 μg of 1,25-DHCC, or 5 mg of dihydrotachysterol).

Hypocalcaemia associated with renal failure requires individually tailored therapy in order to avoid secondary hyperparathyroidism, or hypercalcaemia which will result in a further reduction in renal function. Renal physicians should be consulted for determination of the best form of therapy.

Case Examples

Phenytoin Therapy

A 70-year-old lady was started on Dilantin (sodium phenytoin) therapy following craniotomy for bilateral subdural haematomas. Over a period of years, the following results were obtained:

Year		1978	1980	1982	
Plasma	Ca	2·10	1·77	1·32 mmol/l	(2·05–2·55)
	PO_4	0·84	0·92	1·47 mmol/l	(0·6–1·25)
	Alb	32	35	37 g/l	(30–50)
	AP	96	286	600 u/l	(30–110)

Initiation of therapy with vitamin D and calcium supplements enabled correction of the hypocalcaemia.

Comment

Sodium phenytoin has the ability to 'induce' hepatic microsomal enzyme systems, a property shared by other drugs, including ethanol and phenobarbitone. As a result of this enzyme induction, metabolism of some drugs and hormones, including vitamin D metabolites, is markedly increased. This situation may cause a relative deficiency of 1,25-DHCC, and consequent biochemical findings of an 'osteomalacia-like' state. Note the markedly elevated plasma AP levels.

Pancreatitis

A 60-year-old known alcoholic male was admitted to hospital with a 2-day history of severe epigastric pain radiating through to the back, and associated vomiting. Clinical examination revealed an unkempt man, with the clinical stigmata of alcoholism, as well as epigastric rigidity, marked abdominal tenderness and guarding. Biochemical analysis revealed.

Plasma	Ca	1·82 mmol/l	(2·20–2·55)
	PO$_4$	0·41 mmol/l	(0·7–1·25)
	Alb	38 g/l	(39–48)
	AP	79 u/l	(30–110)
	Amylase	1200 u/l	(70–300)

Following conservative management with nasogastric suction and i.v. therapy, the patient's condition settled, with normalization of most of the biochemical parameters.

Comment
As previously mentioned, the hypocalcaemia in these cases can be due to:
1. Formation of calcium soaps
2. Release of glucagon
3. Hypomagnesaemia.

Hypoparathyroidism
An 80-year-old man was admitted to hospital for preoperative assessment following recurrence of a squamous-cell carcinoma of the larynx, which had been treated 2 years previously by laryngectomy and left hemi-thyroidectomy.

Clinically, the patient had stridor, as a result of mucous obstruction of the tracheostomy. A large right-sided paratracheal mass was evident.

Biochemical investigation revealed:

Plasma	Ca	1·44 mmol/l	(2·05–2·55)
	PO$_4$	2·00 mmol/l	(0·6–1·25)
	Alb	40 g/l	(30–50)
	AP	198 u/l	(30–110)

Repeat clinical examination was unable to reveal any evidence of tetany. Following verification of the plasma biochemistry results, treatment with oral calcium supplements and 1,25-DHCC (calcitriol) was instituted. One month later, the biochemical results were as follows:

Plasma	Ca	1·93 mmol/l	(2·05–2·55)
	PO$_4$	1·18 mmol/l	(0·6–1·25)
	Alb	42 g/l	(30–50)
	AP	99 u/l	(30–110)

The patient was also started on cytotoxic therapy and radiotherapy with reduction in the size of the tumour mass.

Comment
The hypoparathyroid state in this patient was the result of parathyroid gland ablation due to surgical clearance of the left side of the neck, followed by infiltration of the malignancy into the right side of the neck. The plasma i-PTH in this patient was still detectable, indicating the inaccuracy of the i-PTH assay method at low plasma levels.

Renal Failure

A 27-year-old man with severe bilateral polycystic renal disease had the following biochemical results:

Plasma			
	Ca	1·86 mmol/l	(2·05–2·55)
	PO_4	2·14 mmol/l	(0·6–1·25)
	Alb	40 g/l	(30–50)
	AP	152 u/l	(30–110)
	Urea	35 mmol/l	(3·0–8·0)
	Creat	0·65 mmol/l	(0·06–0·12)
	i-PTH	12 u/l	(2–6)

Comment

Hypocalcaemia in renal failure may be due to the following:

1. Hyperphosphataemia (as a result of ↓ GFR) leads to metastatic calcification as well as decreased Ca uptake in the gut due to ↑ PO_4 secretion in the gut
2. Reduced 1-α-hydroxylase activity in the damaged kidneys
3. Peripheral resistance to the action of PTH due to 'uraemic' toxins

As a result of the hypocalcaemia, PTH secretion is stimulated, yet calcium levels remain low due to ineffective action of PTH on bone. Because the PTH COOH-terminal is metabolized by the kidney, levels of this hormone fragment are further elevated in renal failure.

Elevated plasma AP levels reflect increased osteoblastic activity as a result of decreased production of 1,25-DHCC, and the increased PTH activity.

PHOSPHATE

Homeostasis

The total body phosphate content of the average adult male is of the order of 25 000 mmol, which is distributed as follows:

Bone	~80%
Soft tissues	~15%
Extracellular	~0·1%

Since most of the body phosphate is intracellular (intracellular : extracellular concentration ratios are approximately 100 : 1), the plasma PO_4 concentration is not a reliable indicator of the total body content. The functions of phosphorus include:

1. Maintenance of cell wall integrity
2. Enzyme regulation
3. Energy storage (ATP)
4. Oxygen transport (2,3-DPG)
5. H^+ buffer (HPO_4/H_2PO_4)

The plasma levels of inorganic phosphate are of the order of $0.7–1.25$ mmol/l, of which:

1. $12–15\%$ is protein bound
2. 85% is in the free form

At normal blood pH ($7.35–7.45$), the ratio of $HPO_4 : H_2PO_4$ is about $4 : 1$.

Input

Phosphates are widely distributed in all foods, being a major prerequisite for survival of plant and animal life. The average daily oral intake is approximately $20–40$ mmol, of which about 80% is absorbed, mainly in the duodenum. Because of the wide distribution in food, an inadequate phosphate intake is rare where subjects are on normal diets. In fasting hospitalized patients, particularly those on hyperalimentation with increased glucose loads, hypophosphataemia can be pronounced.

Distribution

The intracellular concentration of phosphate approaches 100 mmol/l, and is the most abundant intracellular anion. The major proportion of the intracellular phosphorus is in the organic form, (e.g. phosphoprotein, phospholipid and nucleic acid), whilst only a small fraction is in the inorganic form. The control of intracellular phosphate levels appears to be related to the rate of glycolysis and the acid–base status of the individual, i.e. alkalosis and glycolysis both result in increased cell PO_4 uptake.

Output

The major mechanism for the control of plasma $[PO_4]$ is renal excretion. Of the $100–200$ mmol of PO_4 filtered by the glomeruli daily, approximately 85% is reabsorbed in the proximal tubule, the remainder being excreted in the urine. The renal excretion of this ion is influenced by the following:

Increased excretion:

1. $\uparrow$ PTH
2.   Increased ECV
3.   Increased PO_4 intake
4.   Calcitonin
5.   Adrenaline

Decreased excretion:

1.   Thyroxine
2.   Growth hormone
3.   Decreased PO_4 intake

The function of vitamin D in the renal control of phosphate excretion is controversial with both decreased and increased renal excretion having been claimed.

Hyperphosphataemia

Consequences

There appear to be no specific clinical sequelae consequent to a high plasma PO_4 level. However, persistent hyperphosphataemia influences calcium homeostasis, and this may result in metastatic calcification and inhibition of intestinal calcium absorption.

Causes

The aetiology of hyperphosphataemia may be related to disorders of input, redistribution and output as listed in *Table 6.5*.

Table 6.5. Causes of hyperphosphataemia

Factitious
  Haemolysis
  Sample separation delay
	Output (renal)
	  Hypoparathyroidism
	  Pseudohypoparathyroidism
	  Acromegaly
	  Renal failure (acute/chronic)

Physiological Infants/children	

Input
  Oral phosphate ingestion (antacids)
  Intravenous phosphate
  Vitamin D overdose
	Miscellaneous
	  Tumoral calcinosis
	  Cortical hyperostosis

Redistribution
  Tissue destruction
  Acidosis	

Haemolysis

Haemolysis, which results in the release of PO_4 from red cells, is the most frequent cause of hyperphosphataemia. A similar effect is seen in blood samples where there has been a significant delay in separation of the plasma from the cells.

Input

Excessive intake of PO_4 is rarely a cause of hyperphosphataemia, unless there is a concomitant defect in renal function. Neonates fed cow's milk may develop significantly elevated plasma PO_4 levels because of the high concentrations of PO_4 in this fluid. Occasionally, phosphate enemas (for constipation) have resulted in hyperphosphataemia.

Overdosage of vitamin D, or its metabolites, can result in significantly increased PO_4 absorption from the gut, with consequent hyperphosphataemia.

Redistribution

Any significant destruction of cellular integrity will release intracellular PO_4 into the extracellular space, with possible hyperphosphataemia. This is particularly evident in tumour destruction, such as is sometimes seen in leukaemia and in chemotherapy (or radiotherapy) of tumours.

Acidosis, either respiratory or metabolic, will result in increased extracellular PO_4 levels. This effect, due to cellular PO_4 release, often occurs in diabetic ketoacidosis (prior to treatment) and in lactic acidosis.

Output
Apart from specimen artefacts, disorders of renal function are the commonest cause of hyperphosphataemia.

Renal Failure
In progressive renal insufficiency, the fraction of PO_4 excreted by the surviving nephrons increases. At GFR levels less than 20 ml/min, however, this protective mechanism is unable to maintain normophosphataemia. The possible effects of the increased plasma $[PO_4]$ are:
1. Hypocalcaemia (metastatic calcification, ↓ absorption due to ↓ 1,25-DHCC)
2. Increased PTH secretion (secondary hyperparathyroidism)
3. Metastatic calcification
4. Inhibition of renal 1-α-hydroxylase activity, thereby decreasing levels of 1,25-DHCC

Hypoparathyroidism
In the absence of PTH, phosphate excretion decreases until a new steady state level of plasma PO_4 is attained. In Type 1 pseudohypoparathyroidism, a similar effect occurs, due to resistance of the kidney to PTH action.

Acromegaly
Growth hormone appears to result in increased renal tubular reabsorption of PO_4, which may cause hyperphosphataemia if the hormone is present in excess. This mechanism may also explain the increased levels of plasma $[PO_4]$ in children.

Diagnosis/Evaluation
A simple outline for evaluation of increased plasma PO_4 levels is shown in *Fig.* 6.6. In practice, however, the majority of cases will be due to factitious causes or to renal insufficiency. The other causes of hyperphosphataemia are rare.

Treatment
Decreased gastrointestinal intake of phosphate by use of specific PO_4-binding agents, e.g. aluminium hydroxide, is the most frequent therapeutic manoeuvre for the treatment of hyperphosphataemia. This can result in significant plasma levels of aluminium, however, and consequent aluminium toxicity. Frequently, this binder causes constipation, and the addition of Mg salts will counteract this effect but, in turn, can result in hypermagnesaemia.

Saline expansion of the extracellular space will also increase renal excretion of PO_4, if renal function is adequate.

Commonly, plasma PO_4 levels in chronic renal failure are controlled by haemodialysis or peritoneal dialysis.

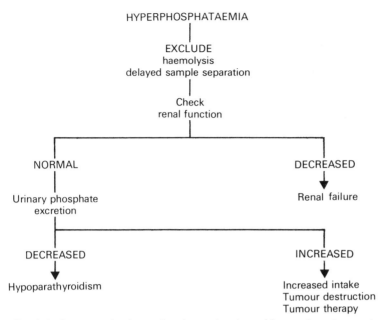

HYPERPHOSPHATAEMIA

EXCLUDE
haemolysis
delayed sample separation

Check
renal function

NORMAL

Urinary phosphate
excretion

DECREASED

Hypoparathyroidism

DECREASED

Renal failure

INCREASED

Increased intake
Tumour destruction
Tumour therapy

Fig. 6.6. Suggested scheme for the evaluation of hyperphosphataemia.

Case Examples

Lactic Acidosis

A 27-year-old female suddenly collapsed at work following 3 days of persistent headaches. Cardiopulmonary resuscitation was instituted, together with infusion of HCO_3^-. On admission to hospital, initial biochemical analysis revealed:

Plasma	Na	144 mmol/l	(137–145)
	K	3·3 mmol/l	(3·1–4·2)
	Cl	85 mmol/l	(98–106)
	HCO_3	21 mmol/l	(22–32)
	AG	41 mEq/l	(10–18)
	Ca	2·47 mmol/l	(2·20–2·55)
	PO_4	3·65 mmol/l	(0·7–1·25)
	Alb	41 g/l	(39–48)
	AP	72 u/l	(30–110)
	Lactate	16·8 mmol/l	(0·7–1·8)

Despite intensive therapy, the patient died within a few hours of admission. Autopsy revealed a ruptured 'berry' aneurysm on the anterior communicating artery near the brain.

Comment

Although cardiopulmonary resuscitation on this patient had been performed, a marked lactic acidosis had developed. The acidosis suppresses glycolysis, with release of intracellular PO_4 into the extracellular space, resulting in hyperphosphataemia.

Renal Failure

A 70-year-old lady, with known chronic renal failure had the following biochemical results:

Plasma			
	Na	124 mmol/l	(132–144)
	K	3·6 mmol/l	(3·1–4·8)
	Cl	90 mmol/l	(98–108)
	HCO_3	12 mmol/l	(21–32)
	Urea	60 mmol/l	(3·0–8·0)
	Creat	0·68 mmol/l	(0·06–0·12)
	Ca	1·82 mmol/l	(2·05–2·55)
	PO_4	2·69 mmol/l	(0·6–1·2)
	Alb	31 g/l	(30–52)
	AP	120 u/l	(30–110)

Comment

As a result of decreased glomerular filtration rate (usually < 20 ml/min), reduced renal excretion of PO_4 occurs. Acidosis can also result in hyperphosphataemia by causing an extracellular shift of PO_4.

Hypoparathyroidism

A 58-year-old lady had a parathyroid adenoma removed at operation. Post-operatively, her clinical progress was uncomplicated, but biochemical evaluation 2 weeks later revealed:

Plasma			
	Ca	1·50 mmol/l	(2·05–2·55)
	PO_4	2·22 mmol/l	(0·6–1·2)
	Alb	46 g/l	(30–52)
	AP	89 u/l	(30–110)

Comment

The removal of a parathyroid adenoma is often followed by a period of hypoparathyroidism, since recovery of function by the remaining glands may take as long as 6 months. Failure of PTH secretion results in hypocalcaemia, and decreased renal excretion of PO_4, with consequent hyperphosphataemia.

Hypophosphataemia

Consequences

Because of the importance of phosphorus in energy storage, metabolic processes and cellular structure, hypophosphataemia affects a number of organ systems, particularly as a result of decreased levels of ATP and 2,3-diphosphoglyceric acid (2,3-DPG). Examples include:

1. Paraesthesia, ataxia, coma
2. Haemolysis (↓ 2,3-DPG)
3. Muscle weakness, rhabdomyolysis
4. ↓ Platelet aggregation

5

5.   Infection ($\downarrow$ leucocyte phagocytosis)
6.   Skeletal abnormalities (e.g. osteomalacia)
     Usually, the clinical sequelae of hypophosphataemia are not detected until the plasma PO_4 level falls below 0·1 mmol/l. It must be recalled, however, that plasma PO_4 levels are a poor reflection of total body PO_4 stores.

Causes
There are a number of causes of hypophosphataemia, but only a few are associated with profound hypophosphataemia ($<0·2$ mmol/l). *Table* 6.6 lists the causes of significant hypophosphataemia.

Table 6.6. Causes of hypophosphataemia

Input	Alcoholism*
Antacids	'Hungry bone' syndrome
Pregnancy	*Renal*
Redistribution	Vitamin D deficiency
Nutritional refeeding	Renal tubular defect
Alkalosis	Hyperparathyroidism
respiratory*	Hypomagnesaemia
metabolic	*Miscellaneous*
diuretics	Haemodialysis
Vitamin D defect	Hypothyroidism
Hyperparathyroidism	Recovery from severe burns
Diabetic ketoacidosis	
(treatment)*	

(*Note*: Conditions marked with an asterisk may cause profound hypophosphataemia)

Input
Because of the wide distribution of phosphate in food, hypophosphataemia due to a low dietary intake is rare. In hospitalized patients, however, significant hypophosphataemia may result if fasting regimes are maintained, particularly in the presence of infusions of high concentrations of carbohydrate ($\uparrow$ cellular PO_4 uptake). Fructose infusions also bind large amounts of PO_4 intracellularly as fructose-1-PO_4.
     Ingestion of binding agents, such as $Al(OH)_2$, $Mg(OH)_2$, or $AlCO_3$, may result in inhibition of gut absorption of ingested PO_4.

Redistribution
The major effectors of intracellular PO_4 distribution appear to be acid–base status, plasma insulin and glycolytic rate.
     Changes in plasma PO_4 (and K^+) are related particularly to the activity of the glycolytic pathway, since 1 mole of glucose requires 4 moles of PO_4 for metabolism. As the intracellular PO_4 concentration is small, increases in the rate of glycolysis may rapidly deplete free intracellular PO_4 concentrations, causing a PO_4 shift from the extracellular fluid and consequent hypophosphataemia.

In alkalosis, particularly acute respiratory alkalosis, the induction of activity of the enzyme phosphofructokinase results in a marked increase in glycolysis. The consequent PO_4 shift into the cells may result in a rapid, profound hypophosphataemia.

Prior to therapy, diabetic ketoacidotic patients can have elevated plasma PO_4 levels, with marked phosphaturia. On institution of treatment, however, as a direct effect of insulin, and increased glycolysis, PO_4 moves intracellularly, and the plasma PO_4 may fall precipitously.

Alcoholism, particularly following a 'binge', results in the interaction of a number of effects to promote hypophosphataemia:

1.   Nutritional ($\downarrow PO_4$ intake)
2.   Respiratory alkalosis, as a result of pain or delirium tremens (PO_4 moves intracellularly)
3.   Increased glycolysis following clearance of ketones, i.e. alcoholic ketosis (PO_4 moves intracellularly)
4.   Refeeding, resulting in increased demand in production of phosphoprotein, phospholipid, etc.
5.   Use of antacids for gastritis (binds PO_4 in the gut)

Output

As a result of a marked stress reaction, severe burns cause retention of salt and water, with hypervolaemia and oedema. On clearance of this excess fluid, phosphaturia occurs, with increased loss of PO_4. Concomitantly, increased anabolism increases demand for PO_4 in the manufacture of complex PO_4-containing molecules.

A number of other effectors, by their actions on the kidney, may promote hypophosphataemia to a moderate degree. Disorders of PTH and vitamin D metabolism resulting in hypophosphataemia are described under calcium metabolism. The specific renal tubular defect, Fanconi syndrome, results in low plasma PO_4 levels due to marked phosphaturia.

Diagnosis/Evaluation

The commonest cause of hypophosphataemia is alkalosis (respiratory and metabolic). Causes of profound hypophosphataemia may be rapidly identified by a review of the clinical and biochemical findings, including specific drug therapy (e.g. antacids). Examination of the urinary excretion of PO_4 may reveal renal defects in PO_4 handling, as compared to intracellular redistribution, where the renal PO_4 excretion is reduced. An outline is shown in *Fig.* 6.7.

Treatment

If the plasma PO_4 level is less than 0·4 mmol/l, i.v. replacement is recommended. Several commercial preparations are available containing mixtures of KH_2PO_4 and Na_2HPO_4. The recommended dose is 0·08 mmol/kg of PO_4 over 6 h, followed by remeasurement of the plasma PO_4 level. In cases where the

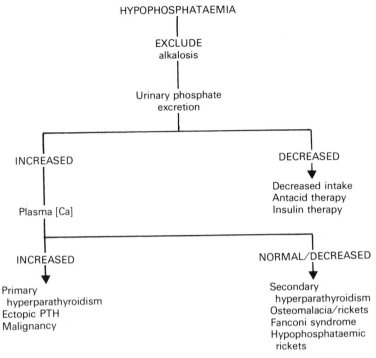

HYPOPHOSPHATAEMIA

EXCLUDE
alkalosis

Urinary phosphate
excretion

INCREASED

Plasma [Ca]

INCREASED

Primary
 hyperparathyroidism
Ectopic PTH
Malignancy

DECREASED

Decreased intake
Antacid therapy
Insulin therapy

NORMAL/DECREASED

Secondary
 hyperparathyroidism
Osteomalacia/rickets
Fanconi syndrome
Hypophosphataemic
 rickets

Fig. 6.7. Suggested scheme for the evaluation of hypophosphataemia.

hypophosphataemia is symptomatic, or if prolonged PO_4 wastage has occurred, then the dosage may be increased to 0·16 mmol/kg. If hypercalcaemia coexists, however, the PO_4 infusion will need to be decreased for fear of metastatic calcification. The maximum dose of PO_4 in an adult should not exceed 15 mmol.

Complications of PO_4 infusions include:
1. Hypocalcaemia
2. Metastatic calcification
3. Hyperkalaemia, hypernatraemia (as a result of infusion of these elements along with the PO_4)

Oral phosphate supplements are rarely required because of the ubiquitous distribution of PO_4 in food. They may be used, however, in the treatment of hypercalcaemia, i.e. binding of calcium in the gut, thereby decreasing absorption.

Case Examples

Respiratory Alkalosis

A 29-year-old man, with a past history of psychosis, was admitted to hospital complaining of severe chest pain, and paraesthesia in the upper extremities. Clinical examination was unrewarding apart from a marked increase in respiratory rate of 30/min. Arterial blood gas estimation revealed the following:

pH	7·60	(7·35–7·45)
H^+	25 nmol/l	(33–45)
PCO_2	28 mmHg	(35–45)
PO_2	128 mmHg	(80–110)
HCO_3	27 mmol/l	(22–31)

Biochemical analysis at the time revealed:

Plasma	Ca	2·50 mmol/l	(2·20–2·55)
	PO_4	0·23 mmol/l	(0·7–1·25)
	Alb	46 g/l	(39–48)
	AP	97 u/l	(30–110)

Reassurance of the patient that he was not dying of a 'heart attack' resulted in normalization of respiratory rate and plasma PO_4.

Comment

A frequent isolated finding, hypophosphataemia, occurs very rapidly following hyperventilation and respiratory alkalosis. Normalization of blood pH results in rapid return of the plasma $[PO_4]$ to normal, The clinical finding of paraesthesia in these cases is believed to be the result of decreased free plasma Ca levels as a consequence of the change in $[H^+]$—($\downarrow[H^+]$ causes $\downarrow$ [Ca]).

Alcoholism

A 46-year-old known alcoholic male was admitted to hospital complaining of persistent vomiting following a 'binge'. Clinical examination revealed an unkempt man, with the stigmata of chronic alcohol abuse. Treatment included dextrose–saline infusion with potassium supplements, and i.m. thiamine. During the evening the patient became restless and disorientated, suggesting a diagnosis of delirium tremens. Biochemical results the next day showed:

Plasma	Na	130 mmol/l	(137–145)
	K	2·4 mmol/l	(3·1–4·2)
	Cl	72 mmol/l	(98–106)
	HCO_3	42 mmol/l	(22–32)
	Urea	4·7 mmol/l	(3·0–8·0)
	Ca	2·10 mmol/l	(2·20–2·55)
	PO_4	0·12 mmol/l	(0·7–1·25)
	Alb	27 g/l	(34–45)
	AP	221 u/l	(30–110)
	AST	109 u/l	(10–45)

Comment

The development of a profound hypophosphataemia is often seen in alcoholic patients following therapy. The probable mechanisms include:
1. Poor nutrition ($\downarrow PO_4$ intake)
2. Metabolic alkalosis (vomiting)
3. Respiratory alkalosis (delirium tremens)
4. $\uparrow$ Glycolysis as a result of refeeding (e.g. glucose infusion)

The increased AP in this patient is due to alcoholic liver disease, as indicated by the increase in aspartate aminotransferase (AST). The hypokalaemia reflects persistent vomiting, which causes a metabolic alkalosis and K^+ to shift intracellularly (p. 66).

Diabetic Ketoacidosis

A 19-year-old girl developed polyuria, polydipsia and polyphagia over a period of 4 weeks. She became severely ill as a result of intercurrent septicaemia, and was admitted to hospital in a ketoacidotic state. Initial biochemical parameters, and those 24 h after therapy (i.v. saline, KCl and insulin) are shown:

Plasma				
Na	140	145 mmol/l	(132–144)
K	3·5	3·5 mmol/l	(3·1–4·8)
Cl	103	125 mmol/l	(98–106)
HCO_3	7	15 mmol/l	(21–32)
Urea	11·9	9·7 mmol/l	(3·0–8·0)
Glu	53·0	18·0 mmol/l	(3·0–5·5)
Ca	2·42	2·20 mmol/l	(2·05–2·55)
PO_4	1·54	0·1 mmol/l	(0·6–1·25)
Alb	36	31 g/l	(30–50)
AP	125	85 u/l	(30–110)

Continued management of the diabetes and the septicaemia resulted in full recovery. Plasma phosphate levels slowly returned to normal over a period of 5 days.

Comment

Patients with diabetic ketoacidosis usually present with a mild hyperphosphataemia, which rapidly falls on initiation of therapy with insulin. The hypophosphataemia is due to intracellular uptake of PO_4 for use in the stimulated (effect of insulin) glycolytic pathway. Prior to therapy, the hyperphosphataemia (and the osmotic diuresis due to glucose) results in increased renal phosphate clearance, so that total body phosphate stores are already depleted on admission.

MAGNESIUM

Magnesium, which is the second most abundant intracellular cation (after K^+), is particularly important as an activator of numerous enzyme systems in the body. It is also associated with regulation of neuromuscular activity.

The average adult contains approximately 750–1000 mmol of Mg, of which 50% is adsorbed to the hydroxyapatite of bone. Of the remaining 50%, 90% is distributed intracellularly within the soft tissues.

Plasma magnesium levels, as measured by atomic absorption spectroscopy, are of the order of 0·7–0·95 mmol/l in fasting young adults. In plasma, Mg exists as:

1. 'Free'   55%
2. Protein bound   33% (mainly albumin)
3. Complexes   12% (phosphate, citrate)

The intracellular distribution of Mg^{2+} is not homogeneous, being mainly present in microsomes, with lesser amounts in mitochondria. At least 80% of intracellular Mg^{2+} is bound to protein.

Homeostasis

Input

Magnesium is found in green vegetables and meats. The average daily intake is about 10–15 mmol, and of this approximately 50% is absorbed (mainly in the duodenum). The mechanism of absorption appears to be energy dependent, and is inhibited by excessive PO_4 ingestion and also in steatorrhoea. In the human, dietary calcium appears to inhibit Mg uptake.

Distribution

Magnesium is taken up into cells by an energy-dependent mechanism. Calcium transport mechanisms, which involve Mg, are thought to be involved in this process. Intracellular Mg levels are of the order of 20 mmol/l (plasma levels are of the order of 0·7–0·95 mmol/l).

Output

Apart from losses of magnesium in intestinal secretions, the main site of Mg excretion from the body is via the kidney. Of the 100–150 mmol of Mg^{2+} filtered by the glomeruli daily, approximately 3–5% is excreted in the urine, resulting in urinary Mg^{2+} levels of 2·5–5 mmol/d. The major site of Mg^{2+} reabsorption in the kidney is in the ascending limb of the loop of Henle. At this site, Mg^{2+} reabsorption is closely related to calcium reabsorption.

Controllers of renal Mg^{2+} handling include:

Increased excretion:
1. ECV expansion
2. Alcohol
3. Glucose
4. Diuretics (frusemide)
5. Hypercalcaemia
6. Vitamin D
7. Calcitonin
8. Thyroxine
9. Diabetes mellitus

Decreased excretion:
1. PTH

Hypermagnesaemia

Consequences

The major effects of hypermagnesaemia are those of neuromuscular irritability. At plasma [Mg] greater than 2·5 mmol/l, abolition of deep tendon reflexes occurs. Paralysis and hypotension can occur at levels greater than 5 mmol/l.

Causes

A list of the causes of hypermagnesaemia is given in *Table* 6.7.

Table 6.7. Causes of hypermagnesaemia

Intake	Output
Oral Mg	Chronic renal failure
Mg-containing antacids	Acute renal failure
Eclampsia (Mg treatment)	Hypoadrenalism
i.v. Mg supplements	Familial hypocalciuric hypercalcaemia
Rectal enemas	
Purgatives (Mg-containing)	

Input

A high magnesium intake, in the form of oral purgatives (or enemas), may be associated with significantly increased gut absorption of magnesium.

Distribution

In acidosis, particularly diabetic ketoacidosis, a moderate hypermagnesaemia may result as a consequence of an extracellular shift of magnesium.

Output

The commonest cause of hypermagnesaemia is decreased renal excretion due to acute renal failure or severe chronic renal failure.

In familial hypocalciuric hypercalcaemia (p. 145), the defect of divalent cation transport results in hypermagnesaemia in association with hypercalcaemia generally, hypomagnesaemia occurs in most cases of hypercalcaemia).

Treatment

Cessation of any magnesium-containing drug therapy, and antagonism of the toxic effects of magnesium by calcium gluconate infusion, is of value in symptomatic cases. In prolonged situations of hypermagnesaemia, dialysis is the treatment of choice.

Case Examples

Antacid Abuse

A 76-year-old man, with a long history of peptic ulceration, was admitted to hospital complaining of malaise and epigastric discomfort. Clinical examination revealed an unkempt man, with mild epigastric tenderness. Neurological examination was unremarkable apart from depressed ankle and knee tendon reflexes. Biochemical analysis revealed:

Plasma	Na	147 mmol/l	(132–144)
	K	5·0 mmol/l	(3·1–4·8)
	Cl	103 mmol/l	(93–108)
	HCO₃	33 mmol/l	(21–32)
	Urea	6·5 mmol/l	(3·0–8·0)
	Creat	0·14 mmol/l	(0·06–0·12)
	Ca	1·94 mmol/l	(2·05–2·55)
	PO₄	0·75 mmol/l	(0·6–1·2)
	Mg	2·82 mmol/l	(0·7–0·95)
	Alb	46 g/l	(30–50)
	AP	118 u/l	(30–110)

Further history taking revealed that the patient ingested large amounts of magnesium carbonate in an attempt to relieve his 'indigestion'.

Comment

The hypermagnesaemic alkalosis as a result of ingestion of $MgCO_3$ is evident in this case. The hypocalcaemia may be due to the suppressive effect of Mg on the release and activity of PTH.

Renal Failure

Routine screening in a 69-year-old man with chronic renal failure revealed:

Plasma	Na	131 mmol/l	(132–144)
	K	6·3 mmol/l	(3·1–4·2)
	Cl	94 mmol/l	(98–106)
	HCO₃	15 mmol/l	(21–32)
	Urea	49·6 mmol/l	(3·0–8·0)
	Mg	1·44 mmol/l	(0·7–0·95)

Comment

In severe renal failure (GFR < 20 ml/min), plasma magnesium levels are often raised. In acute renal failure, plasma [Mg] is elevated initially, but falls during the polyuric phase of the disease.

Hypomagnesaemia

Consequences

The major consequences of hypomagnesaemia are neuromuscular and mental disturbances. Clinical findings can include hyper-reflexia, ataxia, tetany, carpopedal spasm and tremors. Mental irritability, depression, apathy and weakness may also be prominent. ECG findings include prolongation of Q–T interval and abnormal T-waves.

Causes

The finding of hypomagnesaemia has become more frequent in hospital populations as physicians have become aware of the significance of this cation (and therefore requested measurement of plasma Mg levels). The advent of certain drugs has also increased the frequency of significant hypomagnesaemia. A short list of causes of hypomagnesaemia is given in *Table* 6.8.

Table 6.8. Causes of hypomagnesaemia

Factitious	Renal tubular acidosis
EDTA contamination	Diabetic ketoacidosis therapy
(non-AAS analysis)	Alcoholism
Input	Drugs
Malnutrition	gentamicin
Malabsorption	cis-platinum
Small bowel resection	Hyperaldosteronism
Output	Hyperthyroidism
Acute renal failure (polyuric phase)	Acute pancreatitis
Hypercalcaemia	

Input

Although magnesium is widely distributed in food, hypomagnesaemia may result from an inadequate diet, or from the malabsorption syndromes, e.g. intestinal resection and coeliac disease. Hypomagnesaemia can also occur during prolonged parenteral nutrition if magnesium supplements are not incorporated in the infusions.

Output

Excessive losses of gastrointestinal fluids may result in magnesium depletion as a result of the high Mg concentrations of gut secretions. Nasogastric suction, fistulas and purgatives have all been implicated.

The most frequent cause of hypomagnesaemia results from increased renal excretion. This is often seen in 'loop acting' diuretic therapy (e.g. frusemide), which inhibits Mg reabsorption in the renal tubule. It can also occur during the diuretic phase of acture renal failure.

Many hypercalcaemic states are associated with hypomagnesaemia, as a result of suppression of PTH secretion, and competitive interaction between the divalent cations in the renal tubule. The notable exception appears to be familial hypocalciuric hypercalcaemia, where 50% of cases are noted to be hypermagnesaemic as well as hypercalcaemic. Thiazide diuretic therapy of long duration also may result in hypomagnesaemia, as well as hypercalcaemia (p. 140).

Alcoholism is associated with hypomagnesaemia, possibly as a result of a direct effect of alcohol on the renal tubule (↑ excretion), as well as associated malnutrition, diarrhoea and metabolic acidosis.

Several drugs, particularly gentamicin and tobramycin, cause magnesuria as well as kaliuresis and calciuresis. The mechanism is uncertain. Cis-platinum, a relatively recent cytotoxic agent causes frequent hypomagnesaemia, as a result of renal Mg wasting.

Treatment

The significant feature of magnesium replacement therapy is the marked renal loss of Mg^{2+} during therapy, with over 50% of the administered metal appearing in the urine. Consequently, replacement therapy must allow for this loss.

In most oral replacement schedules, 10 mmol of $MgSO_4$ are given 4 times daily. Diarrhoea is a potential complication with this form of therapy.

In situations of significant hypomagnesaemia (plasma $Mg < 0.3$ mmol/l), i.v. infusion of Mg^{2+} is the therapy of choice. In acute replacement, 0.15 mmol/kg may be given over 1 h for each 0.1 mmol/l the plasma Mg is less than 0.7 mmol/l.

For chronic replacement, allowing for 50% urinary losses, 0.4–0.8 mmol/kg may be given over the first 24 h. If the plasma $[Mg^{2+}]$ level has risen, but is still low at the end of this period, further replacement is given at a reduced rate (e.g. 0.2–0.4 mmol/kg). The usual formulation of i.v. Mg supplements is 50% $MgSO_4$ (i.e. 20 mmol/10 ml). Note that in renal disease, dosage schedules should be reduced by at least half, and frequent monitoring of plasma Mg instituted.

Case Examples

Cis-platinum Therapy

A 76-year-old lady with disseminated carcinoma of the breast had been given cytotoxic therapy, which had included cis-platinum. A few days following therapy, repeated blood examination revealed a persistent hypocalcaemia as indicated:

Plasma			
	Na	136 mmol/l	(137–145)
	K	3.5 mmol/l	(3.1–4.2)
	Cl	105 mmol/l	(98–106)
	HCO_3	23 mmol/l	(22–32)
	Urea	1.9 mmol/l	(3.0–8.0)
	Creat	0.10 mmol/l	(0.05–0.12)
	Ca	1.58 mmol/l	(2.20–2.55)
	PO_4	0.46 mmol/l	(0.7–1.25)
	Mg	0.27 mmol/l	(0.7–0.95)
	Alb	29 g/l	(39–48)
	AP	68 u/l	(30–110)

Replacement therapy with i.v. $MgSO_4$ resulted in a plasma Mg level of 1.08 mmol/l after 2 days. Eight days later repeat blood examination revealed normalization of the plasma Ca as shown (renal function remained unaltered):

Plasma			
	Ca	2.30 mmol/l	(2.20–2.55)
	PO_4	0.69 mmol/l	(0.7–1.25)
	Alb	32 g/l	(39–48)
	AP	93 u/l	(30–110)

Comment

The occurrence of hypomagnesaemia following cis-platinum therapy has been estimated to occur in approximately 50% of cases. Often, the deficiency is detected by a persistent hypocalcaemia which does not respond to therapy. The aetiology of the hypocalcaemia appear to be related to inhibition of PTH release and impaired peripheral response to the hormone due to Mg deficiency. In this particular case, the possibility of inadequate calcium input, or volume expansion, as reflected by the low plasma urea may have made significant contributions to the low plasma [Ca].

The aetiology of the hypophosphataemia may reflect the effect of i.v. glucose infusion, as well as possible respiratory alkalosis due to pain from the patient's condition.

Diabetic Ketoacidosis

A 35-year-old female, a known diabetic for 10 years, was admitted to hospital in diabetic ketoacidosis following an infection. Among a number of biochemical changes, the following were noted:

Plasma	Glu	34·7 mmol/l	(3·0–5·5)
	Ca	2·18 mmol/l	(2·05–2·55)
	PO_4	1·37 mmol/l	(0·6–1·25)
	Mg	1·03 mmol/l	(0·7–0·95)
	Alb	39 g/l	(30–50)
	AP	250 u/l	(30–110)

Following therapy for her condition, which did not include replacement of Mg, repeat analyses 2 days later revealed:

Plasma	Ca	2·22 mmol/l	(2·05–2·55)
	PO_4	0·25 mmol/l	(0·6–1·25)
	Mg	0·64 mmol/l	(0·7–0·95)
	Alb	34 g/l	(30–50)
	AP	230 u/l	(30–110)

Comment

Ths osmotic diuresis resulting from glycosuria causes increased Mg loss in the urine. In untreated diabetic ketoacidosis, plasma [Mg] are often slightly elevated, possibly as a result of acidosis. On treatment, however, magnesium moves intracellularly, and any depletion of the cation will become evident. Some authors suggest that insulin resistance may result from hypomagnesaemia, but few clinicians specifically replace magnesium losses in diabetic ketoacidosis.

Further Reading

Agus Z. S., Wasserstein A. and Goldfarb S. (1982) Disorders of calcium and magnesium homeostasis. *Am. J. Med.* **72**, 473–488.

Austin L. A. and Heath III, H. (1981) Calcitonin: physiology and pathophysiology. *N. Engl. J. Med.* **304**, 269–278.

Ebel H. and Gunther T. (1980) Magnesium metabolism: a review. *J. Clin. Chem. Clin. Biochem.* **18**, 257–270.

Kao P. C. (1982) Parathyroid hormone assay. *Mayo Clin. Proc.* **57**, 596–597.
Marx S. J., Spiegel A. M. and Levine M. A. (1982) Familial hypocalciuric hypercalcaemia: the relation to primary parathyroid hyperplasia. *N. Engl. J. Med.* **307**, 416–426.
Ritz E. (1982) Acute hypophosphataemia. *Kid. Int.* **22**, 84–94.
Singer F. R., Bethune J. E. and Massry S. G. (1977) Hypercalcaemia and hypocalcaemia. *Clin. Nephrol.* **7**, 154–162.
Stewart A. I., Horst R., et al. (1980) Biochemical evaluation of patients with cancer-associated hypercalcaemia. *N. Engl. J. Med.* **303**, 1377–1388.

7

Renal disease

Definitions

Clearance

The renal clearance of a substance (x) is the amount of blood, or plasma, completely cleared of that substance by the kidney in a given time, e.g. ml/min. It is calculated from the following formula:

$$\text{Clearance of x (ml/min)} = \frac{U_x \times V}{P_x}$$

Where U_x = urinary concentration of x (mmol/l); P_x = plasma concentration of x (mmol/l); V = volume of urine (ml/min).

    If a substance, after glomerular filtration, passes through the renal tubules without being added to (no tubular secretion), or subtracted from (no tubular reabsorption), its clearance will equal the glomerular filtration rate (GFR). Such a substance is inulin. In the routine clinical situation the clearance of creatinine is considered to approximate the GFR. However, the clearance of creatinine is slightly greater than that of inulin because a small amount of creatinine is secreted by the renal tubules.

Fractional Excretion (FE)

The renal fractional excretion of a substance (x) is that percentage of the total amount filtered by the glomeruli that is finally excreted in the urine:

$$FE_x = \frac{\text{x (mmol) excreted}}{\text{x (mmol) filtered}} \times 100\%$$

$$\text{amount excreted/min} = V \times U_x$$

$$\text{amount filtered/min} = GFR \text{ (l/min)} \times P_x$$

Where U_x = urinary concentration of x (mmol/l); P_x = plasma concentration of x (mmol/l); V = volume of urine (l/min)

    If GFR = creatinine clearance (cr cl)

171

Then:

$$FE_x = \frac{V \times U_x}{1} \times \frac{1}{cr\ cl \times P_x}$$

$$= \frac{V \times U_x}{1} \times \frac{P_{cr}}{U_{cr} \times V} \times \frac{1}{P_x}$$

$$= \frac{U_x}{P_x} \times \frac{P_{cr}}{U_{cr}}$$

Normal Renal Physiology

The major role of the kidney is the maintenance of the extracellular, and indirectly the intracellular, fluid volume and composition. This regulation is dependent on the normal function of the glomeruli and tubules of the approximately one million nephrons that are present in each healthy adult kidney. In the normal adult around 150 litres of glomerular filtrate are presented daily to the renal tubules from which approximately 1·5 litres of urine are formed. The final volume and composition of the urine depends on tubular function.

The kidney also plays an important role in vitamin D metabolism (p. 134), acts as an endocrine organ (renin-angiotensin system, p. 240, and is involved in erythrocyte production (erythropoietin synthesis).

Glomerular Filtration

The normal adult glomerular filtration rate (GFR) is of the order of 130–180 litres a day (90–120 ml/min, 1·5–2·0 ml/s). The composition and volume of the filtrate varies with a number of factors (glomerular permeability, colloidal osmotic pressure, renal blood flow). One of the most important factors that affects filtrate formation is the renal blood perfusion rate or renal blood flow (RBF). Under normal circumstances approximately 20% of the cardiac output is delivered to the kidneys (about 1 litre/min). The renal blood flow rate can be kept relatively constant by renal auto-regulation in the presence of a variety of circulatory disorders; however if there is a very low cardiac output or a large fall in blood pressure the renal blood vessels will constrict, resulting in a decrease in RBF and GFR and an inadequate excretion of urea, creatinine and other waste products. this condition is termed the 'prerenal state' or prerenal uraemia (PRU).

Tubular Function

The four main functions of the renal tubules are:
1. Retention of essential metabolites
2. Controlled excretion of waste products
3. Regulation of water and electrolyte balance
4. Regulation of acid–base balance

There is a degree of overlap between some of these functions, e.g. phosphate ions are a waste product as well as an essential metabolite; however it is convenient to discuss tubular function under these four headings.

Retention of Essential Metabolites

Important non-electrolyte substances such as amino acids and glucose are almost completely reabsorbed in the proximal renal tubule by specific, active transport mechanisms. These substances do not appear in the urine in significant quantities unless there is a defect in their transport mechanism, damage to the tubular epithelium, or the plasma levels are so high that the tubule reabsorptive capacity is exceeded.

Controlled Excretion of Waste Products

The kidney plays the major role in the excretion of creatinine, urea, uric acid, phosphate, sulphate and many drugs.

Creatinine

Creatinine is derived from the muscle energy storage component, creatine phosphate. All creatinine filtered by the glomeruli passes through the renal tubules without any significant reabsorption, but a small amount is added to the forming urine by tubular secretion. The amount secreted increases with rising plasma levels of creatinine (e.g. renal failure) and therefore the renal creatinine clearance rate in such situations is usually higher than the GFR as measured by inulin clearance. The amount of creatinine excreted daily is a function of the muscle mass, and in the adult is around 8–25 mmol.

Urea

A major portion of the filtered urea is reabsorbed by the renal collecting ducts. The amount reabsorbed depends on the rate of urine flow, being around 40% at high rates (~ 10 ml/min) and 60% at low rates ($\sim 0 \cdot 5$ ml/min). This tubular reabsorption results in the urea clearance rate (about 1-1·5 ml/s) being much lower than the GFR or the creatinine clearance rate. The reabsorbed urea plays an important role, along with sodium, in maintaining the high osmolal gradient between the renal interstitial tissue and the collecting duct urine (i.e. it is important for ADH action and water reabsorption). The amount of urea excreted daily in the normal adult averages 400–600 mmol.

Urate

The renal clearance of urate, which is about 10% of the inulin clearance rate, involves both tubular reabsorption and secretion. Around 98% of the filtered urate is reabsorbed in the proximal nephron (2% allowed through) and an amount, equal to about 8% of that filtered, is secreted by the tubules. Thus, of the amount excreted, about 20% comes from the glomerular filtrate and 80% from renal tubular secretion. The daily excretion rate depends on dietary purine intake, but is of the order of 4–10 mmol.

Phosphate

Some 70–90% of the filtered phosphate is reabsorbed in the proximal renal tubule. This reabsorption is influenced by the level of circulating parathyroid hormone

(PTH), i.e. $\uparrow$ PTH $\longrightarrow$ $\downarrow$ PO_4^{2-} reabsorption and $\downarrow$ PTH $\longrightarrow$ $\uparrow$ PO_4^{2-} reabsorption. The urinary phosphate is a major urinary buffer and is necessary for the excretion of hydrogen ions (see below). Between 15 and 50 mmol of phosphate are excreted daily.

Regulation of Water and Electrolyte Balance

Water

Of the 150 litres of fluid filtered each day by the glomeruli only about 1% (approximately 1500 ml but depends on fluid intake) appears as urinary water.

About 50–70% of the filtered water is reabsorbed along with sodium in the proximal renal tubule (obligatory). This reabsorption is isotonic and therefore the fluid leaving this portion of the nephron has the same osmolality as that of plasma. In the ascending limb of the loop of Henle, which is impermeable to water, sodium chloride is reabsorbed, leaving a dilute urine (50–100 mmol/kg). The final volume and concentration of the urine is regulated by the rate of water reabsorption in the collecting ducts which in turn is regulated by ADH (p. 18).

The water content of urine is dependent on four factors:

1. Normal delivery of fluid to the diluting segment (ascending limb of the loop of Henle), i.e. normal GFR and proximal tubule reabsorption.
2. Reabsorption of NaCl in the diluting segment.
3. Functional collecting duct cells.
4. Normal ADH secreting mechanism.

Sodium

Less than 1% of the the filtered sodium appears in the urine, i.e. of the 20 000–25 000 mmol filtered daily all except 100–200 mmol are reabsorbed by the renal tubules. Reabsorption occurs in four areas of the nephron: proximal tubule, ascending limb of the loop of Henle, distal tubule, collecting duct.

   Proximal tubule: 50–70% actively reabsorbed along with water

   Ascending loop of Henle: 20–30% passively reabsorbed consequent to active Cl^- reabsorption

   Distal tubule: 5–10% reabsorbed—influenced by aldosterone (p. 22).

   Collecting duct: up to 5–8% reabsorption depending on intake—influenced by aldosterone and the postulated natriuretic hormone (p. 22).

Potassium

About 600–700 mmol of potassium are filtered daily, but only some 10–14% of this amount ($\sim$50–100 mmol) is finally excreted in the urine. A major portion of the filtered potassium ($\sim$95%) is reabsorbed in the proximal tubule and the ascending limb of the loop of Henle. The bulk of the potassium appearing in the urine is secreted by the distal nephron which is under the influence of aldosterone. The rate of potassium secretion by the distal tubule is controlled by a number of factors (p. 54) of which the most important are:

1.   Intracellular potassium concentration of the distal tubular cells—
       ↑ concentration (↑ aldosterone, alkalosis)⟶ ↑ rate of secretion.
2.   Rate of urine flow through the distal tubule (↑ secretion with ↑ flow rate).

Chloride

Sodium and chloride reabsorption are closely linked. In the proximal tubule Cl^- is passively reabsorbed following active Na^+ reabsorption whilst in the ascending limb of the loop of Henle there is active Cl^- reabsorption and passive Na^+ reabsorption. Some chloride is also reabsorbed along with sodium in the distal tubule and collecting ducts.

Calcium

Approximately 200 mmol of ionized calcium (Ca^{2+}) are filtered daily, and of this 60–70% is reabsorbed in the proximal tubule. This uptake is closely linked to Na^+ reabsorption. Around 20–30% of filtered calcium is reabsorbed in the ascending limb of the loop of Henle and 2–5% is taken up in the distal tubules and collecting ducts. Parathyroid hormone increases calcium reabsorption in the distal nephron but has no affect on that occurring in the proximal tubule.

In the proximal tubule calcium reabsorption is closely related to that of sodium so that factors that influence Na^+ reabsorption (e.g. ↑ reabsorption with ↓ blood volume) similarly affect calcium uptake.

The daily urine excretion of calcium is around 2·5–7·5 mmol and represents about 3–5% of the filtered calcium.

Magnesium

Of the 50–100 mmol of filtered magnesium some 2–5% appears in the urine: 20–30% is reabsorbed in the proximal tubule, 50–60% in the ascending limb of the loop of Henle and 1–5% in the distal nephron. Recent evidence suggests that parathyroid hormone increases magnesium reabsorption in the ascending limb of the loop of Henle.

Regulation of Acid–base Balance

The kidney, in concert with the lungs and extracellular buffers (p. 88), plays a major role in acid–base homeostasis. The kidney is responsible for:
1.   Excretion of non-volatile acids formed as a by-product of metabolism
       (50–100 mmol of H_2SO_4, H_3PO_4, lactic acid, etc.)
2.   Excretion of excess alkali (as HCO_3^-)
3.   Compensation of respiratory acid–base disorders by manipulating the
       extracellular bicarbonate concentration (p. 86)
       These three functions are carried out by increasing or decreasing the rate at which the following two mechanisms operate:
1.   Tubular reabsorption of HCO_3^-
2.   Tubular excretion of H^+
       Both of these mechanisms are in turn dependent on the ability of the nephron to secrete hydrogen ions into its lumen.

Reabsorption of Bicarbonate (see also p. 91)

In the normal adult approximately 4000 mmol of HCO_3^- are filtered each day by the glomeruli. About 90% of this is reabsorbed in the proximal tubule, and the remainder being taken up by the distal nephron. However, this uptake of HCO_3^- cannot be achieved in a simple fashion because it is a complex anion which has difficulty in traversing the tubular epithelium in its original form.

In the proximal tubular cell (*Fig.* 7.1) water and CO_2, assisted by the action or carbonic anhydrase, form H^+ and HCO_3^-. The H^+ is secreted into the tubular lumen in exchange for filtered Na^+.

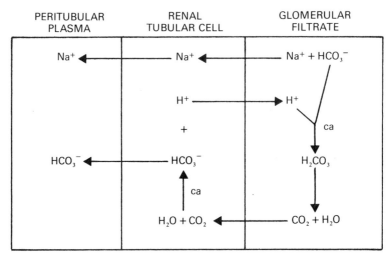

Fig. 7.1. Bicarbonate reabsorption in the proximal renal tubule. ca, carbonic anhydrase.

Within the lumen, under the influence of carbonic anhydrase (present on the luminal surface of the tubular cells), the H^+ reacts with filtered HCO_3^- to form water and CO_2. This CO_2 diffuses back into the tubular cell to combine with water and forms more H^+ and HCO_3^-.

The reabsorbed Na^+, and the cell-generated HCO_3^-, pass out of the cell back to the renal bloodstream, i.e. for each H^+ exchanged with Na^+ one HCO_3^- is generated in the cell and one HCO_3^- is removed from the glomerular filtrate. Thus HCO_3^- is reabsorbed from the filtrate by an indirect mechanism.

N.B. Although some 4000 mmol of H^+ are secreted daily by the proximal tubule there is no loss of this (excretion) in the urine.

The 10% of filtered HCO_3^- which escapes proximal reabsorption is returned to the blood by a similar mechanism in the distal tubules.

When the amount of HCO_3^- filtered exceeds the tubular reabsorptive capacity (plasma level of 28–30 mmol/l) it will appear in the urine, e.g. bicarbonaturia associated with the metabolic alkalosis of vomiting (p. 191).

Excretion of H⁺ (*see also* p. 89)

Each day some 50–100 mmol of H^+, representing endogenous production of non-volatile acids, are excreted by the distal nephron (mainly the collecting ducts) in the urine.

The rate and amount of H^+ secreted by the nephron are limited by the H^+ concentration gradient across the tubule cell membrane between the urine forming in the lumen and the cell cytoplasm. If the $[H^+]$ of the luminal fluid rises above 0·03–0·1 mmol/l (pH of 4·5–4·0) the secretion of H^+ will cease (i.e. the distal nephron is unable to generate a blood : urine H^+ concentration gradient above 1 : 1000 or a urine pH below 4·0–4·5). Thus if the urine consisted of pure water and 1 litre was excreted per day the amount of H^+ excreted would only be 0·03–0·1 mmol, which is only a fraction of the amount required to be excreted each day (50–100 mmol).

This H^+ gradient problem is overcome by the presence in the urine of two substances which trap the H^+ : the urinary buffers phosphate and ammonia (*Fig. 7·2*). Other substances in the urine are also capable of binding H^+, e.g. creatinine and urate, but are not quantitatively important in acid–base homeostasis.

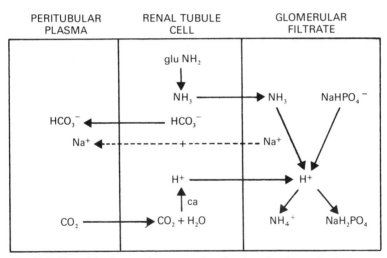

Fig. 7.2. Renal hydrogen ion excretion in the distal renal tubule. ca, carbonic anhydrase.

An important urinary buffer is disodium hydrogen phosphate (Na_2HPO_4), which accounts for about half of the total H^+ excreted. This component is measured in the urine as titratable acidity (TA). The other major H^+ carrier is ammonia. It is generated in the renal tubular cells from amino acids, principally glutamine, and diffuses freely into the tubular lumen. Here it acts as a strong base and removes H^+ by forming ions (NH_4^+) which are then excreted in the urine.

The amount of H^+ removed by phosphate buffer is limited by the amount of phosphate filtered by the glomeruli. In contrast the amount of NH_3 synthesized by the cell can be increased some tenfold, if increased buffering is required, e.g. in conditions such as ketosis and lactic acidosis.

The secretion of H^+ by the distal tubule, as in the proximal tubule, results in generation of HCO_3^- and reabsorption of Na^+ (*Fig.* 7.2). The difference between these two tubular mechanisms is as follows: in the proximal tubule there is no loss of H^+ from the body, and the generated HCO_3^- replaces HCO_3^- removed from the blood by the glomerular filtrate; in the distal tubule the H^+ is excreted from the body and the generated HCO_3^- increases the plasma level. This HCO_3^- replaces the extracellular HCO_3^- lost (consumed) during buffering action, as occurs when acid (H^+A^-) is added from cellular metabolism, i.e. $H^+A^- + NaHCO_3 \longrightarrow Na^+A^- + H_2CO_3 \longrightarrow Na^+A^- + H_2O + CO_2$.— $NaHCO_3$ is replaced by Na^+A^-, and CO_2 is excreted by the lung.

Chronic Renal Failure

Chronic renal failure occurs when disease causes a slow (months, years) decrease in the number of functional nephrons, and the kidney is no longer able to maintain a normal cellular environment.

The earliest biochemical feature is increased plasma levels of urea and creatinine. This is usually referred to as uraemia (literally 'urine' in the blood).

In the early phase of the disease the remaining healthy nephrons increase their 'work-load' by increasing their individual excretory capacity, and therefore are able to maintain the internal environment. This adaptation is due to the ability of the nephrons to increase their fractional excretion (p. 171) of substances normally removed from the body by the kidney (urea, creatinine, phosphate, etc.). This adaptation finally fails to maintain the internal environment when some 70–80% of nephrons are non-functional.

As chronic renal failure progresses and glomerular filtration rate declines, the increase in the plasma level of various analytes follows a characteristic pattern (*Table* 7.1).

Table 7.1. Plasma levels of various analytes in progressive chronic renal disease

Creatinine clearance (ml/s)		Plasma analyte increased
1·0–2·0	(120 ml/min)	Nil
0·5–1·0	(30–60 ml/min)	Creatinine, urea
0·3–0·5	(20–30 ml/min)	K^+, H^+ ($\downarrow$ $[HCO_3^-]$)
0·2–0·3	(10–20 ml/min)	Phosphate, urate

Sodium Homeostasis

Patients with chronic renal failure (CRF), despite a declining GFR, are able to maintain sodium balance by increasing its fractional excretion (FE_{Na^+}). A normal adult with a GFR of 1.7 ml/s (100 ml/min, 144 litres/day) and a plasma $[Na^+]$ of 140 mmol/l filters about 20 000 mmol of sodium daily. If the intake and renal excretion of sodium is 100 mmol/day ($\sim$6g) then the FE_{Na^+} is 0.5%. If the GFR falls to 0.25 ml/s (15 ml/min, 21.6 litres/day) and the sodium intake is still 100 mmol/day then to remain in balance the FE_{Na^+} must be increased to 3.3%. The mechanism for increasing the FE_{Na^+} in CRF is unclear, but may be related to urea-induced osmotic diuresis and possibly also the postulated natriuretic hormone.

By increasing the FE_{Na^+} patients in CRF are able to maintain sodium balance. However, this adaptive process is limited as the FE_{Na^+} cannot be increased above 25%. When this level is reached the dietary intake of sodium has to be decreased or sodium overload will occur.

Most patients in CRF are in sodium balance until the later stages of the disease when positive balance may occur. In some patients, particularly those with tubulo-interstitial disease (hydronephrosis, polycystic kidneys, etc.), renal sodium wasting may occur, resulting in a negative sodium balance and, if water intake is increased, hyponatraemia.

Water Homeostasis

As CRF worsens with destruction of renal architecture, and damage to tubules and collecting ducts continues, the ability of the kidney to concentrate, and dilute, the urine is progressively lost. The inability to concentrate urine occurs early in the disease, followed later by the inability to dilute the urine. In the later stages of the disease the urine osmolality, despite varying fluid intake, becomes fixed at around the plasma value ($\sim$300 mmol/kg). Most patients, however, are usually able to vary urine osmolality between 250 and 350 mmol/kg, depending on their fluid intake.

It should be borne in mind, however, that adults have to excrete, via the kidney, some 600 mmol of osmotically active substances each day. If the urine osmolality is fixed at 300 mmol/kg then the urine output, and therefore the oral intake of fluid, has to be around 2 litres a day ($600/300 = 2$), in order to excrete the 600 mmol of particles.

Potassium Homeostasis

The patient with progressive CRF remains in potassium balance for a long period due to:
1.   Increased renal fractional excretion of potassium (FE_{K^+})
2.   Increased excretion of potassium into the large bowel

Fractional excretion: The normal adult on a daily potassium intake of 50–100 mmol has a FE_{K^+} of 10–15%. To compensate for nephron loss in CRF the FE_{K^+} of the functional nephrons will increase up to 200–300%. Only when the GRF falls to 0.25–0.5 ml/s will potassium be retained and hyperkalaemia occur.

Colonic excretion: Under normal circumstances about 10% of ingested potassium is excreted in the faeces. In renal failure up to 30–40% of the oral intake may be excreted by this route. This increase is due to potassium secretion by the colonic epithelium, which may be related to increased aldosterone secretion (hyperkalaemia is a potent stimulus to aldosterone secretion).

Potassium retention and hyperkalaemia, as noted above, tend not to occur until there has been a significant fall in the GFR. If hyperkalaemia occurs at higher levels of GFR it is usually due to mechanisms other than decreased renal excretion, e.g. increased intake, acidosis. Some patients with moderate renal failure (plasma [creatinine] <0.2 mmol/l) may develop hyperkalaemia in the absence of severe acidosis or increased potassium intake. This may be due to damage to the distal tubular cells (e.g. tubulo-interstitial disease). In some cases, particularly diabetics, there may be a defect in aldosterone secretion (*see* Syndrome of hyporeninaemic hypoaldosteronism, p. 59).

Acid–base Homeostasis

Acidosis, like hyperkalaemia, usually does not occur in CRF until there is a significant decrease in GFR (to 0.25–0.5 ml/s). The limiting factor in severe renal disease appears, not to be the inability of the renal tubule to secrete H^+, but the lack of H^+ binders, phosphate and ammonia, in the tubular fluid.

As the GFR declines the FE of phosphate rises which will be reflected by an increase in the FE of titratable acid (TA). However, there is a limit to this increase and eventually the total amount excreted as TA falls. Similarly, there is an increase in NH_3 production by individual nephrons early in renal disease, but eventually there are too few ammonia-producing cells and NH_4^+ excretion declines. The final result is a kidney that can secrete H^+ (pH of urine can be lowered to ~ 4.5) but cannot excrete it from the body. This inability to excrete H^+ results in a decrease in plasma $[HCO_3]$ (inability of the kidney to regenerate bicarbonate).

In addition to the problem of H^+ excretion, patients with CRF often have a proximal tubule bicarbonate leak which manifests itself when the plasma level is raised during bicarbonate therapy. The mechanism of this leak is unclear. It has been suggested that it may be due to increased circulating PTH which has been shown, in experimental animals, to decrease proximal tubule bicarbonate reabsorption.

The metabolic acidosis of CRF may be of two types: hyperchloraemic (normal anion gap) metabolic acidosis (HCMA), and high anion gap acidosis (p. 105). HCMA tends to occur early in CRF, especially if there is significant tubular dysfunction (e.g. tubulo-interstitial disease) and indicates that there is sufficient glomerular function to excrete acid anions (SO_4^{2-}, PO_4^{2-}, etc.) but insufficient tubular function to excrete H^+. As the renal disease progresses the declining glomerular function results in acid anion retention and the acid–base defect becomes a high anion gap metabolic acidosis (p. 90).

An interesting feature of metabolic acidosis of CRF is that the plasma bicarbonate level does not usually fall below 13–15 mmol despite a positive H^+ balance of 20–40 mmol/day. This is most likely due to the release of bone buffer ($CaCO_3$). The demineralization of bone that occurs during the acidosis of CRF supports this theory.

Calcium and Phosphate Homeostasis

Advanced CRF is associated with a positive phosphate and a negative calcium balance, which results in hyperphosphataemia, hypocalcaemia and bone disease. An outline of the pathophysiology is shown in *Fig.* 7.3.

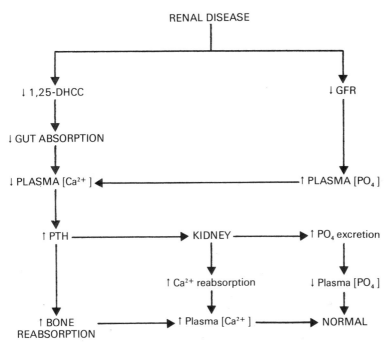

Fig. 7.3. Calcium and phosphate homeostasis in chronic renal failure prior to decomposition and the development of hyperphosphataemia and hypocalcaemia. 1,25-DHCC; 1,25-dihydroxycholecalciferol.

The negative calcium balance is due to decreased gut absorption as a consequence of deficient 1,25-dihydroxycholecalciferol (1,25-DHCC) production by the diseased kidney. As the ionized calcium (Ca^{2+}) level falls it stimulates parathyroid hormone (PTH) secretion which mobilizes calcium from bone and increases renal Ca^{2+} reabsorption. This action returns the plasma [Ca^{2+}] back to normal levels. However, as the disease progresses and less calcium becomes available from gut absorption and bone resorption, the plasma [Ca^{2+}] (and total plasma calcium) falls. This hypocalcaemia is usually mild (1·80–2·00 mmol/l) and rarely results in symptoms (tetany, etc.). However, the negative calcium balance and increased PTH secretion will result in bone disease (renal osteodystrophy).

Phosphate balance is maintained by increasing its FE until the GFR falls to ~0·3 ml/s, when balance becomes positive and hyperphosphataemia occurs. Increased circulating PTH is responsible for this increase in FE (decreased tubular reabsorption). Hyperphosphataemia affects calcium homeostasis by decreasing the level of ionised calcium (in vivo precipitation).

PTH secretion, and its plasma level, is increased early in CRF due to the fall in $[Ca^{2+}]$. However, although very high plasma levels have been reported to occur in renal disease, this is due mainly to an increase in the C-terminal fragment PTH (p. 153). This fragment is biologically inactive and is normally removed from the body by glomerular filtration followed by metabolism in the renal tubule cells. A fall in GFR results in its retention in plasma.

Magnesium Homeostasis

Magnesium, like most of the analytes discussed above, remains in balance in renal failure due to increased FE until there is a fairly low GFR. The plasma level begins to rise when the GFR declines to 0·25–0·30 ml/s or earlier if the patient's magnesium intake is increased (e.g. magnesium-containing antacid therapy).

Case Examples

Mild Chronic Renal Failure

A 62-year-old female was admitted to hospital for repair of a vaginal prolapse. The preoperative plasma electrolytes were 'normal' but a raised urea and creatinine was noted. Prior to discharge renal function was investigated.

Plasma			
	Na	136 mmol/l	(132–144)
	K	4·2 mmol/l	(3·2–4·8)
	Cl	105 mmol/l	(98–108)
	HCO_3	24 mmol/l	(23–33)
	Urea	15·0 mmol/l	(3·0–8·0)
	Creat	0·21 mmol/l	(0·06–0·12)
	Anion gap	11 mEq/l	(7–17)
	Ca	2·34 mmol/l	(2·15–2·55)
	PO_4	1·22 mmol/l	(0·6–1·25)
	AP	99 u/l	(30–120)
	Alb	42 g/l	(32–50)
Creatinine clearance		0·60 ml/s	(1·5–2·0).

Comment

On the basis of plasma creatinine (P_{cr}) levels renal failure may be divided into mild (P_{cr}: <0·2 mmol/l), moderate (P_{cr}: 0·2–0·4 mmol/l) and severe (P_{cr}: >0·4 mmol/l). In mild, uncomplicated CRF with a creatinine clearance of around 0·5 ml/s the only plasma abnormalities are usually raised urea and creatinine levels.

Before there is a rise in the plasma level of creatinine and urea approximately 50–60% of the renal tissue has to be non-functional (creatinine clearance of around 0·7–0·8 ml/s). However, in lesser degrees of renal insufficiency, if there is a concomitant disorder causing a decreased GFR (shock, haemorrhage, dehydration), or an increase in urea synthesis (high protein meal, haemorrhage into gut), the plasma urea level may rise above the upper reference limit ($\sim$8·0 mmol/l).

Moderate CRF with Acidosis and Hyperkalaemia

A 48-year-old female presented to her local doctor complaining of tiredness. A blood examination revealed a normocytic, normochromic anaemia with a haemoglobulin level of 7·5 g/dl. Her plasma biochemistry revealed mild to moderate renal failure. She was later considered to have analgesic nephropathy.

Plasma	Na	141 mmol/l	(132–144)
	K	5·2 mmol/l	(3·2–4·8)
	Cl	111 mmol/l	(98–108)
	HCO_3	19 mmol/l	(23–33)
	Urea	36·0 mmol/l	(3·0–8·0)
	Creat	0·35 mmol/l	(0·06–0·12)
	Anion gap	16 mEq/l	(7–17)
	Ca	2·25 mmol/l	(2·15–2·55)
	PO_4	1·56 mmol/l	(0·6–1·25)
	AP	125 u/l	(30–120)
	Alb	37 g/l	(32–50)
	PTH (C-term)	10 u/l	(2·0–6·0)
Creatinine clearance		0·25 ml/s	(1·5–2·0)

Comment

In the early stages of analgesic nephropathy the disease is limited to the renal medulla so that tubular function is compromised before glomerular function. In the above case this situation is reflected by the hyperchloraemic (normal anion gap) metabolic acidosis and hyperkalaemia.

The normal anion gap acidosis in this patient suggests that tubular dysfunction ($\downarrow$ excretion of H^+ by distal nephron) is relatively greater than glomerular dysfunction (ability to excrete acid anions).

The hyperchloraemia is a consequence of the inability to excrete H:

$\downarrow$ Tubular H^+ secretion $\longrightarrow$ $\downarrow$ Na^+–H^+ exchange and Na^+ reabsorption $\longrightarrow$ Na^+ loss (with acid anions) in urine $\longrightarrow$ $\downarrow$ extracellular volume $\longrightarrow$ $\uparrow$ proximal tubule reabsorption of Na^+ as NaCl.

Thus the Na^+ lost in the urine as Na^+. (acid-anion)$^-$ is replaced by $Na^+.Cl^-$ and so the extracellular chloride concentration is increased.

The hyperkalaemia in this patient represents a mixture of decreased renal secretion (distal tubule dysfunction) and acidosis (potassium leak from cells—p. 58).

Severe Chronic Renal Failure

A 40-year-old male was admitted from a country hospital with a history of vomiting, progressive malaise and weakness. He had been found to have polycystic renal disease 6 years previously, after he had been involved in a motor vehicle accident and ruptured his spleen.

Plasma	Na	133 mmol/l	(132–144)
	K	5·4 mmol/l	3·2–4·8)
	Cl	98 mmol/l	(98–108)
	HCO_3	15 mmol/l	(23–33)

Urea	54·0 mmol/l	(3·0–8·0)
Creat	1·13 mmol/l	(0·06–0·12)
Anion gap	25 mEq/l	(7–17)
Ca	1·69 mmol/l	(2·15–2·55)
PO$_4$	2·80 mmol/l	(0·6–1·25)
AP	160 u/l	(30–120)
Alb	30 g/l	(32–50)
PTH (C-term)	17 u/l	(2–6)
Creatinine clearance	0·05 ml/s	(1·5–2·0)

Comment

The classic textbook picture of biochemical findings in CRF (hyperkalaemia, high anion gap acidosis, hyperphosphataemia and hypocalcaemia) is only seen in the latter stages of the disease.

The low total plasma calcium in the above case is due not only to the renal failure (↓ 1,25-DHCC, hyperphosphataemia) but also to the low plasma albumin level. As noted earlier raised plasma PTH level is due to increased secretion and decreased excretion of the catabolic products (C-terminal fragment rises with falling GFR). The increased alkaline phosphatase indicates increased osteoblastic activity in the skeleton (uraemic osteodystrophy).

The high anion gap in the above case indicates that the glomerular filtration rate is insufficient to clear the plasma of the non-volatile acid anions (cf. the previous patient).

Chronic Renal Failure: Haemodialysis

The biochemistry results shown below are those of a patient undergoing haemodialysis. The dialysis fluid contained: Na$^+$—137 mmol/l, K$^+$—1·0 mmol/l, Cl$^-$—102 mmol/l, Mg^{2+}—0·25 mmol/l, acetate—40 mmol/l, osmolality—288 mmol/kg. The 1245 h specimen was inadvertently taken from the venous side of the dialyser.

Date	08/10	08/10	08/10	
Time (h)	0930	1245	1315	
Plasma Na	145	137	140 mmol/l	(132–144)
K	4·6	1·0	2·6 mmol/l	(3·2–4·8)
Cl	105	99	95 mmol/l	(98–108)
HCO$_3$	22	2	26 mmol/l	(23–33)
Urea	35·0	4·5	15·5 mmol/l	(3·0–8·0)
Creat	1·16	0·20	0·56 mmol/l	(0·06–0·12)
Ca	2·50	—	2·84 mmol/l	(2·15–2·55)
PO$_4$	3·16	—	1·33 mmol/l	(0·6–1·25)
AP	126	—	153 u/l	(30–120)
Alb	37	—	44 g/l	(32–50)

Comment

This case indicates some of the biochemical features associated with haemodialysis.

1.   The second set of results (venous side of the dialyser) shows the effect on the plasma analytes of one passage of the blood through the dialyser, and

should be compared with the third set of results taken 30 min later: i.e.
- *a.* Removal of potassium
- *b.* Exchange of blood $HCO_3{}^-$ for acetate ion (anion gap of blood leaving dialyser is 37 mEq/l)
- *c.* Removal of urea and creatinine
2. Hypokalaemia: This often occurs in the post-dialysis period due to the removal of K^+ by dialysis. Although hypokalaemic, these patients rarely become potassium depleted because in most cases only a small amount has been removed from the extracellular fluid, and equilibrium with the intracellular K^+ has not had time to occur.
3. Plasma Bicarbonate Increase: Acetate ions, from the dialysis fluid, cross into the patient's bloodstream and are readily metabolized by all tissues of the body to $HCO_3{}^-$. If the patient has poor tissue blood perfusion (e.g. cardiac insufficiency) acetate metabolism may be retarded and the patient will exhibit a high anion gap due to accumulated acetate ions.
4. Hypercalcaemia: This does not occur in all patients, but most will show an increase in their plasma calcium level. Possible causes include:
- *a.* Infusion of calcium from the dialysis fluid: Some dialysis fluids are manufactured using tap water which may contain significant quantities of calcium.
- *b.* Fall in level of extracellular phosphate concentration.
- *c.* Increased activity of PTH on bone. (It has been suggested that hypocalcaemia of CRF may be due in part to 'uraemic' toxins preventing the full expression of PTH at the bone level.)
5. Plasma Albumin Increase: In this patient the rise in plasma albumin reflects a decreased extracellular water content—removal during dialysis.
6. Fall in Plasma Levels of Creatinine, Urea, Phosphate: The average fall in the levels of these analytes after 5–6 hours of haemodialysis is:

Creatinine	40–50%
Urea	50–60%
Phosphate	50–60%

Acute Renal Failure

Acute renal failure usually describes a condition where there is acute suppression of urinary output (to less than 400 ml/day—oliguria). Not all patients with acute renal failure present with oligura, so it is perhaps better to apply the term to those patients showing an acute rise (hours, days) in plasma levels of urea or creatinine or both.

For the formation of urine and adequate excretion of metabolic waste products the kidney must: (1) receive an adequate blood supply, (2) must function normally; and (3) the urine must be able to escape from the body. Using these three conditions as a starting point it is helpful to simply classify acute renal failure into:

prerenal uraemia (PRU), acute renal parenchymal disease or acute tubular necrosis (ATN), and obstructive nephropathy or postrenal uraemia.

Prerenal Uraemia (PRU)

The essential factor in this condition is a decreased GFR in an otherwise normal kidney, which results in decreased urine output and retention of metabolic waste products (urea and creatinine). The fall in GFR is usually due to hypovolaemia and subsequent decreased renal blood perfusion. As mentioned earlier, the kidney, by autoregulation, is able to maintain its blood supply despite a variety of circulatory problems. However, in severe volume depletion the renal blood vessels constrict and renal blood flow is compromised, resulting in suppression of GFR.

All conditions associated with extracellular volume depletion (*Table* 7.2) have the potential to proceed to PRU. The commonest causes are haemorrhage, shock and gastrointestinal fluid loss.

Table 7.2. Causes of prerenal uraemia (PRU)

Extracellular Volume (ECV) Depletion
  Haemorrhage
  Burns
  GI loss: vomiting, diarrhoea
  Renal loss: diuretics, osmotic diuresis, Addison's disease, salt-losing nephritis

Normal or Increased ECV with Ineffective Intravascular Volume
  Shock
  Congestive cardiac failure
  Nephrosis
  'Third space' fluid loss: pancreatitis, ascites, crush injury

---

The normal physiological response to volume depletion and inadequate renal perfusion results in characteristic features which are diagnostic of the condition:

Hypovolaemia

Hypovolaemia $\longrightarrow$
1. $\uparrow$ Renal NaCl reabsorption $\longrightarrow$
  a. $\downarrow$ Urinary $[Na^+]$ (<20 mmol/l)
  b. $FE_{Na^+} < 1\%$
  c. $\downarrow$ Urinary $[Cl^-]$ (<20 mmol/l)
2. $\uparrow$ ADH secretion $\longrightarrow$
  a. $\downarrow$ Urinary output (<500 ml/day)
  b.   Concentrated urine:
       Urine : plasma (U/P) osmol = >1
       Urine : plasma (U/P) urea = >20
       Urine : plasma (U/P) creat = >20

In patients who are vomiting or who are on gastric suction the high levels of plasma bicarbonate (metabolic alkalosis) reached may exceed the proximal tubular reabsorptive capacity. This may be associated with urinary bicarbonate loss (as $NaHCO_3$) and a high (>20 mmol/l) urinary sodium concentration. In these cases the urinary FE_{Na^+} may be greater than 1%. These two features are usually associated with ATN (*Table* 7.3), but an inspection of the urinary chloride concentration (U [Cl^-]) and urine: plasma osmolality ratio (U/P osmol) will reveal the status of tubular function. A U[Cl^-] less than 20 mmol/l and a U/P osmol greater than 1·3 indicates intact tubular function.

Table 7.3. Differentiation of ATN from PRU

	PRU	ATN
Urine [Na^+] mmol/l	<20	>20
Fractional excretion of Na (%)	<1	>1
Urine [Cl^-] mmol/l	<20	>20
Urine/plasma osmolality	$>1·3$	$<1·3$
Urine/plasma urea	>20	<14
Urine/plasma creatinine	>20	<14
Urine sediment	Normal	Cell debris, red cells, casts etc.

Conditions causing PRU may progress to acute tubular necrosis (ATN), so it is important to make an early assessment of renal function in these disorders and treat them promptly.

Acute Tubular Necrosis (ATN)

Acute tubular necrosis is an acute, potentially reversible, renal disease due to ischaemic or toxic insult to the kidney, which characteristically results in scattered areas of tubular necrosis. Not all cases will show this renal pathology, and various other terms such as 'vasomotor nephropathy' and 'lower nephron nephrosis' have been used to describe the condition.

The commonest causes of ATN are renal ischaemia (progression of PRU, *see Table* 7.2) and toxic insult to the kidney (haem pigments, bacterial toxins, heavy metals, etc.). Acute oliguria may also be due to other types of renal disease, e.g. acute glomerulonephritis, occlusion of renal blood vessels, interstitial nephritis, urate nephropathy, urinary tract obstruction.

Despite many theories, the pathophysiology of this condition is still unclear. Possibilities include:

1. Intrarenal blood flow redistributed from cortex to medulla (blood shunted away from the glomeruli).
2. Obstruction of tubular lumina with cellular and other debris.
3. Diffusion of urine back into the blood through damaged tubular epithelium.

The presentation and severity of this condition varies from severe renal injury with corticol necrosis and no recovery of renal function, to minimal injury with mild renal failure and early recovery. In between these two extremes lies the classic picture of oliguria which lasts 1–2 weeks followed by a diuretic phase and a slow recovery of renal function.

The biochemical features of the oliguric phase of ATN (*Table* 7.3) can be explained in terms of decreased GFR and tubular dysfunction:

1. Decreased GFR $\longrightarrow$
    a. Low urine output (oliguria)
    b. Retention of waste products (urea, etc.)
2. Tubular dysfunction $\longrightarrow$
    a. $\downarrow$ NaCl reabsorption $\longrightarrow$ $\uparrow$ U $[Na^+]$, FE_{Na^+} and $[Cl^-]$
    b. Resistance to ADH $\longrightarrow$ dilute urine $\longrightarrow$ U/P osmol ~ 1
    c. Retention of K^+, H^+ $\longrightarrow$ hyperkalaemia, acidosis

The urinary sediment is an important diagnostic feature which differentiates ATN from PRU; it is normal in PRU but contains cell debris, erythrocytes, amorphous material and casts in ATN.

If the patient survives the 7–14 days of the oliguric phase, recovery with diuresis usually occurs. During diuresis the urine output increases daily and reaches a maximum at around 5–7 days. Early in the diuretic phase the GFR remains low, and often the plasma urea level rises further before finally falling. The major physiological problem encountered is the uncontrolled urinary loss of water and electrolytes in the period prior to the tubules regaining normal function.

Fluid and Electrolytes in ATN

Water

The extracellular volume in those patients presenting with ATN will depend on the aetiology. If the ECV is decreased it should be replenished with the appropriate fluid (saline, plasma, whole blood). However, the major problem with water homeostasis in these patients is that of diminished renal excretion. During the oliguric phase water balance may be maintained by giving the patient 500 ml plus the volume of the previous day's urine output. The 500 ml derives from normal skin and mucous membrane losses (800–1000 ml/day) minus the water gained endogenously from metabolism (approximately 400–500 ml). In the diuretic phase careful attention to water balance is necessary because of the potentially large urinary losses that may occur.

Sodium

In the anuric phase renal sodium excretion is low, and unless the intake is kept to a minimum (~ 20 mmol/day) volume expansion and hypertension may occur. In the diuretic phase sodium losses may be considerable, and intake should be increased accordingly to preclude sodium depletion and consequent hypovolaemia.

Potassium

Hyperkalaemia is a serious and common complication of ATN. Not only is there reduced renal potassium excretion, but there is often increased input into the extracellular compartment due to tissue damage and hypercatabolic states. Severe increases in extracellular potassium may be associated with cardiotoxicity and prompt treatment of hyperkalaemia is essential (p. 60).

Hydrogen Ion

Decreased renal excretion of H^+ and acid anions results in a high anion gap metabolic acidosis. Treatment depends on the severity of the acidosis, but care should be taken with sodium bicarbonate infusion because of the possibility of sodium overload.

Calcium and Phosphates

In the anuric phase plasma $[PO_4^{2-}]$ rises ($\downarrow$ GFR) and plasma $[Ca^{2+}]$ tends to fall ($\uparrow$ plasma $[PO_4^{2-}]$, $\downarrow$ 1,25-dihydroxycholecalciferol, (?) bone resistance to PTH). The plasma calcium rarely falls below 1·8 mmol/l and rarely produces symptoms. Plasma phosphate levels usually do not rise above 5 mmol/l, but may go higher if there is muscle destruction or haemolysis.

During the diuretic phase hypercalcaemia may occur. This temporary rise in plasma calcium probably reflects a transient overactivity of the parathyroid glands, i.e. the low plasma Ca^{2+} of the oliguric phase results in secondary hyperparathyroidism and increased secretion of PTH. The resolution of this hyperparathyroidism may lag behind the normalization of the hypocalcaemic factors as renal function returns towards normal.

Postrenal Uraemia: Obstructive Nephropathy

Obstructive nephropathy is the term applied to functional and structural disturbances of the kidney as a consequence of obstruction to the urine outflow. The obstruction may be bilateral and complete, or unilateral with the other kidney functioning normally. If the obstruction is bilateral and complete, absolute anuria will be present, if incomplete the urine output may be diminished, normal, or more usually, increased (polyuria).

In the chronic situation there is a reduction in GFR and tubular dysfunction (? back pressure of urine in the tubule). The reduced GFR results in retention of waste products (urea, creatinine, uric acid), whilst the tubular dysfunction is manifested by:
1. Reduced urine concentrating ability
2. Impaired sodium reabsorption
3. Impaired potassium excretion
4. Impaired urinary acidification

Reduction Concentrating Ability

This is due to (*a*) decreased sodium reabsorption in the ascending limb of the loop of Henle (diluting segment), (*b*) solute (urea) diuresis, and (*c*) insensitivity of the collecting ducts to ADH. Therefore in partial obstruction there may be an increased output of urine isotonic with plasma (urine:plasma osmolality ~1).

Impaired Sodium Reabsorption
Experimental evidence suggests that this is due to decreased reabsorption of NaCl in the ascending limb of the loop of Henle. The urinary sodium concentration is usually high (>20 mmol/l) as is the FE_{Na^+} ($>1\%$).

Impaired Potassium Secretion
This is due to a transport defect in the distal tubule. The consequent potassium retention usually results in hyperkalaemia and this is often associated with metabolic acidosis.

Hydrogen Ion Retention
An acidosis, usually out of proportion to the degree of renal insufficiency, often occurs. It is usually hyperchloraemic (normal anion gap) in nature and is due to distal tubular dysfunction ($\downarrow$ renal H^+ tubular excretion). As the disease progresses acid anions are retained and a high anion gap will develop.

With relief of obstruction there usually develops a diuresis. This increased output of urine, which is usually iso-osmotic with plasma, is due to:
1.   Urea diuresis (clearance of retained urea)
2.   Defect in sodium reabsorption $\longrightarrow$ solute diuresis
3.   Tubule unresponsiveness to ADH
This diuresis, which may last for several days, often results in daily urine output of 8–12 litres. During this period, until tubular function is regained, there may be: (*a*) sodium loss ($\downarrow$ tubular reabsorption), (*b*) metabolic acidosis ($\downarrow$ distal nephron H^+ secretion), and (*c*) hyperkalaemia ($\downarrow$ distal tubular secretion). Throughout this period the patient's fluid and electrolyte balance should be watched carefully as any upset may have life-threatening consequences.

Case Examples

Prerenal Uraemia: Gut Obstruction
A male aged 53 years was admitted to hospital with a 3-day history of colicky abdominal pain and vomiting. He was dehydrated and given an infusion of 2 litres of normal saline and 2 litres of 5% dextrose in the 7 h prior to laparotomy at 1200 h on 16/04.

Date		16/04	16/04	
Time (h)		0400	1100	
Plasma	Na	137	140 mmol/l	(132–144)
	K	3·4	2·8 mmol/l	(3·2–4·8)
	Cl	90	105 mmol/l	(98–108)
	HCO_3	31	28 mmol/l	(23–33)
	Urea	22·4	11·0 mmol/l	(3·0–8·0)
	Creat	0·22	0·14 mmol/l	(0·16–0·12)
	Osmol	313	303 mmol/kg	(281–295)

Urine biochemistry on admission (0400 h):

Urine	Na	16 mmol/l	FE_{Na^+}	0·2%
	Cl	12 mmol/l	U/P Osmol	1·8
	Urea	464 mmol/l	U/P Urea	20·6
	Creat	11·8 mmol/l	U/P Creat	53
	Osmol	576 mmol/kg		

Comment

This patient's urine biochemistry, and derived parameteres, suggest that the increased levels of plasma urea and creatinine were due to PRU (*see Table* 7.3). This diagnosis is confirmed by the response to rehydration, i.e. fall in plasma and creatinine levels.

Of all the diagnostic parameters in *Table* 7.3 the FE_{Na^+} is the most reliable in the differentation of PRU from ATN—except in some cases of vomiting associated with severe metabolic alkalosis (*see below*).

Prerenal Uraemia: Pyloric Stenosis

A male aged 56 years was admitted to hospital with pyloric obstruction (3-day history of severe vomiting). On examination he was moderately dehydrated with a blood pressure of 120/60 (supine) and a pulse rate of 126. Over the first 8h he was infused with 4·5 litres of normal saline containing 2 g of KCl (26 mmol) per litre.

Date		05/11	06/11	
Time (h)		2200	0630	
Plasma	Na	125	133 mmol/l	(132–144)
	K	2·1	3·2 mmol/l	(3·2–4·8)
	Cl	70	95 mmol/l	(98–108)
	HCO_3	>40	34 mmol/l	(23–33)
	Urea	18·6	8·8 mmol/l	(3·0–8·0)
	Creat	0·18	0·08 mmol/l	(0·06–0·12)
	Osmol	280	289 mmol/kg	(281–295)

Urine biochemistry on admission (2200 h):

Urine	Na	82 mmol/l	FE_{Na^+}	1·18%
	K	24 mmol/l	U/P Osmol	2·57
	Cl	<10 mmol/l	U/P Urea	25·5
	HCO_3	43 mmol/l	U/P Creat	55·5
	Urea	475 mmol/l		
	Creat	10·0 mmol/l		
	Osmol	720 mmol/kg		

Comment

This patient shows several features characteristic of gastric vomiting:

1. Metabolic alkalosis— ↑ plasma $[HCO_3^-]$ (loss of H^+ in vomitus)
2. Hypochloraemia (loss of Cl^- in vomitus)
3. Dehydration
4. Hypokalaemia (loss of K^+ in vomitus and urine)

5. High urinary $[HCO_3^-]$ ($\uparrow$ plasma $[HCO_3^-] \longrightarrow \uparrow$ filtered HCO_3 $\longrightarrow$ flooding of proximal tubule reabsorption mechanism $\longrightarrow$ loss of HCO_3^- in urine

6. High urinary $[Na^+]$ ($>20\,mmol/l$) and FE_{Na^+} ($>1\%$) (Na^+ loss with HCO_3^- loss)

The FE_{Na^+} and urinary sodium concentration in this case are characteristic of ATN. All other urinary and derived parameters suggest PRU, which is confirmed by the patient's response to intravenous saline infusion. In patients with vomiting and metabolic alkalosis the best discriminator between PRU and ATN is the urinary chloride concentration (PRU: $<20\,mmol/l$; ATN: $>20\,mmol/l$). The urinary sodium and derived parameters involving urinary sodium concentration are unreliable in this situation.

Acute Tubular Necrosis

A male patient aged 47 years was admitted with a history of acute abdominal pain, vomiting and jaundice. He was given a diagnosis of acute pancreatitis associated with cholelithiasis. After laparotomy, during which a cholecystectomy was performed and several stones removed from the common bile duct, he had a sustained drop in blood pressure. This was treated with blood transfusion followed by infusion of normal saline. His blood pressure responded to this therapy but his urine output fell to approximately $5\,ml/min$. The first set of electrolytes results shown below were taken 5 h after the operation.

Date		13/12	14/12	
Time (h)		1345	0730	
Plasma	Na	146	139 mmol/l	(132–144)
	K	4·2	5·9 mmol/l	(3·2–4·8)
	Cl	94	104 mmol/l	(98–108)
	HCO_3	21	16 mmol/l	(23–33)
	Urea	34·4	45 mmol/l	(3·0–8·0)
	Creat	0·45	0·58 mmol/l	(0·06–0·12)
	Osmol	337	— mmol/kg	(281–295)

Urine electrolytes and derived values at 1345 h on 13/12:

Urine	Na	50 mmol/l	FE_{Na^+}	4·8%
	Cl	57 mmol/l	U/P Osmol	0·96
	Urea	100 mmol/l	U/P Urea	2·9
	Creat	3·2 mmol/l	U/P Creat	7·1
	Osmol	325 mmol/kg		

Comment

The urine biochemistry and the derived parameters in this case suggest ATN (see Table 7.3). This was confirmed by the rising plasma levels of urea, creatinine and potassium despite restoration of blood volume and stabilization of the blood pressure. The urine output remained at 5–6 ml/h.

Obstructive Nephropathy: Benign Prostatic Hyperplasia

A male aged 72 years was admitted with a 6-week history of urinary incontinence and dull lower abdominal pain. On examination there was bladder distension and bilateral flank tenderness. He was catheterized and several litres of urine was obtained. A diagnosis of benign prostatic hypertrophy and obstructive nephropathy was made. The plasma electrolytes on admission and 2 days after relief of obstruction are shown below.

Date		20/04	22/04	
Plasma	Na	137	142 mmol/l	(132–144)
	K	5·1	5·0 mmol/l	(3·2–4·8)
	Cl	107	112 mmol/l	(98–108)
	HCO$_3$	16	17 mmol/l	(23–33)
	Urea	20·7	15·5 mmol/l	(3·0–8·0)
	Creat	0·64	0·29 mmol/l	(0·06–0·12)
	Anion gap	19	18 mEq/l	(7–17)
	Osmol	314	312 mmol/kg	(281–295)
Urine	Osmol	362	350 mmol/kg	

Comment

This patient shows several biochemical features commonly found in obstructive nephropathy which result from: (*a*) decreased GFR, and (*b*) tubular dysfunction.

1. Retention of urea and creatinine—↓ GFR
2. Hyperkalaemia—↓ distal tubular secretion
3. Metabolic acidosis—↓ distal nephron H$^+$ excretion

These patients, depending on the length and severity of the obstruction, often have a normal anion gap (hyperchloraemic) acidosis which progresses to a high anion gap acidosis as the GFR falls. In this case the anion gap is at the upper limit of the reference range suggesting compromised glomerular secretion of acid anions.

4. Defect in urinary concentrating ability—tubular dysfunction and insensitivity to ADH. This patient has a moderately increased plasma tonicity which normally would result in a more concentrated urine, e.g. urinary osmolality of around 400–600 mmol/kg.

After the relief of obstruction, providing renal damage is not severe, restoration of renal function can be expected within 1–2 months.

Renal Acidosis

The kidney's main function in acid–base homeostasis is the reabsorption of filtered bicarbonate and excretion of hydrogen ions. The feature common to both of these functions is renal tubular secretion of hydrogen ion, or, more specifically H$^+$ and Na$^+$ exchange across the tubule cell membrane. In the proximal tubule this is coupled with HCO$_3$$^-$ reabsorption and there is no net loss of H$^+$ from the body (no H$^+$ excretion). The hydrogen ions secreted by the distal tubule, provided there is adequate tubular fluid H$^+$-binding substances (phosphate, ammonia— p. 90), are excreted from the body, and are associated with generation of bicarbonate ions.

Aldosterone appears to play an important but undefined role in the distal tubular Na$^+$–H$^+$ exchange. Its action may be indirect by virtue of its effect on plasma potassium levels (hyperkalaemia, which is associated with suppressed aldosterone secretion, results in decreased ammonia production by the renal tubules); or it may be necessary for normal cation exchange in the distal tubule.

Failure in any of the above mechanisms results in renal acidosis, *Table* 7.4.

Table 7.4. Causes of renal acidosis

Decreased Proximal Reabsorption of $HCO_3{}^-$
    a. Proximal (Type 2) renal tubular acidosis
    b. Uraemia acidosis

Decreased Distal H^+ *Excretion*
    a. Distal (Type 1) renal tubular acidosis
    b. Uraemic acidosis

Mineralocorticoid Deficiency
    a. Type 4 renal tubular acidosis

All of the renal acidoses reflect tubular dysfunction. This may be part of a generalized renal disease associated with a very low GFR (uraemic acidosis), or due to a primary tubular disorder with a normal, or near-normal, GFR (renal tubular acidosis, RTA).

Uraemic Acidosis

The acidosis of renal failure is usually of the high anion gap variety, but in early chronic renal failure there may occur a normal anion gap (hyperchloraemic) acidosis. These two varieties reflect differing degrees of tubular and glomerular dysfunction. If the tubules are severely damaged, but the glomerular function is sufficient to excrete acid anions, the acidosis will be associated with a normal anion gap. As the disease progresses and GFR falls the acid anions will be retained and a high anion gap will result.

The mechanism of decreased tubular H^+ excretion in renal failure is due, not to an inability of the remaining nephrons to secrete H^+, but to a lack of tubular fluid H^+ trapping mechanisms. The decreased rate of ammonia synthesis and secretion, due to too few functional tubules, appears to be the main deficiency.

Most patients with chronic renal failure also have decreased proximal bicarbonate reabsorption (mechanism uncertain). This deficiency only manifests itself when the patient's plasma bicarbonate is raised, e.g. sodium bicarbonate therapy. It therefore limits the efficacy of bicarbonate treatment in these patients.

Patients with chronic renal failure maintain a stable plasma bicarbonate level of 13–15 mmol/l despite a positive H^+ balance of 20–40 mmol/day. This is thought to be due to intracellular buffering and, particularly, the buffering action of bone (calcium carbonate).

Renal Tubular Acidosis (RTA)

The characteristic feature of RTA is the defective secretion of H^+ by the renal tubules in the presence of a normal or near-normal glomerular filtration rate.

The acidosis is hyperchloraemic (normal anion gap) in nature and can present in two major forms: distal tubular and proximal tubular.

The distal (Type 1) form is associated with an inability to lower the urine pH maximally even in the presence of low plasma bicarbonate concentration. In the proximal tubular form (Type 2) there is an inability of the kidney to retain administered bicarbonate despite a low plasma bicarbonate level.

Both of these conditions may be associated with hypokalaemia due to increased renal potassium secretion. RTA associated with hyperkalaemia occurs in conditions associated with mineralocorticoid deficiency and has been designated Type 4. The term Type 3 has been used to describe a condition of Type 1 RTA associated with bicarbonate wasting which occurs mainly in infants and children.

Distal RTA (Type 1)

Of the two major forms of RTA, Type 1 is the most severe and is associated with the more serious complications. This condition is due to an inability of the distal nephron (mainly collecting ducts) to secrete H^+ and, unlike Type 2 RTA which is self limiting, it is progressive with a positive H^+ balance.

Most of the features of this disorder—hypokalaemia, bone disease, hypercalciuria, volume depletion—can be explained in terms of the ineffective Na^+–H^+ exchange in the distal nephron. This decreased exchange is due to an inability of the distal nephron to secrete H^+ and maintain a high H^+ concentration gradient (1 : 1000) between the tubular cell and tubular fluid.

$\downarrow Na^+$–H^+ exchange $\longrightarrow$

1. H^+ retention $\longrightarrow$ acidosis ($\downarrow$ plasma $[HCO_3{}^-]$ $\longrightarrow$ bone dissolution (bone buffer) $\longrightarrow$ bone calcium release $\longrightarrow$ hypercalciuria $\longrightarrow$ nephrocalcinosis and nephrolithiasis

2. $\uparrow$ Renal Na^+ excretion $\longrightarrow$
    a. Hypovolaemia $\longrightarrow$ $\uparrow$ aldosterone
    b. $\uparrow$ Distal tubule urine flow
    a+b $\longrightarrow$ $\uparrow K^+$ excretion $\longrightarrow$ hypokalaemia

3. $\downarrow H^+$ excretion $\longrightarrow$ alkaline urine in presence of a metabolic acidosis

Causes

Type 1 RTA may exist as an isolated (primary) defect or more commonly as a complication of autoimmune disease or nephrocalcinosis (*Table* 7.5).

Diagnosis/Evaluation

A common presentation is hypokalaemia with muscle weakness, but the clinical picture can be variable with differing degrees of:

1. Muscle weakness (hypokalaemia)
2. Nephrocalcinosis
3. Nephrolithiasis (recurrent)
4. Bone disease (osteomalacia, rickets)
5. Extracellular volume depletion (Na^+ loss)
6. Failure to thrive (infants and children)

Table 7.5 Causes of distal RTA

Primary
  Familial
  Sporadic

Secondary
  Autoimmune disease
    systemic lupus erythematosus
    chronic active hepatitis
    cryoglobulinaemia

  Nephrocalcinosis

  Drugs
    amphotericin B
    toluene
    analgesics

  Renal disease
    transplanted kidney
    analgesic nephropathy
    pyelonephritis
    obstructive nephropathy

The definitive diagnosis (*Table* 7.6) rests on the recognition of the characteristic features of the disease:
1.   Hyperchloraemic acidosis
2.   Hypokalaemia
3.   Urine pH > 6.0 despite low plasma $[HCO_3^-]$
4.   Fractional excretion of HCO_3^- ($FE_{HCO_3}-$) $< 3\%$ at normal and low levels of plasma $[HCO_3^-]$
5.   Inability to increase H^+ excretion (titratable acidity and ammonium despite acidosis (e.g. NH_4Cl loading test)
6.   Response to administration of small amounts of sodium bicarbonate (1–2 mmol/kg/day) with amelioration of hypokalemia, hypercalciuria and acidosis.

Management
Therapy with alkali is necessary in almost all cases in order to diminish bone disease and prevent potassium wasting. Hypokalaemia is a serious complication of this disorder and can be life threatening, e.g. respiratory failure may occur which will superimpose a respiratory acidosis on the already present metabolic acidosis. In the acute presentation it is necessary to administer potassium before or with bicarbonate therapy as diminution of acidaemia is associated with passage of K^+ into the cells and a worsening of the hypokalaemia. The amount of bicarbonate required by these patients is small in comparison with Type 2 acidosis and is of the order of 2–3 mmol/kg/day.

Proximal RTA (Type 2)
Type 2 RTA is characterized by a decreased tubular reabsorption of bicarbonate. This defect, which involves mainly, but not exclusively, the proximal tubule, results

Table 7.6. Biochemical differentiation of renal tubular acidosis

	Uraemic	Type 1	Type 2	Type 4
GFR	↓↓↓	N ⟶ ↓	N ⟶ ↓	N ⟶ ↓↓
Plasma K	N ⟶ ↑	N ⟶ ↓	N ⟶ ↓	↑ ⟶ ↑↑
Urine pH during acidosis	<5·4	>6·0	<5·4	<5·4
$FE_{HCO_3^-}$ with:				
plasma $[HCO_3^-]$ ↓	Nil	<3%	Nil	Nil
plasma $[HCO_3^-]$ N	0–3%	<3%	>15%	5–10%
Bicarbonate requirement mmol/kg/day	1–3	1–3	>5	0–3

$FE_{HCO_3^-}$ = fractional excretion of bicarbonate.

in large amounts of HCO_3^- passing to the distal nephron. Here it floods the distal bicarbonate reabsorptive capacity and is lost in the urine. The ability of the distal tubule to excrete H^+ is not affected.

Unlike Type 1 RTA, Type 2 is self-limiting and not associated with positive H^+ balance. Once the plasma bicarbonate level falls below a certain limit (14–16 mmol/l) the proximal tubule is able to reabsorb all that is presented to it and bicarbonate disappears from the urine. At this point urinary pH, ammonium excretion and titratable acidity become normal and a steady state is achieved, i.e. renal H^+ excretion now balances body H^+ production even though the plasma bicarbonate level is depressed.

Most patients with this disorder also have other defects of the proximal renal tubule which may include defects in phosphate, glucose, amino acid and urate reabsorption (Fanconi syndrome). Occurrence as an isolated disorder is rare, but may arise in a transient form in infants, and may also be seen in adults on acetazolamide (Diamox) therapy.

The plasma potassium concentration in Type 2 RTA is often normal but may fall to hypokalaemic levels if correction of the acidaemia by bicarbonate is attempted. The mechanism is probably due to increased distal nephron urine flow rate which will increase renal potassium secretion (↑ plasma $[HCO_3^-]$ ⟶ ↑ filtered $NaHCO_3^-$ which exceeds the proximal reabsorptive capacity ⟶ loss of $NaHCO_3$ (and water) through the distal nephron ⟶ ↑ K^+ secretion ⟶ potassium depletion).

Causes

The childhood forms of this disease are :(a) primary, transient bicarbonate wasting in infants (usually male), and (b) the Fanconi syndrome which is associated with such disorders as cystinosis, tyrosinaemia and hereditary fructose intolerance. In adults Type 2 RTA may occur: (a) in heavy metal intoxication (copper in Wilson's disease, lead poisoning); (*b*) associated with carbonic anhydrase inhibition (acetazolamide); (*c*) after renal transplant; (*d*) in vitamin D deficiency with hypocalcaemia and increased PTH secretion; (*e*) in Sjögren's syndrome and in myelomatosis (*Table* 7.7).

Table 7.7. Causes of proximal RTA

Primary
  Infants (transient)
  Familial
  Sporadic

Secondary
  Inborn errors of metabolism
    cystinosis
    tyrosinaemia
    Lowe's syndrome
    hereditary fructose intolerance
    Wilson's disease
  Heavy metal intoxication
  Drugs
    acetazolamide
    outdated tetracyclines
    sulphonamides
  Hypergammaglobulinaemia
    Sjögren's syndrome
    multiple myeloma
  Renal transplant
  Hypercalcaemia with hyperparathyroidism
    vitamin D deficiency

Diagnosis/Evaluation
The diagnosis of this disease (*see Table* 7.6) depends on the demonstration of:
1. Hyperchloraemic acidosis with or without other proximal tubular disorders
2. Absence of severe hypokalaemia
3. Urine pH $< 5\cdot40$ during acidosis (low plasma bicarbonate levels)
4. $FE_{HCO_3^-} > 15\%$ when plasma $[HCO_3^-]$ is normal, and zero when plasma bicarbonate is low
5. Normal distal nephron H^+ excretion
6. Need for a large amount of exogenous bicarbonate to normalize the plasma level, and aggravation of hypokalaemia during its adminstration
7. Absence of bone disease, nephrocalcinosis and nephrolithiasis

Management
Therapy in adults without bone disease is probably unnecessary. Infants who fail to thrive will require bicarbonate therapy. In these cases potassium should be added to the therapy to preclude the development of hypokalaemia.

Type 4 RTA

This term (Type 4) has been used to describe patients with:
1. Hyperchloraemic metabolic acidosis
2. Mild to moderate renal impairment
3. Hyperkalaemia
4. Mineralocorticoid deficiency

During acidosis these patients have an acidic urine (pH <5.4) which is bicarbonate free. Their renal ammonia excretion rate is reduced even when the urine is very acidic. This reduced ammonia excretion may be related to hyperkalaemia which has been shown, in experimental animals, to decrease renal tubular ammonia production. A possible sequence of events is:

$\downarrow$ aldosterone $\longrightarrow \downarrow K^+$ excretion $\longrightarrow$ hyperkalaemia $\longrightarrow \downarrow NH_3$ production $\longrightarrow$ inability to excrete H^+ load.

Causes

Clinical disorders associated with Type 4 RTA are:
1. Addison's disease
2. Adrenal enzyme deficiencies
    C21 hydroxylase
    corticosterone methyl oxidase
3. Syndrome of hyporeninaemic hypoaldosteronism (SHH)
4. Tubulo-interstitial disease
    pyelonephritis
    renal transplant

A similar biochemical syndrome may occur during the use of potassium-sparing diuretics (spironolactone, amiloride, triamterene).

Recently it has been suggested that Type 4 RTA be classified into five subgroups (McSherry, 1981) depending on renal function, age and a number of other factors.

Diagnosis/Evaluation

This is discussed in the section dealing with mineralocorticoid disorders (p. 249).

Case Examples

Renal Tubular Acidosis: Type 1

A male aged 60 years was admitted to hospital with severe weakness of the upper and lower limbs which had been progressive over the previous 3 weeks. His plasma electrolytes on admission showed severe hypokalaemia and hyperchloraemic metabolic acidosis. He was given a provisional diagnosis of RTA and infused with 5% dextrose containing potassium and bicarbonate supplements.

He was later diagnosed as RTA secondary to Sjögren's syndrome. The biochemistry below shows the relevant plasma and urine results on admission and the plasma values 2 weeks later after stabilization on 9 g (~ 100 mmol) of sodium bicarbonate daily.

Date		31/11	9/12	
Plasma	Na	137	138 mmol/l	(132–144)
	K	1·7	3·5 mmol/l	(3·2–4·8)
	Cl	120	108 mmol/l	(98–108)
	HCO_3	8	21 mmol/l	(23–33)
	Urea	8·4	6·5 mmol/l	(3·0–8·0)
	Creat	0·18	0·12 mmol/l	(0·06–0·12)
	Anion gap	11	12 mEq/l	(7–17)
Urine	Na		43 mmol/l	
	K		42 mmol/l	
	HCO_3		4 mmol/l	
	Creat		9·4 mmol/l	
	pH		7·3	
	$FE_{HCO_3^-}$		0·9%	

Comment

In Type 1 RTA the decreased Na^+–H^+ exchange ($\downarrow H^+$ secretion) in the distal nephron results in:

1. $\downarrow$ Renal excretion of $H^+ \longrightarrow \downarrow$ plasma $[HCO_3^-]$ and $\uparrow$ urine pH ($> 5\cdot40$)
2. $\downarrow$ Renal reabsorption of $Na^+ \longrightarrow$

a. Na^+ depletion $\longrightarrow$ hypovolaemia $\longrightarrow \uparrow$ aldosterone
b. $\uparrow$ Distal tubule flow rate
$a + b \longrightarrow \uparrow$ renal K^+ secretion $\longrightarrow K^+$ depletion and hypokalaemia

The sodium ions lost in the urine are balanced by the simultaneous loss of acid anions (SO_4^{2-}, PO_4^{2-} etc.). The resulting hypovolaemia increases the reabsorption of NaCl in the proximal tubule and ascending limb of the loop of Henle. The overall effect is hyperchloraemia because the retained $Na^+ . Cl^-$ replaces plasma $Na^+ . (acid anion)^-$.

The diagnosis of Type 1 RTA in this patient was made on the basis of a hyperchloraemic acidosis associated with: (*a*) severe hypokalaemia, (*b*) alkaline urine pH in the presence of metabolic acidosis, and (*c*) fractional excretion of HCO_3^- less than 3%. Further studies included estimation of the renal excretion rates of titratable acidity and ammonium which were both subnormal in the presence of systemic acidosis.

Proximal (Type 2) RTA: Acetazolamide Therapy

The plasma electrolytes shown below are those of a 66–year-old female who was treated for glaucoma with 250 mg of acetazolamide (Diamox) three times daily.

Plasma	Na	139 mmol/l	(132–144)
	K	2·8 mmol/l	(3·2–4·8)
	Cl	112 mmol/l	(98–108)
	HCO_3	19 mmol/l	(23–33)
	Urea	6·4 mmol/l	(3·0–8·0)
	Creat	0·11 mmol/l	(0·06–0·12)
	Anion gap	11 mEq/l	(7–17)

Comment
Acetazolamide is a potent inhibitor of carbonic anhydrase activity, with the predominant effects occurring in the kidney and aqueous humour. In the proximal tubule carbonic anhydrase inhibition suppresses both H^+ secretion and HCO_3^- reabsorption. The unreabsorbed bicarbonate, in the form of $NaHCO_3$, floods the distal nephron which results in:

1. $\uparrow$ Distal tubular flow rate $\longrightarrow \uparrow K^+$ secretion $\longrightarrow \uparrow K^+$ loss in the urine and potassium depletion

2. Loss of Na^+ (with HCO_3^-) in the urine $\longrightarrow Na^+$ depletion $\longrightarrow$ hypovolaemia $\longrightarrow$ increased renal reabsorption of NaCl $\longrightarrow$ retention of Cl^- which balances the lost HCO_3^- (hyperchloraemia). This increased reabsorption of NaCl, in both the proximal tubule and ascending limb of the loop of Henle, limits the diuretic action of this drug (p. 256).

The decreased proximal tubule bicarbonate reabsorption in this condition is not associated with defective reabsorption of any other analytes, and the acidosis is usually of a modest degree (plasma bicarbonate level rarely falls below 18 mmol/l).

Type 4 RTA: Adrenal Failure
The plasma and urinary electrolytes shown below are those of a male aged 57 years who was admitted to hospital after his general practitioner discovered that his plasma potassium level was 7·5 mmol/l. The patient gave a vague history of malaise and weakness. Appropriate investigations led to a diagnosis of Addison's disease.

Plasma	Na	125 mmol/l	(132–144)
	K	7·0 mmol/l	(3·2–4·8)
	Cl	102 mmol/l	(98–108)
	HCO_3	16 mmol/l	(23–33)
	Urea	17·1 mmol/l	(3·0–8·0)
	Creat	0·18 mmol/l	(0·06–0·12)
	Anion gap	14 mEq/l	(7–17)
Urine	Na	74 mmol/l	
	K	43 mmol/l	
	pH	5·0	

Comment
The term Type 4 RTA has, in the past, been reserved for those patients with hyperkalaemia and HCMA associated with selective aldosterone deficiency, and some degree of nephron loss, e.g. syndrome of hyporeninaemic hypoaldosteronism, SHH, (p. 59). However, primary adrenal failure is now recognized as one of the causes of this disorder and represents a subgroup which is associated with a normal GFR (McSherry, 1981).

It has been suggested that the decreased H^+ excretion associated with mineralocorticoid deficiency results from an inadequate NH_3 production as a consequence of hyperkalaemia. However, there is experimental evidence, at least in the dog and the isolated turtle bladder (these cells behave similarly to mammalian renal tubular cells), that aldosterone itself is capable of increasing H^+ secretion.

The biochemical feature of Type 4 RTA is hyperkalaemic, normal anion gap metabolic acidosis, but this has to be differentiated from other causes of the same biochemical pattern, e.g. early uraemic acidosis, and obstructive nephropathy (p. 105). In the above patient the ability to acidify the urine is intact (urine pH of 5·0), but the renal insufficiency is probably inadequate to produce early uraemic acidosis (plasma creatinine level $<0.20\,mmol/l$). The diagnosis of obstructive nephropathy would be made on clinical grounds.

Polyuria

Polyuria is defined as an increased volume of urine per unit of time. The urine output of a normal adult obviously varies with fluid intake and climatic conditions (insensible loss), but is of the order of 1–2 litres a day. What minimum volume of urine output per unit time constitutes polyuria is a subjective matter and largely depends on the patient's past experience. For want of a better definition many physicians define polyuria as urine volume greater than 3 litres a day.

Consequences

The clinical and biochemical features of polyuria depend upon the primary disorder, e.g. diabetes insipidus, diabetes mellitus, chronic renal failure, etc. The polyuria of diabetes insipidus is 'pure' water loss, and if this loss is not replaced it can lead to hypernatraemic dehydration (p. 25). A similar situation may develop during a solute diuresis due to non-electrolyte solute (osmotic diuresis due to glucose or urea). This situation differs from that of a pure water loss because varying quantities of sodium are lost as well as (p. 25). In the case of solute diuresis due to sodium, the loss of quantities of both sodium and water may result, if replacement is inadequate, in an isotonic or hyponatraemic dehydration.

Causes

A simple diagnostic approach to the causes of polyuria can be made on the basis of the urinary osmolality; two general types can be recognized: (1) water diuresis with a osmolality less than 200 mmol/kg, and (2) solute diuresis with a osmolality similar to that of the plasma ($\sim 300\,mmol/kg$) (*Table* 7.8).

Diagnosis/Evaluation (*see also Fig.* 7.4)

From a laboratory point of view the first test in the work-up of a patient with polyuria should be a urine osmolality estimation. Patients with a water diuresis (diabetes insipidus, compulsive water drinking) will have an osmolality less than 200 mmol/kg with the level approaching maximum dilution ($\sim 50\,mmol/kg$). On the other hand, patients with a solute diuresis will have a level approaching that of the plasma ($\sim 300\,mmol/l$) or slightly above. In the latter case the urinary osmolality usually falls within the range: plasma osmolality $\pm 50\,mmol/kg$.

Table 7.8. Classification of polyuria

Water Diuresis (defective ADH-renal axis)
  ↓ *ADH secretion*
    a. Physiological: compulsive water drinking
    b. Pathological: neurogenic diabetes insipidus
  Defective ADH action (nephrogenic diabetes insipidus)
    a. Congenital
    b. Acquired:
      renal disease—pyelonephritis, amyloid, myeloma, polycystic kidney, obstructive
        uropathy, analgesic nephropathy
      electrolyte disorders—hypercalcaemia, hypokalaemia
      drugs—lithium, demeclocycline, methoxyflurane
Solute Diuresis
  Sodium
    ↑ Intake: dietary, iatrogenic
    ↑ Renal loss—diuretic therapy, renal salt-losing disease, renal tubular acidosis,
      mineralocorticoid deficiency
  Urea
    ↑ Production—hypercatabolic states
    Renal disease—CRF, post-obstruction, post-ATN
  Glucose
    Diabetes mellitus

Solute Diuresis

If a solute diuresis is suggested by the above test then further investigations should include: plasma glucose (diabetes mellitus), plasma urea (renal disease), plasma electrolytes (sodium diuresis), urine glucose and electrolytes (*Fig.* 7.4).

Water Diuresis

This condition is due to a defect in the ADH–renal axis, i.e. physiological suppression of ADH release (increased water intake), pathological suppression of ADH release (neurogenic diabetes insipidus), defective action of ADH at the renal level (nephrogenic diabetes insipidus). Further investigations are made after an overnight (at least 12 h) abstinence from fluid.

After 12 h of fluid deprivation the patient's urine osmolality is measured. If the level reaches 800 mmol/kg, or above, the ADH–renal axis is considered intact and the test terminated. Patients with this response are classified as belonging to the high water intake group (e.g. compulsive water drinkers). N.B. In some case of prolonged water overload the renal concentration mechanism may be defective due to a dissipation of the normal medullary osmotic gradient ('washed' out), and the kidney may not respond to ADH. This will produce a response similar to that of nephrogenic diabetes insipidus (*see below*).

If the patient's urine osmolality is less than 800 mmol/kg then the test is continued as follows:

The patient remains on the nil-per-mouth regimen and the urine osmolaltiy is measured hourly until it reaches a plateau, i.e. the difference between two

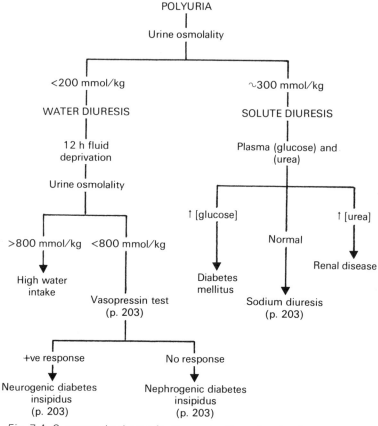

Fig. 7.4. Suggested scheme for the evaluation of polyuria.

successive results is less than 30 mmol/kg. At this stage 5 units of aqueous vasopressin are given subcutaneously and the urine osmolality then estimated again at hourly intervals for a further 2–3 hours.

A post-injection rise in urine osmolality to 800 mmol/kg or more is typical of neurogenic diabetes insipidus. If the post-injection osmolality does not change the kidney is deemed to be at fault, i.e. nephrogenic diabetes insipidus.

Intermediate values can also be obtained, e.g. a significant rise in osmolality to a value less than 800 mmol/kg prior to vasopressin injection, followed by a post-injection rise to above 800 mmol/kg may indicate incomplete neurogenic diabetes insipidus.

When a patient is undergoing a fluid deprivation test it is advisable, especially in children, to weigh them regularly and stop the test if the weight falls by more than 5%.

Management

Treatment of the polyuric syndromes will vary with the aetiology and severity of the condition. Only brief notes are given below.

Neurogenic Diabetes Insipidus

Specific therapy: vasopressin—aqueous, vasopressin tannate in oil, synthetic vasopressin (1-desamino-8-arginine vasopressin, DDAVP).

Adjunctive therapy: chlorpropamide (acts by (*a*) enhancing the action of any circulating native ADH, (*b*) enhancing release of ADH from posterior pituitary); clofibrate (acts by enhancing the release of pituitary ADH); thiazide diuretics (thought to act through a diuretic-induced hypovolaemia, i.e. ↑ renal Na^+ loss ⟶ hypovolaemia ⟶ enhanced sodium and water reabsorption in the proximal renal tubule ⟶ ↓ delivery of fluid to diluting segment ⟶ ↓ renal excretion of 'free' water).

Nephrogenic Diabetes Insipidus

Treat underlying disease, thiazide therapy.

Solute Diuresis

Treat underlying disease.

Case Example

A 24-year-old female presented with a 3-year history of thirst, polydipsia and polyuria. Other features included hypothyroidism (secondary to a low thyroid stimulating hormone) and amenorrhoea. A water deprivation and vasopressin test gave the following results:

Time (h)	Urine Osmol (mmol/kg)	Plasma Osmol (mmol/kg)
0600	235	299
0700	244	—
0800	243	—
0900	255	—
1000	281	—
1100	277	325
5 units of aqueous vasopressin		
1200	640	—
1300	795	322

Comment

The above test indicates neurogenic diabetes insipidus, i.e. a low urine osmolality, in the presence of plasma hypertonicity, which responded to vasopressin. The variations in the urine osmolality values reflect, in part, the inherent analytical error of the method of analysis (5–10%).

The nature of this patient's primary pathology is undecided, but appears to involve the hypothalamus. She responded satisfactorily to DDAVP therapy.

Further Reading

Espinel C. H. (1980) Differential diagnosis of acute renal failure. *Clin. Nephrol.* **13**, 73–77.

McSherry E. (1981) Renal tubular acidosis in childhood. *Kidney Int.* **20**, 799–809.

Moses M. and Notman D. D. (1982) Diabetes insipidus and syndrome of inappropriate secretion of antidiuretic hormone (SIADH). *Adv. Intern. Med.* **27**, 73–100.

Quintanilla A. P. (1980) Renal tubular acidosis. *Postgrad. Med.* **67**, 60–73.

Sebastian A. and Morris R. C. (1977) Renal tubular acidosis. *Clin. Nephrol.* **7**, 216–230.

8

Digestive tract disorders

Introduction

With a normal intake of food and water about 8–10 litres of fluid reach the upper intestine daily, the major portion coming from digestive tract secretions—saliva, gastric juice, bile, pancreatic juice, succus entericus. Of the 8–10 litres per day of fluids entering the small intestine some 7·5–9·5 litres are absorbed. Overall during passage through the gut the fluid is modified in both composition and volume and finally less than 200 ml are excreted daily via the faeces (*Fig.* 8.1, *Table* 8.1).

In the stomach the parietal cells secrete hydrochloric acid (HCl) into the lumen at a concentration of 140–160 mmol/l which lowers the pH of the gastric fluids to around 1–2 (10–100 mmol/l of H^+). During HCl production HCO_3^- is generated within the parietal cells and secreted back into the blood.

That is, CO_2, from the blood, diffuses into the parietal cells and reacts with water, in the presence of carbonic anhydrase (ca), to form H_2CO_3 and then H^+ and HCO_3^-. The HCO_3^- diffuses back into the blood in exchange for Cl^- which is then secreted into the gastric lumen along with H^+. In the normal adult approximately 200–300 mmol of HCl are secreted daily, and therefore the same amount of HCO_3^- is secreted back into the blood. It is this bicarbonate that constitutes the postcibal 'alkaline tide'. The secretion of HCl is controlled by vagal impulses; and gastrin, which is secreted in response to gastric distension, changes in luminal pH, and the chemical products of protein digestion.

During meals, therefore, the fluid entering the small intestine is acidic and the blood leaving the stomach is alkaline ($\uparrow [HCO_3^-]$). The acidic gastric fluid is neutralized in the upper small intestine by the alkaline bile and pancreatic juice. Consequently the potential acid–base disturbance generated by the stomach is offset by a reverse process occurring in the intestine.

The mechanism of electrolyte absorption in the small gut is ill-defined. Recent evidence suggests that H^+ and HCO_3^- are formed in the absorbing cells under the influence of carbonic anhydrase:

$$(CO_2 + H_2O \xrightarrow{\text{ca}} H_2CO_3 \longrightarrow H^+ + HCO_3^-).$$

The H^+ is then secreted into the gut lumen in exchange for Na^+, and the HCO_3^- is

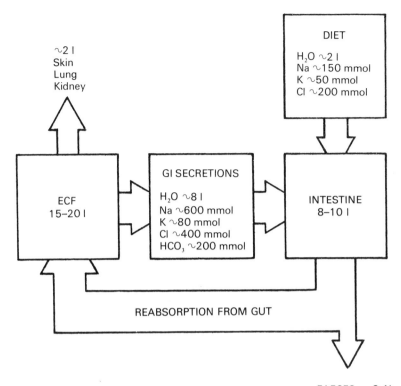

Fig. 8.1. Daily water and electrolyte flux in the digestive tract. The values are approximate only.

Table 8.1. Approximate composition of gastrointestinal secretions. Note that gastric juice is high in H^+ (loss $\longrightarrow$ alkalosis) and small bowel secretions are high in HCO_3^- (loss $\longrightarrow$ acidosis)

	Vol/24 h		Concentration (mmol/l)			
	(l)	pH	Na^+	K^+	Cl^-	HCO_3^-
Saliva	1	7–8	60	15	30	40
Gastric juice	2	1–2	80	10	150	—
Bile	1	7–8	150	10	50	30
Pancreatic juice	2	7–8	110	10	40	100
Succus entericus	2	7–8	140	5	110	25

exchanged for luminal Cl^-. In the lumen the secreted H^+ and HCO_3^- combine, first forming H_2CO_3 and then CO_2. The CO_2 is reabsorbed and re-enters the H^+/HCO_3^- generating reaction. Potassium ions probably passively diffuse across the gut mucosa as a result of an electrochemical gradient.

In the large intestine there is further absorption of water, Na^+ and Cl^-; there also appears to be active secretion of HCO_3^-, perhaps in exhange for Cl^-. Under normal conditions potassium ions are absorbed in this area, however, in some circumstances they may also be secreted, e.g. hyperaldosteronism ($\uparrow Na^+-K^+$ exchange in most epithelial cells), renal failure ($\uparrow$ plasma $[K^+] \longrightarrow \uparrow$ secretion of aldosterone).

Vomiting

From the biochemical and metabolic point of view there are two types of vomiting; that from above the pylorus (prepyloric), and that from below the pylorus (postpyloric). These two forms are both associated with a loss of water and sodium which results in hypovolaemia, and a loss of K^+ in the vomitus and in the urine (secondary hyperaldosteronism consequent to hypovolaemia). However, the acid–base disturbances arising from the two types of vomiting are different.

Prepyloric vomiting

In this condition (*see* examples, pp. 30 and 114) there is extensive loss of HCl from the stomach which results in a metabolic alkalosis ($\uparrow$ plasma $[HCO_3^-]$), and hypochloraemia, i.e. the HCO_3 generated by the parietal cells during H^+ secretion is not neutralized by the subsequent passage of acid gastric contents into the small intestine (*see above*). The hypovolaemia, resulting from fluid loss, maintains the alkalosis by increasing proximal renal tubular HCO_3^- reabsorption (p. 112). In this type of vomiting the patient may lose 200–300 mmol of H^+ daily and at the same time generate a similar amount of HCO_3^-.

Postpyloric Vomiting

If vomiting occurs from below the pylorus the vomitus usually contains upper small bowel contents (pancreatic and biliary secretions) and therefore the loss of H^+ from the stomach will be partly balanced by the loss of HCO_3^- from the small intestinal fluid. Thus, instead of the dramatic hypochloraemia and hyper-bicarbonataemia seen in prepyloric vomiting, these patients usually present with a lesser degree of metabolic alkalosis or, occasionally, with a normal plasma chloride and bicarbonate level.

Case Example

Vomiting: Small Gut Obstruction

A 43-year-old male was admitted to hospital with a 4-day history of vomiting and 'crampy' abdominal pains. On examination he had a swollen, tender abdomen, dry skin and tongue, a pulse rate of 106/min, and a blood pressure of 110/70. On admission his urine output was about 4–5 ml/h.

Over the first 12 h after his admission he was treated conservatively with gastric suction and intravenous fluids (7 litres of fluid: 4 of 5% dextrose, 3 of normal saline, 100 mmol of KCl). At operation 10 cm of gangrenous small bowel, due to volvulus, were removed. The two sets of electrolyte results shown below are those on admission and 11 h after the i.v. therapy. Urine output just prior to operation had risen to 50 ml/h.

Time		0400 h	1500 h	
Plasma	Na	151	142 mmol/l	(132–144)
	K	3·1	3·9 mmol/l	(3·2–4·8)
	Cl	107	105 mmol/l	(98–108)
	HCO$_3$	29	25 mmol/l	(23–33)
	Urea	3·7	3·1 mmol/l	(3·0–8·0)
	Creat	0·14	0·10 mmol/l	(0·06–0·12)
Urine	Na	<5	— mmol/l	
	K	42	— mmol/l	

Comment

The two notable features of the admission electrolytes of this patient are the hypernatraemia and the normal plasma bicarbonate level.

The hypernatraemia indicates hypertonic dehydration (p. 24), i.e. water depletion of the extracellular fluid is relatively greater than the sodium depletion. This arises because the majority of gut secretions have a sodium concentration much lower than that of the ECF, and so a significant loss of these fluids would result in a water loss that is greater than the salt loss. However, most patients with excessive loss of gut fluid present with a low to normal plasma sodium concentration. This reflects the patient's ability to drink tap water but disinclination to eat and thus take in salt. The intake of 'salt-poor' fluid with continued secretion of ADH (hypovolaemia, stress) results in either the normalization of the plasma sodium or hyponatraemia.

The normal plasma bicarbonate level in the above case reflects postpyloric vomiting, i.e. loss of H$^+$ in the gastric juice coupled with the loss of HCO_3^- in the pancreatic juice and bile.

The low urinary [Na$^+$] indicates that there has been renal sodium conservation by undamaged tubules (p. 186). The high urinary [K$^+$] (>20 mmol/l), occurring in the presence of hypokalaemia, reflects an increased renal K$^+$ secretion as a consequence of hyperaldosteronism that is secondary to hypovolaemia.

The second set of electrolyte results and the increasing urine output indicates that the intravenous therapy was adequate and highlights the amount of fluid, and potassium, that can be lost during vomiting.

Diarrhoea

Diarrhoea, characterized by an increased frequency of stools containing excessive water, is due, in most cases, to increased solute in the gut lumen, and may result from either decreased gut absorption or increased gut secretion. The solute involved is often sodium, but may include other substances, such as fatty acids (malabsorption), organic anions (carbohydrate malabsorption), chloride (chloride diarrhoea), potassium (villous adenoma of the colon), therapeutic substances ($MgSO_4$, lactulose).

The high water content of the stools of diarrhoea is a result of the solute-generated osmotic gradient between the gut lumen and the extracellular fluid. The high solute content of the gut draws water (and salts) from the extracellular fluid until the osmolality of the gut and extracellular fluids is similar ($\sim$ 280–300 mmol/kg).

Although defective gut absorption and excessive gut secretion may both play a role in an individual patient with diarrhoea, three main types of diarrhoea are usually recognized:
1.   Osmotic diarrhoea
2.   Secretory diarrhoea
3.   Diarrhoea due to defective ion absorption

Osmotic Diarrhoea

This is due to the accumulation in the gut of non-ionic osmotically active particles, e.g.
1.   Poorly absorbed solute—some laxatives
2.   Maldigestion—lactase deficiency (lactose), lipase deficiency (lipids)
3.   Malabsorption of non-electrolytes—mucosal disease, glucose transport defect (glucose and other sugars)

In these situations the high osmotic activity of the luminal contents causes water (and sodium) withdrawal into the gut. As this fluid passes through the colon some of the water and sodium is reabsorbed, leaving a diarrhoea fluid with a content that is low in sodium and high in the offending solute.

A helpful test to distinguish between osmotic diarrhoea and the secretory variety (discussed below) is to determine the osmolal gap of the diarrhoea fluid. This osmolal gap is the difference between the measured osmolality (by osmometer) and the calculated osmolality.

$$\text{Calculated osmolality} = 2 \times ([Na^+] + [K^+])\,\text{mmol/kg}.$$

In secretory diarrhoea the major solutes are the salts of sodium and potassium, and therefore the measured osmolality will be similar to the calculated osmolality (osmolal gap < 20 mmol/kg). In osmotic diarrhoea there is a large osmolal gap due to the low sodium level and high level of the offending solute.

Secretory Diarrhoea

This is due to an excessive gastrointestinal secretion of solute which usually originates in either the small bowel or the colon. In these cases the main solute is sodium (main cation of gut secretions) and, unlike osmotic diarrhoea, the calculated osmolality approximates the measured osmolality.

The causes of this type of diarrhoea are numerous and include the following: toxic insult to the gut mucosae (bacterial toxins—*Escherichia coli, Vibrio cholerae*), damage to the mucosae (regional enteritis, ulcerative colitis), hormonal (Zollinger–Ellison syndrome, VIPoma).

Defective Ion Absorption

This is a rare cause of diarrhoea, but the best example of this type is chloride diarrhoea in which there is defective gut absorption of Cl^-. In these cases the normal gut exchange of Cl^- for HCO_3^- (*see above*) does not occur, but Na^+ exchange for H^+ proceeds normally. This results in a metabolic alkalosis ($\uparrow$ plasma $[HCO_3^-]$) rather than the metabolic acidosis (*see below*) which is often associated with severe diarrhoea.

Consequences of Diarrhoea

The loss of diarrhoea fluid which is rich in Na^+, K^+ and HCO_3^- (bile, pancreatic juice), results in:

1. Water depletion $\longrightarrow$ hypovolaemia
2. Na^+ depletion—in terms of ECF composition the water loss is usually relatively greater than the sodium loss and thus initially a hypertonic dehydration occurs. If the patient replaces the fluid deficit with tap water, and does not take in sodium, the result will be to convert the hyper-natraemia to either normonatraemia or hyponatraemia
3. K^+ depletion—potassium may be lost in the diarrhoea fluid ($[K^+]$ often high, ~ 100 mmol/l) and also in the urine if there is significant hypovol-aemia, i.e. secondary hyperaldosteronism
4. HCO_3^- loss—if there is significant loss of bicarbonate a metabolic acidosis of the normal anion gap variety occurs (p. 105).

Case Examples

Severe Diarrhoea: Bacillary

The results below are those of a 3-year-old child (13·5 kg) who presented with severe diarrhoea of 3 days' duration. On admission he had dry skin and mucous membranes, and an estimated fluid deficit of around 10% of body weight. He was infused with 2·5% dextrose in half-normal saline with potassium and bicarbonate supplements. The second set of results are those on the day following admission and after an infusion of about 700 ml of the dextrose–saline solution, and approximately 20 mmol each of potassium and bicarbonate.

Date		02/01	03/01	
Plasma	Na	136	133 mmol/l	(132–144)
	K	2·5	3·7 mmol/l	(3·2–4·8)
	Cl	112	105 mmol/l	(98–108)
	HCO_3	14	19 mmol/l	(23–33)
	Urea	6·1	3·2 mmol/l	(3·0–8·0)
	Creat	0·11	0·06 mmol/l	(0·06–0·12)
	Anion gap	12	13 mEq/l	(7–17)

Comment

A feature of severe diarrhoea is a hyperchloraemic (normal anion gap) metabolic acidosis which is often associated with hypokalaemia. There are other causes of this electrolyte pattern (p. 105) but in the case of diarrhoea there should be no confusion about this diagnosis as it is usually evident on clinical grounds. An important point to remember about the metabolic acidosis of diarrhoea is that the body bicarbonate deficit can only be replaced, physiologically, by the generation of new bicarbonate by the kidney. This mechanism takes some days to realize its maximum potential and therefore parenteral bicarbonate therapy is usually necessary.

Laxative Abuse

The laboratory results listed below are those of a 46-year-old female admitted for investigation of chronic diarrhoea.

Plasma	Na	139 mmol/l	(132–144)
	K	2·8 mmol/l	(3·2–4·8)
	Cl	100 mmol/l	(98–108)
	HCO_3	28 mmol/l	(23–33)
	Creat	0·09 mmol/l	(0·06–0·12)
Urine	Na	25 mmol/l	
	K	6 mmol/l	
Faecal	Na	25 mmol/l (<10)	
	K	146 mmol/l (<10)	

Comment

The hypokalaemia and low urinary potassium concentration in this patient suggest an extrarenal cause for her potassium depletion. Although this patient denied any self-medication, an examination of her stools and urine revealed phenol-phthalein. The reason for the massive loss of potassium in the faeces of patients who abuse laxatives is unclear but it appears to be associated with an increased secretion of colonic mucus with a high potassium content. Diarrhoea association with a high faecal potassium content may also occur in some cases of villous adenoma of the colon (p. 67).

Bowel Obstruction

Intestinal obstruction may be due to mechanical causes—volvulus, hernia, adhesive bands—or functional (ileus) as a result of peritonitis, pancreatitis, occlusive vascular disease, etc.

Consequences

In mechanical obstruction the progress of the gut contents is halted, the proximal bowel distends, and absorption becomes compromised. After several hours of obstruction absorption ceases and sodium and water are then secreted into the lumen. Later, vomiting of the bowel contents occurs.

During obstruction several litres of fluid may become sequestered in the bowel lumen. This loss of fluid from the extracellular space may result in severe hypovolaemia and lead to shock. The plasma electrolyte picture is variable. Early in the course of the disorder the plasma electrolyte concentrations are normal (isotonic dehydration). However, the patients usually become thirsty and drink tap water which will result, if there is no concomitant intake of salt, in hyponatraemia. The acid–base status varies from metabolic alkalosis early in the disease (severe vomiting), to mild and to moderate metabolic acidosis later on (loss of HCO_3^-, compromised renal function, starvation ketosis).

Gut Fistulae

Fistulae are abnormal communications between two hollow viscera (internal), or between a hollow viscera and the skin (external). The metabolic consequences depend upon the anatomical site.

External Fistulae

Gastric
Loss of gastric juice $\longrightarrow$ similar biochemical picture to that of vomiting (*see above*).

Duodenal/jejunal/pancreatic
Loss of fluid containing significant quantities of HCO_3^- will result in hyperchloraemic metabolic acidosis.

Ileum
Ileostomies may discharge up to 1 litre of sodium-rich fluid daily; significant HCO_3^- loss may also occur.

Internal Fistulae

Upper and Lower Bowel
These result in a rerouting of intestinal contents and consequently a malabsorption syndrome. Overgrowth of bacteria may occur in the upper bowel which will further contribute to the malabsorption problem.

Gut and Bladder
Communication between the colon and the bladder results in the entry of urine into the large bowel and a characteristic electrolyte picture which is also seen following ureterosigmoidostomy.

Example
The laboratory results shown below were those of a male patient aged 50 years who had a vesicocolic fistula as a consequence of bladder carcinoma.

Plasma	Na	145 mmol/l	(132–144)
	K	3·6 mmol/l	(3·2–4·8)
	Cl	126 mmol/l	(98–108)
	HCO$_3$	12 mmol/l	(23–33)
	Urea	13·6 mmol/l	(3·0–8·0)
	Creat	0·09 mmol/l	(0·06–0·12)

Comment

When chloride-rich urine comes in contact with the colonic mucosa the Cl^- is reabsorbed by the gut mucosa cells in exchange for extracelluar HCO_3^-. The bicarbonate ions are then evacuated with the bowel contents. This results in a hyperchloraemic metabolic acidosis (p. 105). Often these patients will have a hypokalaemia due to increased colonic secretion of K^+. The high plasma urea in the above patient, associated with a normal creatinine level, suggests reabsorption of urea from the urine by the colon rather than renal failure.

Liver Disease and Electrolytes

Severe liver disease, such as hepatic failure or advanced cirrhosis, may be associated with hyponatraemia, hypokalaemia and acid–base disturbances.

Hyponatraemia

Hyponatraemia can result from the liver disease *per se* (p. 43), or may be a result of diuretic therapy (p. 256).

Hypokalaemia

Like hyponatraemia, hypokalaemia may be due to diuretic therapy (p. 259) or to the liver disease itself. In the latter case there is potassium loss via the kidney, which is thought to be due to a secondary hyperaldosteronism as a consequence of hypovolaemia (hypoalbuminaemia). Vomiting, if present, will also play a part in potassium depletion.

Acid–base Disturbance

A wide variety of acid–base disturbances may be associated with chronic liver disease.

Metabolic Alkalosis

This can arise from either vomiting or diuretic therapy (especially thiazides, p. 256).

Respiratory Alkalosis

Hyperventilation, possibly due to some circulating toxins, is common in terminal liver failure.

Renal Tubular Acidosis

The association of cirrhosis and hyperchloraemia metabolic acidosis has been described with increasing frequency over the past few years. When it occurs the acidosis is usually mild (plasma bicarbonate of around 15–20 mmol/l), and rarely produces significant symptoms. It is thought to be due to a decreased delivery of Na^+ to the distal renal tubule as a consequence of the increased proximal tubule reabsorption of NaCl, the latter being a characteristic of cirrhosis, i.e. ↑ Proximal Na^+ reabsorption $\longrightarrow$ ↓ Na^+ delivery to distal renal tubule $\longrightarrow$ ↓ Na^+–H^+ exchange $\longrightarrow$ retention of H^+ and metabolic acidosis.

9

Diabetes mellitus

Definitions

Tricarboxylic Acid (TCA) Cycle
Also known as the Krebs cycle and the citric acid cycle. This is the main energy-producing process of the cell. Initially acetyl-CoA (derived from glycolysis, or β-oxidation of fatty acids) reacts with oxaloacetic acid to produce citric acid. This is followed by series of reactions which produce energy (ATP), and CO_2, from the two carbon atom skeleton of acetyl-CoA.

Glycolysis
The oxidation of glucose to pyruvate with the formation of small amounts of ATP. The oxygenation status of the organism may alter this process. In the aerobic state pyruvate is further metabolized to acetyl-CoA. This is then incorporated into the tricarboxylic acid (TCA) cycle with the formation of energy (ATP). In the anaerobic state pyruvate is converted to lactate as the transformation to acetyl-CoA cannot proceed in the absence of molecular oxygen. This may result in lactic acidosis (p. 109) if hypoxia is severe.

Glycogenolysis
The enzymatic breakdown of glycogen to glucose.

Gluconeogenesis
The formation of glucose from non-carbohydrate sources, e.g. amino acids.

Glycogenesis
The formation of glycogen from glucose.

β-Oxidation of Fatty Acids
The conversion of long chain fatty acids to acetyl-CoA which then enters the TCA cycle.

Lipolysis
Degradation of triglycerides to glycerol and fatty acids.

Lipogenesis

Synthesis of triglycerides from glycerol and fatty acids. The fatty acids may be derived from glucose via acetyl-CoA.

Ketone Bodies

Substances derived from acetyl-CoA, and usually associated with excessive fatty acid oxidation. Two of the three major ketone bodies are acids: acetoacetic acid (AcAc) and β-hydroxybutyric acid (BOHB). These two acids may be interconverted by the mitochondrial enzyme β-hydroxybutyrate dehydrogenase. The third ketone body, acetone, is produced by irreversible non-enymatic decarboxylation of acetoacetic acid.

Glucose Metabolism

The pathways of carbohydrate metabolism are intimately linked with those of protein and lipids; and the interaction between these three substances allows the maintenance of 'normal' blood glucose levels ($3 \cdot 0 - 5 \cdot 5$ mmol/l in the fasting state) even in the presence of a carbohydrate-free diet. Although brain tissue can adapt to ketone utilization, the usual source of energy for this tissue, red cells, white cells and renal tubule cells, is glucose derived directly from the blood. Other tissues, e.g. liver and skeletal muscle, are capable of storing glucose as glycogen and utilizing this store when necessary.

The major metabolic pathways involving glucose are briefly illustrated in *Fig.* 9.1. From this figure it can be seen that:

1. Glucose may be:
   a. Converted to glycogen (glycogenesis)
   b. Converted to fat (lipogenesis)
   c. Converted to energy via glycolysis, formation of acetyl-CoA, and further metabolism in the TCA cycle
2. Glucose may be derived from:
   a. Glycogen (glycogenolysis)
   b. Amino acids (gluconeogenesis)
3. Acetyl-CoA (converted by TCA cycle to energy) may be derived from:
   a. Glucose (glycolysis)
   b. Fatty acids (β-oxidation)

Control of Blood Glucose

The blood glucose concentration results from the cumulative action of a number of hormones, some of which increase the level, whilst others decrease it. Glucose control, however, represents only a part of these hormone interactions, and other metabolic activities, including that of lipids and proteins, can be altered by changes in the blood levels of these hormones.

The main hormones concerned with glucose homeostasis are insulin, glucagon, adrenaline, cortisol and growth hormone.

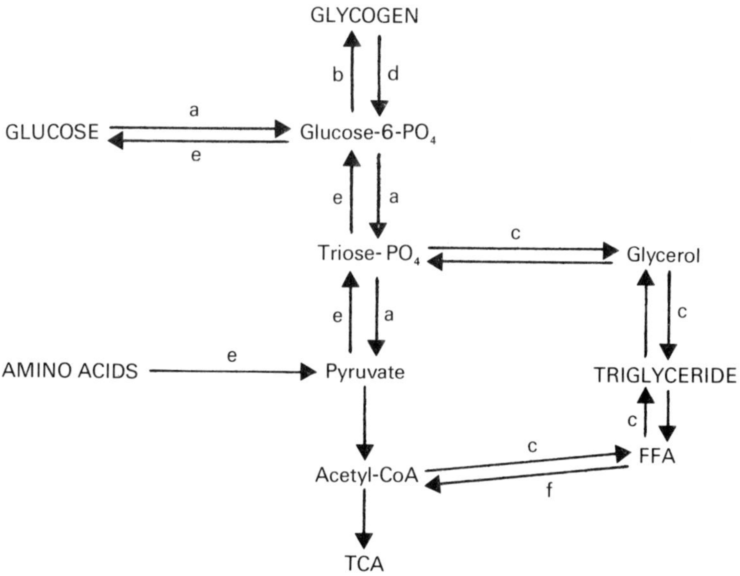

Fig. 9.1. Interrelations of glucose, glycogen, amino acids and trigly-cerides. FFA, free fatty acids; a, glycolysis; b, glycogenesis; c, triglyceride synthesis; d, glycogenolysis; e, gluconeogenesis; f, β-oxidation of fatty acids. TCA, tricarboxylic acid cycle.

Insulin

This is a 51 amino acid, two-chain polypeptide hormone (mol. wt 5800 daltons), which is produced by the β-cells of the pancreatic islets of Langerhans. It is initially produced as a prohormone (pro-insulin) which is then cleaved releasing the active insulin molecule, and an inactive 35 amino acid polypeptide (C-peptide).

Regulation of Insulin

The plasma glucose concentration is the most important factor controlling insulin secretion   ($\uparrow$ [glucose] $\longrightarrow$ $\uparrow$ secretion   and $\downarrow$ [glucose] $\longrightarrow$ $\downarrow$ secretion).   A number of other substance which can also affect its secretion rate include: gastric hormones (secretin, gastrin), somatostatin, growth hormone and obesity (insulin resistance).

Action of Insulin

The major action of insulin is the lowering of the plasma glucose concentration by the following mechanisms:

1.   Increased cell uptake of glucose, e.g. muscle and adipose tissue. Liver cells do not require insulin for glucose uptake
2.   Stimulation of: glycolysis, glycogenesis, lipogenesis
3.   Inhibition of gluconeogenesis, glycogenolysis. Other actions include:
   a.   Inhibition of ketogenesis
   b.   Stimulation of protein synthesis from amino acids
   c.   Increased cell uptake of potassium and phosphate ions

Glucagon

This single chain 29 amino acid peptide (mol. wt 3485 daltons) is synthesized by the α-cells of the pancreatic islets. Its action, which appears to be mediated intra-cellularly by adenylate cyclase, results in:

1.   Increased liver glycogenolysis (hyperglycaemic)
2.   Increased gluconeogenesis (hyperglycaemic)
3.   Increased ketogenesis (hyperketonaemic)

   The activity of glucagon as a hyperglycaemic and hyperketonaemic agent appears to occur only in the presence of insulinopaenia.

Adrenaline

Adrenaline increases the plasma glucose level by suppressing insulin secretion and increasing glucagon secretion. This action is of prime importance in episodes of hypoglycaemia as adrenaline is usually the first hormone to respond in this 'stress' situation.

Cortisol

Cortisol increases the plasma glucose concentration by increasing hepatic pro-duction and suppressing its cell uptake. The increased hepatic production results from increased protein catabolism (gluconeogenesis).

Growth Hormone

The secretion of growth hormone is stimulated by hypoglycaemia and suppressed by hyperglycaemia. It has a number of effects on glucose metabolism including;

1.   Decreased glycogenolysis
2.   Decreased transport of glucose into cells
3.   Decreased cell glucose utilization.

   Its overall effect is to raise the plasma glucose concentration.

   Thus the blood glucose level reflects the interaction of several hormones:

1.   *Insulin* decreases the blood glucose level.
2.   *Cortisol, Adrenaline, Growth Hormone* and *Glucagon* all tend to increase the level. These hormones are often collectively referred to as the 'diabetogenic' or 'counter regulatory' hormones.

Ketone Metabolism

   In low insulin states (e.g. diabetes mellitus) fat deposits are mobilized and energy is derived predominantly from the β-oxidation of fatty acids. The free fatty acids released from these stores are carried to the liver, where they are transported across the cell membrane, and then activated in the cytosol to form fatty acyl-CoA. These fatty acid derivatives then cross into the mitochondria where they are metabolized to acetyl-CoA.

   Acetyl-CoA is normally cleared by two major pathways:

1.   Conversion to energy in the tricarboxylic acid (TCA) cycle.

2.   Fatty acid synthesis. This reaction involves combination of acetyl-CoA with oxaloacetate to form citrate which then exits from the mitochondria. In the cytosol the citrate is converted back to acetyl-CoA and under the influences of insulin forms malonyl-CoA, an intermediate in the pathway to long-chain fatty acids.

A small amount of acetyl-CoA is converted via a third pathway to the ketone bodies, acetoacetate and β-hydroxybutyrate, which are further metabolized by extrahepatic tissues.

Acetoacetate and β-hydroxybutyrate can be interconverted by the enzyme β-hydroxybutyrate dehydrogenase located in the mitochondria, whilst acetone is formed from the non-enzymatic decarboxylation of acetoacetate.

The control of ketogenesis (*Fig.* 9.2) is unclear, but appears to be related to the rate of transfer of fatty acyl-CoA into the mitochondrion which is mediated by

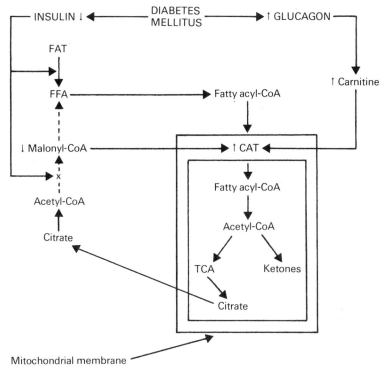

Fig. 9.2. Ketone body metabolism in diabetes mellitus. CAT, carnitine acyl transferase; TCA, tricarboxylic acid cycle. (Reproduced with permission from Walmsley R. N., and White G. H. (1983) *A Guide to Diagnostic Clinical Chemistry*, Melbourne, Blackwell Scientific, p. 210.)

the enzyme carnitine acyl transferase (CAT). The activity of this enzyme appears to be regulated by:
1.   Glucagon: Increases CAT activity by mobilizing carnitine, a necessary cofactor of the enzyme.

2.   Malonyl-CoA: Insulin is necessary for the conversion of acetyl-CoA to malonyl-CoA, an early step in fatty acid synthesis (*Fig.* 9.2). In insulinopaenic states the level of malonyl-CoA falls, and this directly stimulates CAT activity resulting in increased fatty acyl-CoA uptake by the mitochondria, and stimulation of ketogenesis.

3.   Liver glycogen stores (decreased levels stimulate CAT activity).

In insulinopaenic states associated with high circulating levels of glucagon, low levels of malonyl-CoA, and low glucagon stores, the activity of CAT is increased, resulting in increased passage of fatty acyl-CoA into the mitochondria. This is followed by increased synthesis of acetyl-CoA and, as only a limited amount of this substance enters the TCA cycle to produce energy, and because the pathway to fatty acid synthesis is blocked (insulinopaenia), the production of ketone bodies is increased.

Under normal circumstances the ketone bodies, after being released from the liver, are cleared from the plasma by the peripheral tissues (brain, skeletal muscle). If there is excessive production of ketones (insulinopaenia), the rate of clearance by the extrahepatic tissues may be exceeded and ketoacidosis occurs.

The ketone bodies, acetoacetate and β-hydroxybutyrate, are released from the liver to the extracellular fluid in the acid form (H^+K^-) and this results in consumption of the extracellular bicarbonate ion (p. 88). If the ketone production rate exceeds the clearance rate, then a high anion gap metabolic acidosis may result (p. 78),

$$H^+ Ketone^- + NaHCO_3 \longrightarrow Na^+ Ketone^- + H_2CO_3.$$

thus

1. Bicarbonate $[HCO_3^-]$ is $\downarrow$ (metabolic acidosis)
2. $Na^+ Ketone^-$ replaces $NaHCO_3$ and increases the unmeasured plasma anions ($\uparrow$ anion gap).

When ketone bodies are taken up, and metabolized, by the peripheral tissues (under the influence of insulin) they result in bicarbonate generation. Thus the bicarbonate ion, originally removed by the addition of ketone bodies, is now replaced, i.e. the ketone bodies are taken up by the cells in the acid form ($H^+ Ketone^-$). This involves the removal of H from the carbonic acid of the extracellular fluid, and the formation of HCO_3^-:

$$Na^+ Ketone^- + H_2CO_3(H^+HCO_3^-) \longrightarrow H^+ Ketone^- + NaHCO_3.$$

Ketosis may occur in a number of conditions other than diabetes mellitus, e.g. starvation, ethanol and methanol intoxication.

Diabetes Mellitus

Definition

The World Health Organization defines diabetes mellitus as '. . . a state of chronic hyperglycaemia, which may result from many environmental and genetic factors, often acting jointly.'

Classification

The Diabetic Data Group of the National Institute of Health in the USA has proposed a classification of diabetes mellitus which has subsequently been used by the WHO as an interim classification. The clinical classes are divided into three groups:

1.   Type 1—insulin-dependent diabetes mellitus (IDDM). Characterized by: abrupt onset of symptoms, insulinopaenia and dependence on insulin injections, and proneness to ketosis.

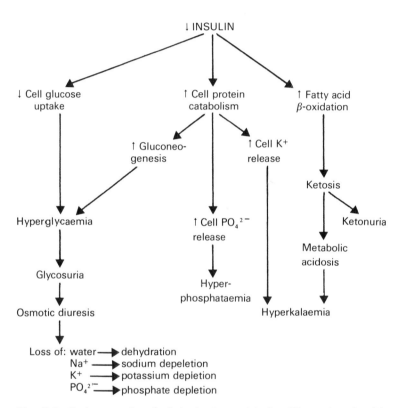

Fig. 9.3. Pathogenesis of diabetic ketoacidosis. (Reproduced with permission from Walmsley, R. N. and White, G. H. (1983) *A Guide to Diagnostic Clinical Chemistry*, Melbourne, Blackwell Scientific, p. 221.)

2.   Type 2—non-insulin-dependent diabetes mellitus (NIDDM). This type frequently presents with minimal or no symptoms. The patients are not dependent on insulin for the prevention of ketosis and are not prone to ketosis.

3.   Diabetes mellitus *secondary* to, or associated with, some other condition (e.g. haemochromatosis, Cushing's disease, phaeochromocytoma, etc.).

Consequences of Insulinopaenia

The biochemical features that may result from insulin deficiency (or relative deficiency) are demonstrated in *Fig.* 9.3, and are discussed in detail in the following section on diabetic ketoacidosis.

Diagnosis

The WHO Special Committee on Diabetes Mellitus, Technical Report No. 646, gives a summary of the diagnostic criteria for diabetes mellitus, and information on this aspect is considered in detail in the report of the National Diabetes Data Group (1979) and will not be considered here.

From the point of view of water and ion metabolism two complications of diabetes mellitus, ketoacidosis and hyperosmolar coma, usually result in severe disturbances. These will be considered in more detail.

Diabetic Ketoacidosis (DKA)

Definition

A metabolic state, as a result of relative insulinopaenia, which results in hyperglycaemia and plasma ketone bodies in excess of 5 mmol/l (normally less than 1 mmol/l).

Causes

Diabetic ketoacidosis is rarely seen in insulin-independent diabetic patients, but is common in insulin-dependent diabetics (IDDM). Evidence from experimental models suggests that for the development of ketoacidosis, besides insulinopaenia, the blood concentrations of the so-called 'counter-regulatory hormones' (growth hormone, cortisol, catecholamines, glucagon) need to be raised. Since the majority of acute presentations of IDDM are associated with infection, it has been suggested that the resulting stress elevates a number of these hormones and results in the development of florid ketoacidosis.

Biochemical Consequences

In diabetic ketoacidosis the increased production of ketone bodies has a marked effect on the patient's acid–base status; and the osmotic diuresis, caused by the increased glucose filtered by the glomeruli, can result in severe inorganic ion and water deficits (*Fig.* 9.3).

The approximate water and ion deficits which can occur are as follows:

water	5000–6000	ml
sodium	400–750	mmol
potassium	300–1000	mmol
chloride	300–400	mmol
bicarbonate	300–500	mmol
calcium	50–100	mmol
phosphate	50–100	mmol

Water

The high extracellular glucose concentration causes an osmotic shift of cell water to the extracellular space resulting in:

a. Intracellular dehydration: The brain responds to this situation by increasing its intracellular osmolality by the formation of 'idiogenic' osmoles (p. 23). On removal of the extracellular osmotic challenge (glucose) these idiogenic osmoles can result in the brain's intracellular fluid being hypertonic to the extracellular fluid. This increases the possibility of cerebral oedema if the extracellular tonicity is suddenly lowered (e.g. infusion of hypotonic fluids).

b. Extracellular solute dilution: The osmotic shift of water to the extracellular space lowers the concentration of its normal solutes, including sodium. This dilutional effect on plasma sodium may result in a hyponatraemia in the presence of a normal, or near-normal, total body sodium. Several formulae have been empirically derived to estimate the plasma $[Na^+]$ which would result if the excess extracellular water moved back into the cells (e.g. with insulin therapy):

Corrected $[Na^+]$ mmol/1 = measured $[Na^+]$ + ([glucose] mmol/1 − 12)/3.

The osmotic diuresis can also result in excessive renal water loss, and (if losses are not replaced) hypovolaemia. The amount of water lost is usually relatively greater than that of sodium, and this will initially lead to hypernatraemic dehydration. However, these patients are usually able to drink fluid (tap water) freely, but are disinclined to eat (take in salt); this often leads to hyponatraemia. As the illness progresses and the patient's fluid intake falls then hypernatraemic dehydration often ensues.

Sodium

As stated above these patients with DKA may present with hyper- or hyponatraemia. Hyponatraemia is the commoner presentation and reflects the action of several mechanisms:

1. Osmotic water shift (*see above*)
2. Loss of Na in urine as a result of osmotic diuresis, and as the accompanying cation of the excreted ketone bodies
3. Associated vomiting (salt loss)
4. Decreased salt intake due to nausea, and debility
5. Factitious (↑ triglycerides)

Regardless of the patient's plasma sodium concentration, all patients with DKA will have some degree of sodium depletion on presentation.

Potassium

Metabolic acidosis and decreased glycolysis (insulinopaenia) cause potassium to move out of the cells and this can result in hyperkalaemia. The increased distal renal tubular flow rate (osmotic diuresis) and secondary hyperaldosteronism (hypovolaemia of dehydration) which often occurs in these patients can induce significant kaliuresis and potassium deficiency. This usually becomes apparent after insulin infusion when the return of the extracellular potassium to the cells converts a presenting hyperkalaemia to hypokalaemia.

On rare occasions patients with ketoacidosis may present with hypokalaemia. This represents a severe potassium deficiency, and occurs in patients who have other causes of potassium depletion, e.g. prolonged persistent vomiting and diarrhoea, previous diuretic therapy.

Glucose

The glucose levels commonly seen in IDDM are of the order of 15–30 mmol/l. Although the aetiology of the hyperglycaemia is obvious, it is often not appreciated that the hepatic output of glucose is increased (up to 3 fold) as a result of gluconeogenesis. This adds significant amounts of glucose to the extracellular fluid.

Ketones/acidosis

Since glucose cannot be utilized as a source of energy ($\downarrow$ cell uptake) the β-oxidation of fatty acids is increased. This can result in the production of massive amounts of ketone bodies (BOHB, AcAc, acetone). This ketone body production rate has been shown in some cases to approach 3400 mmol/d, with approximately 1000 mmol being excreted in the urine (mainly as the sodium salt).

If the patient has poor tissue perfusion (hypovolaemia) and tissue hypoxia, the equilibrium between BOHB and AcAc shifts towards the former, with ratios of 8 – 12 : 1 being recorded. An interesting side effect of this is that although AcAc can be detected by the 'nitroprusside dipstick' test, BOHB does not react with this reagent, so that this test can appear only weakly positive in the presence of a severe ketosis. Following rehydration, and increased tissue perfusion, the equilibrium changes to the more usual ratio of 2 : 1, and the test may then become more positive even though the severity of the ketosis may have decreased.

Consequent to the acidosis, several intracellular ions, such as K^+, PO_4^{2-}, and Mg^{2+} shift to the extracellular fluid. The increased plasma levels of these substances results in increased renal clearance and excretion. This often results in a body deficit which may become apparent during insulin therapy (ions move back into cells).

Phosphate

Phosphate depletion, due to increased cell release ($\downarrow$ insulin) and excretion in the urine, is a common occurrence in DKA. The patients usually present with a normal, or high, plasma concentration which may fall to extremely low levels (e.g. <0.1 mmol/l) with insulin therapy (phosphate moves back into the cells). However, the clinical sequelae of phosphate depletion (p. 158) usually do not occur. Phosphate replacement in these patients is still an unresolved issue, but some clinicians do recommend phosphate repletion during therapy (it is usually given as the potassium salt).

Hyperlipidaemia

The increased release of free fatty acids from adipose tissue, and the presence of the liver-specific enzyme glycerophosphokinase results in increased hepatic production of triglycerides, and increased synthesis of endogenous very low density lipoproteins (VLDL). This may result in hyperlipidaemia which is often apparent on inspection of the patient's plasma.

Diagnosis/evaluation

Patients presenting with clinical features suggestive of ketoacidosis, and heavy glycosuria, should have the following biochemical parameters estimated:

Plasma levels of sodium, potassium, bicarbonate, urea, creatinine and glucose.

Arterial blood gas measurements are useful initially for evaluating the necessity for bicarbonate therapy (some clinicians institute i.v. bicarbonate therapy if the pH is less than 7·20). Blood may be taken for lactate and quantitative ketone estimations (if available). However, these values are usually not clinically useful because of the time delay in analysis. Serial dilutions of the plasma, and estimation of the ketone levels using a 'Ketostix' can give a guide to the plasma levels of AcAc, and consequently an approximation of the total ketones present (e.g. a positive 'Ketostix' result on a plasma dilution of 1 : 16 indicates severe ketoacidosis). Estimations of the plasma concentrations of phosphate and magnesium, which often fall to very low levels after the institution of therapy, are of value only if replacement therapy is to be considered.

After the initial plasma glucose level has been estimated by a specific laboratory method, further estimations, for the monitoring of therapy, may be made using 'dipstick' technology, e.g. Ames 'Dextrostix'.

N.B. The plasma creatinine levels, if measured by the picric acid Jaffe reaction, are often falsely elevated due to positive analytical interference by acetoacetate. This should be considered if these values are used as an indicator of renal function.

Management

The aims of treatment may be summarized as follows:

1. Rehydration (including restoration of intravascular volume in shock)
2. Control of blood glucose (by insulin)
3. Replacement of potassium losses
4. Correction of severe acidosis
5. Replacement of phosphate

In ketoacidosis the first therapeutic consideration is to replace the fluid deficit as this may cause life-threating hypovolaemia. Consequently the initial i.v. therapy should consist of normal saline infusion at the rate of about 2 litres over the first hour, and decreasing to 500 ml/h over the next 4 h. Normal saline is preferred to other i.v. solutions, because it ensures vascular filling, and maintenance of a high extracellular osmolality (inhibits the development of cerebral oedema). If vascular collapse is marked, then plasma expanders such as 'stable plasma protein solution' (SPPS) or crystalloids should be given.

Early potassium replacement is always necessary since insulin infusion will rapidly cause transcellular potassium shifts and a potentially dangerous hypokalaemia. Initial potassium replacement should be at the rate of about 20 mmol/h and accompanied by frequent (at least 2-hourly) estimations of plasma potassium levels. The potassium may be replaced as the chloride salt, although phosphate compounds may be also used with the added advantage of replacing some of the phosphate deficit.

Magnesium replacement therapy has been suggested by some authorities but most clinicians do not specifically treat magnesium deficits.

Insulin therapy is dependent on the protocol that exists within the specific institution. Commonly, i.v. infusions of small amounts of insulin are given using infusion pumps; usually at the rate of 4–8 u/h after an initial 'loading' dose of 10–20 u. Many clinicians prefer low-dose i.m. therapy using a similar dosage regimen. The main advantage of the low-dose insulin regimen is the decreased frequency of rebound hypoglycaemia. There is some evidence, however, that with the low-dose therapy, acidosis takes longer to resolve than with high-dose regimes.

Since insulin may bind to the plastic of the infusion sets, the insulin infusion is often prepared in an albumin solution which precludes this problem, or the infusion set may be 'washed' with a solution of insulin to inhibit further binding.

When the plasma glucose concentration has fallen to around 15 mmol/l, glucose infusion, in the form of 5% dextrose, may be given at a rate of around 100 ml/h. The insulin infusion at this stage should now be maintained at a lower rate (e.g. 2 u/h) so that judicious control of the blood glucose level is maintained. This regime should be continued for about 24 h after which subcutaneous long-acting insulin therapy should be commenced.

The use of bicarbonate therapy in DKA is a controversial issue. Some authorities do not recommend bicarbonate infusions at all, whilst others suggest that if the pH is less than 7·15 bicarbonate should be given with the object of raising the pH to around 7·30, or the plasma $[HCO_3^-]$ to around 15–20 mmol/l.

Case Examples

Diabetic Ketoacidosis

A 34-year-old woman presented to hospital with a three-week history of polyphagia, polyuria, polydipsia and weight loss. In the week previous to presentation, she developed left loin pain and dysuria. Two days before attendance, her husband noticed an unusual odour on her breath, and an increased respiratory rate. On the day of admission, she had become febrile and her mental state deteriorated.

On examination, severe dehydration was evident, with a supine BP of 85/50, and a pulse rate of 120/min. A respiratory rate of 35/min was noted and her breath smelt strongly of acetone. Tenderness was elicited in the left flank. Neurological examination indicated mental clouding, but no localizing signs were evident. Urinalysis revealed positive reactions for blood, protein, nitrites and ketones. Urgent blood electrolyte studies showed:

Plasma			
	Na	119 mmol/l	(132–144)
	K	2·1 mmol/l	(3·1–4·8)
	Cl	88 mmol/l	(93–108)
	HCO_3	4 mmol/l	(21–32)
	AG	29 mEq/l	(10–18)
	Urea	14·1 mmol/l	(3·0–8·0)
	Creat	0·46 mmol/l	(0·06–0·12)
	Gluc	42·5 mmol/l	(3·0–5·5)
	Lactate	3·0 mmol/l	(0·1–2·0)
	PO_4	1·37 mmol/l	(0·6–1·25)

Ketostix estimation on the plasma sample was positive to a 1 : 16 dilution. Arterial blood gas analysis revealed the following;

pH	7·02	(7·35–7·42)
H^+	95 nmol/l	(38–45)
Pco_2	8 mmHg	(35–45)
Po_2	127 mmHg	(80–100)
$AHCO_3$	2 mmol/l	(24–32)

A diagnosis of DKA was made and i.v. therapy initiated with the immediate infusion of 1 litre of normal saline containing 26 mmol of KCl, followed by a further 4 litres of saline containing 285 mmol of KCl over a period of 6 h. In a second i.v. infusion line, insulin therapy was initiated at a rate of 4 u/h.

Once the haemodynamic situation was stabilized, half-normal saline containing 65 mmol/l of potassium was begun at a rate to balance urinary output. Ten hours after admission, when the blood glucose had decreased to 13·5 mmol/l, 5% dextrose (containing 26 mmol/l K^+) was begun at a rate of 100 ml/h. Biochemical results during this period are shown below (time (h) refers to hours after commencement of therapy):

Time (h)		2	5	10	
Plasma	Na	129	130	135 mmol/l	(132–144)
	K	2·8	2·3	3·3 mmol/l	(3·1–4·8)
	Cl	105	111	120 mmol/l	(93–108)
	HCO_3	3	3	8 mmol/l	(21–32)
	AG	24	18	10 mEq/l	(10–18)
	Urea	13·8	15·0	13·5 mmol/l	(3·0–8·0)
	Creat	0·42	0·41	0·26 mmol/l	(0·06–0·12)
	Glu	34·0	27·3	22·3 mmol/l	(3·0–5·5)
	Lactate	3·0	1·3	1·6 mmol/l	(0·1–2·0)
	PO_4	1·37	0·24	0·08 mmol/l	(0·6–1·25)

Comment

This case of severe DKA shows a number of features commonly seen in the disorder:

1.   Hyponatraemia: The possible causes of hyponatraemia are fivefold:

a.   Urinary ketone excretion (loss of Na^+ Ketone$^-$)
b.   Osmotic diuresis (causing ↑ Na^+ loss)
c.   Vomiting (loss of Na^+ in vomitus)
d.   Transcellular water shift due to the osmotic effect of glucose in the ECF (p. 224)
e.   Factitious hyponatraemia (p. 36) from hyperlipidaemia associated with DKA.

2.   Hypokalaemia: The marked hypokalaemia in this case indicated a severe depletion of this ion, which would have become much worse as a result of insulin therapy. Consequently huge doses of potassium were infused, and as the results indicate, even after some 300 mmol had been given, little change in plasma [K^+] was seen. Most patients with DKA initially have increased plasma [K^+] (p. 62). The hypokalaemia in this patient indicated a very severe potassium depletion.

3.   Hypovolaemia: The elevated urea indicates a marked water depletion (prerenal uraemia), as a direct consequence of the osmotic diuresis. Note that the plasma creatinine levels abruptly fall as the ketones are metabolized, clearly showing the interference of AcAc in the analytical method used for creatinine (p. 226).

4.   Ketoacidosis: The severe metabolic acidosis is indicated by the low plasma bicarbonate levels and the compensatory hypocapnoea. Although plasma ketones were not estimated in this case, the initial anion gap acidosis is characteristic of DKA. The plasma lactate values, although slightly elevated (as they are in approximately 50% of cases of DKA), do not account for the increased gap.

As therapy continued, the anion gap decreased, with an increase in plasma [Cl^-], i.e. a hyperchloraemic acidosis developed. As many as 50% of DKA cases show this phenomenon. The development of the hyperchloraemia appears to depend on the state of hydration of the patient. On treatment, or if the patient is able to take in adequate water and thus maintain the plasma volume, the ketones are excreted in huge amounts in the urine (the renal threshold for ketones is of the order of 1 mmol/l). The resulting Na^+ depletion (due to Na^+ Ketone$^-$ loss), however, causes avid Na^+ reabsorption in the proximal tubule, along with the easily reabsorbed chloride anion (i.e. Na^+ lost as Na^+ Ketone$^-$ is replaced by Na^+ Cl$^-$). This results in the development of hyperchloraemic acidosis with marked ketonuria.

5.   Phosphate: Initial plasma phosphate levels showed the expected hyperphosphataemia associated with a severe acidosis. On treatment, however, the plasma phosphate plunged to extremely low levels as a result of activation of glycolytic mechanisms, and consequent movement of PO_4 into the cells.

Although there are theoretical reasons for giving these patients phosphate supplements, very few of them show clinical features of hypophosphataemia. Most clinics, however, do give some phosphate supplementation.

The precipitating cause of the episode of DKA in the above patient was found to be a urinary tract infection, which lead to a left renal abscess.

Diabetic Ketoacidosis

A 15-year-old girl, a known diabetic on insulin therapy for the past 5 years, developed a mild respiratory infection. Home blood glucose monitoring showed increasing levels over a period of 4 days prior to a routine outpatients appointment. When seen in the outpatient department, she was noted to be moderately dehydrated. There was acetone on her breath, and urinalysis revealed a heavy reaction for ketones. Plasma electrolytes showed:

Plasma			
	Na	135 mmol/l	(132–144)
	K	4·2 mmol/l	(3·1–4·8)
	Cl	103 mmol/l	(93–108)
	HCO_3	7 mmol/l	(21–32)
	AG	29 mEq/l	(10–18)
	Urea	7·5 mmol/l	(3·0–8·0)
	Creat	0·19 mmol/l	(0·06–0·12)
	Glu	21·3 mmol/l	(3·0–5·5)

Intravenous therapy was initiated using normal saline, potassium supplementation and low dose insulin infusion. Repeat blood analyses showed no improvement in bicarbonate level, and clinically, the patient was developing respiratory distress. 100 mmol of sodium bicarbonate was infused over 30 min with 26 mmol of potassium in a sidearm of the infusion set. Results before and after the infusion of bicarbonate (approximately 8 h after admission) are shown (time refers to hours after admission, i.e. $NaHCO_3$ was given after the second set of results):

Time (h)		2	6	10		
Plasma	Na	136	135	135	mmol/l	(132–144)
	K	4·9	5·6	4·2	mmol/l	(3·1–4·8)
	Cl	106	115	109	mmol/l	(93–108)
	HCO_3	7	5	12	mmol/l	(21–32)
	Urea	7·0	5·4	4·5	mmol/l	(3·0–8·0)
	Creat	0·15	0·21	0·16	mmol/l	(0·06–0·12)
	Glu	22·9	15·9	14·0	mmol/l	(3·0–5·5)

Comment

The clinical response to the bicarbonate therapy was evidenced by a reduction in respiratory rate, and improved well-being of the patient. Although not evident in this case an increase in plasma sodium ($\uparrow Na^+$ intake with $NaHCO_3$), is often noted with HCO_3^- therapy. The effect of HCO_3^- therapy on the plasma $[K^+]$ is shown by a decrease of some 1·4 mol/l in the plasma level, even though the patient was receiving supplementation. It is usually recommended that for every 100 mmol of sodium bicarbonate infused, at least 15 mmol of potassium should be infused at the same time, over and above that required in usual DKA therapeutic manoeuvres.

The increase in plasma bicarbonate level seen with bicarbonate therapy is variable and depends on the amount of intracellular H^+ ion that requires neutralization.

Diabetic Ketoacidosis

A 38-year-old female, a known IDDM patient for 15 years, was admitted to her local hospital in an unconscious state. Clinical examination revealed moderate dehydration, rapid respirations and only minimal response to painful stimuli, but no localizing signs. Initial biochemical parameters revealed:

Plasma	Na	126 mmol/l	(137–145)
	K	5·9 mmol/l	(3·1–4·2)
	Cl	99 mmol/l	(98–106)
	HCO_3	2 mmol/l	(22–32)
	AG	31 mEq/l	(10–18)
	Urea	14·2 mmol/l	(3·0–8·0)
	Creat	0·38 mmol/l	(0·05–0·12)
	Glu	93·5 mmol/l	(3·8–5·8)

Arterial blood gas measurements performed at the same time were:

pH	6·83	(7·35–7·45)
H^+	148 nmol/l	(38–45)
P_{CO_2}	8 mmHg	(35–45)
P_{O_2}	141 mmHg	(80–110)
$AHCO_3$	1 mmol/l	(22–31)

Intravenous normal saline therapy was initiated, and in view of the very acidotic status of the patient, 350 mmol of sodium bicarbonate were also infused. Four hours later, the patient suffered a cardiac arrest, requiring resuscitation and transfer to a major hospital. Biochemical parameters at the time of the collapse revealed:

Plasma	Na	148 mmol/l	(137–145)
	K	1·4 mmol/l	(3·1–4·2)
	Cl	117 mmol/l	(98–106)
	HCO_3	7 mmol/l	(22–32)
	AG	25 mEq/l	(10–18)
	Urea	7·0 mmol/l	(3·0–8·0)
	Creat	0·32 mmol/l	(0·05–0·12)
	Glu	76 mmol/l	(3·8–5·8)

Repeat arterial blood gas estimation showed the following:

pH	7·04	(7·35–7·45)
H^+	90 nmol/l	(38–45)
P_{CO_2}	36 mmHg	(35–45)
P_{O_2}	64 mmHg	(80–110)
$AHCO_3$	10 mmol/l	(22–31)

Although the hypokalaemia was rapidly corrected, and correction of the diabetic state continued, the patient died of cerebral oedema 3 days later.

Comment

This case shows the startling effect of alteration in acid–base status on plasma potassium, where a decrease in plasma potassium of some 4·5 mmol/l occurred in a period of 3 h, and was the most likely cause of the cardiac arrest. The hypo-kalaemia was a result of:

1.   Insulin infusion (K^+ moves into cells)
2.   Bicarbonate therapy (K^+ moves into cells)
3.   No potassium supplementation

There is still debate on the use of bicarbonate therapy in DKA. Most clinicians accept the premise that in severe acidosis (i.e. pH less than 7·2), cautious use of bicarbonate is of therapeutic benefit. Usually, 100 mmol of sodium bicarbonate are infused (the dose is varied for children, depending on body weight) over 30 min, with extra potassium supplements. After this therapy, acid–base and electrolyte parameters should be reviewed before further alkali therapy is contemplated.

Non-insulin-dependent Diabetes Mellitus (Hyperosmolar Diabetic Coma)

Definition

A significant hyperosmolar diabetic state exists when the plasma tonicity, as a result of increased plasma glucose levels, exceeds 320 mmol/kg. This disorder, which mainly occurs in the elderly, is usually not associated with ketoacidosis.

Clinical Presentation

The detection of diabetes often depends on a history of polyuria, poly-dipsia, polyphagia, weight loss and susceptibility to infections, particularly of the dermis. Commonly, routine screening of urine may reveal the presence of glycosuria, which is then investigated further. Occasionally, however, elderly patients present in an obtunded or comatose state, severely dehydrated, with signs often consistent with a brainstem infarction, such as bilateral flaccid paralysis and upgoing plantar responses. In these patients it is often only on routine urinalysis that the true diagnosis becomes evident, and therapy instituted. For this reason all elderly patients should have properly noted urinalysis or blood glucose estimation performed.

Biochemical Consequences

The major deficiency in hyperosmolar coma is water, with some estimates indicating deficits of up to 25% of total body water. Variable losses of sodium and potassium also occur. Measurement of blood glucose usually reveals extremely high levels which may be greater than 100 mmol/l, with osmolalities often greater than 400 mmol/kg.

As occurs in DKA, the increased plasma osmolality causes water to shift to the extracellular space, but the osmotic diuresis due to glucose results in an increased urine volume and excretion of much of this water.

Idiogenic Osmoles

Extracellular hypertonicity results, in the first instance, in withdrawal of intracellular water and thus cellular contraction (cellular dehydration). If the extracellular hypertonicity persists, the cells increase their tonicity, causing water to be drawn back from the extracellular fluid, and consequently reinstate normal cellular volume. This mechanism is thought to be due to intracellular development of 'idiogenic osmoles'.

The concept of idiogenic osmoles was developed in an attempt to explain the resistance of the brain to dehydration (local increase in intracellular tonicity) in the presence of high ECF tonicity. From studies on lower animal forms, brain levels of amino acids, especially taurine, were shown to increase in this situation, and it was suggested that taurine was involved in brain osmoregulation.

Since taurine seems to have little metabolic activity in the cell, the clearance of this amino acid is slow. Consequently, the development of these idiogenic osmoles as a result of high ECF tonicity may take days to clear. If therapeutic manoeuvres should rapidly drop the ECF osmolality, a reverse water shift will occur, resulting in cerebral oedema, and pressure on the brainstem, with obvious sequelae.

Treatment

The principal aims of therapy are:
1. Correction of hypovolaemia
2. Correction of hyperosmolar state
3. Correction of underlying cause

The basic aim in therapy of hyperosmolar diabetic states is to correct the hyperosmolality without precipitating cerebral oedema. In this context, recalling the concept of idiogenic osmoles, treatment should be prompt, but the hyperosmolar state should be resolved slowly in order to prevent rapid re-entry of water into the brain and consequent cerebral oedema.

Correction of Osmolality

Reports in the recent literature have suggested that hyperosmolar diabetic coma may be treated by volume correction alone. Generally, initial therapy is directed at expansion of the extracellular volume, either with normal saline, or specific plasma expanders (note that the latter will have limited effect since the ECF is already hyperosmolar). Since normal saline has an osmolality of 306 mosmol/kg, the effect of infusion will be a mild to moderate decrease in the extracellular osmolality.

There has been vigorous debate concerning the type of fluid replacement which should be used in hyperosmolar states. In hypertonic states secondary to diabetes, because of the delay in clearance of the brain 'idiogenic osmoles', it has been recommended that the ECF osmolality should be decreased slowly, to allow time for clearance of these osmoles. The suggestion, therefore, is that normal saline should be used to decrease slowly the osmolality of the ECF over a period of 1–2 days. Others recommend that once the vascular space has been stabilized, replacement with 'half-normal' saline in dextrose can be initiated, as a source of water replacement, for rapid repletion of lost body water. As a result of this latter therapy, occasional cases of cerebral oedema (1–5%) with resultant death have been recorded. We feel that it is the osmolality, rather than the hyperglycaemia, that should be monitored, and slowly returned to normal. This should occur over 2–3 days by judicious use of normal and 'half-normal' saline.

Insulin

Insulin therapy in these patients is usually of short duration because, once the glucose level is normalized, the patients rarely require continued insulin therapy for maintenance of the blood glucose level. Often they require no insulin therapy at all, particularly if a drug (e.g. propranolol, thiazide) has precipitated the hyperglycaemic episodes.

The response to insulin therapy is brisk, and rapid changes in blood glucose may occur with minimal amounts of insulin. Consequently, it is suggested that no loading dose be given, and that infusions of insulin should be set at very low levels (e.g. 2 u/h) to ensure that the blood glucose levels do not plummet.

Sodium

The hyperosmolar state results in renal sodium loss as described for DKA. Because the water loss, due to osmotic diuresis, is marked in hyperosmolar coma, the plasma [Na^+] is often normal initially. However, it may be high (as a result of water loss), or low (as a result of dilution of ECF by intracellular water). Calculation of the 'corrected plasma sodium' (p. 224), by allowance for water shifts, will often indicate hypernatraemia, irrespective of the measured plasma [Na^+].

Since the urine in these in these patients usually contains sodium in concentrations of 30–50 mmol/l, sodium depletion is often significant, and sodium replacement with normal saline in the initial therapy is usually required.

Potassium

Potassium losses via the urine may result in deficits approaching 500 mmol, even though the plasma levels are frequently normal on presentation to hospital. Insulin therapy will depress the plasma potassium rapidly (K^+ re-enters the cell) so that the replacement fluid should contain 20–40 mmol/l of potassium salts, depending on the rate of delivery.

Case Examples

Hyperosmolar Diabetic Coma

An unconscious 73-year-old lady was transferred from a nursing home to the Accident and Emergency Department. History from an attendant revealed that the patient had, over the previous fortnight, complained of increasing thirst and polyuria. In the week prior to admission, the patient's mental state had slowly deteriorated and on the morning of admission she was found to be unrousable.

Physical examination revealed a moderately dehydrated lady, with supine BP of 120/60 mmHg, pulse rate 105/min. Neurological examination revealed no response to painful stimuli, bilateral abnormal plantar responses, decreased tendon reflexes, and hypotonia. No localizing features were found. Routine plasma electrolytes revealed:

Plasma	Na	138 mmol/l	(132–144)
	K	3·6 mmol/l	(3·1–4·8)
	Cl	105 mmol/l	(93–108)
	HCO$_3$	32 mmol/l	(21–32)
	Urea	14·7 mmol/l	(3·0–8·0)
	Creat	0·20 mmol/l	(0·06–0·12)

A diagnosis of brainstem cerebrovascular accident was made, and the patient transferred to the ward. On routine urinalysis, a strong reaction to clinistix was found and blood glucose levels were performed:

Plasma	Glu	89·5 mmol/l	(3·8–5·8)
	Osmol	385 mmol/kg	(285–297)

Intravenous therapy with normal saline had already been commenced, but the rate was increased and low dose i.v. insulin therapy instituted at 2 u/h. The patient died approximately 8 h after admission.

Comment
Hyperosmolar coma may mimic the clinical findings of brainstem cerebrovascular accident, so that the correct diagnosis may be missed. In such clinical presentations, the estimation of blood glucose is advisable, so that possible hyperglycaemia is not missed. In the above patient, review of the case notes from the nursing home revealed that routine urinalysis a month previously had detected the presence of glucose.

The presence of the normal plasma sodium concentration in this case demonstrates the inability of this measurement to give an indication of total body sodium. If allowance is made for the osmotic shift of water into the ECF, i.e.

$$\text{Corrected Na} = 138 + (89 - 12)/3$$
$$= 164 \text{ mmol/l,}$$

the degree of hypertonic dehydration in this patient becomes apparent. In hyperosmolar coma, although some sodium is lost through osmotic diuresis, large amounts of Na^+ are not required to accompany the excreted ketones as seen in DKA (*see above*). Consequently, as hypovolaemia develops, renal reabsorption of sodium increases, and hypernatraemia would normally develop. This development is often masked, however, by the osmotic shift of intracellular water to the extracellular space as a result of the high extracellular glucose concentration.

Hyperosmolar Diabetes Mellitus
An 80-year-old lady with a past history of mild congestive cardiac failure (treated with chlorothiazide), presented to the Accident and Emergency Department

complaining of increasing polyuria and an itchy groin rash. Physical examination revealed moderate dehydration and the typical rash of *Candida albicans*. Urinalysis showed a strongly positive response for glucose. Biochemical results obtained at this time were:

Plasma	Na	158 mmol/l	(132–144)
	K	4·0 mmol/l	(3·1–4·8)
	Cl	118 mmol/l	(93–108)
	HCO_3	33 mmol/l	(21–32)
	Urea	16·0 mmol/l	(3·0–8·0)
	Creat	0·15 mmol/l	(0·06–0·12)
	Glu	43·0 mmol/l	(3·0–5·5)
	Osmol	393 mmol/kg	(281–297)

Intravenous normal saline (with K^+ supplements) was instituted immediately, with 3 litres infused in the first 4 h, followed by 1 litre over the next 4 h. At the same time, an insulin infusion of 2 u/h was given. Eight hours after admission, the biochemical results obtained were:

Plasma	Na	170 mmol/l	(132–144)
	K	4·3 mmol/l	(3·1–4·8)
	Cl	130 mmol/l	(93–108)
	HCO_3	32 mmol/l	(21–32)
	Urea	12·0 mmol/l	(3·0–8·0)
	Creat	0·10 mmol/l	(0·06–0·12)
	Glu	8·9 mmol/l	(3·0–5·5)
	Osmol	371 mmol/kg	(281–297)

At this point, the insulin infusion was ceased and 0·45% saline and 5% dextrose infused alternately at rates decreasing from 200 ml/h to 100 ml/h over 2 days. At that time the following results were obtained:

Plasma	Na	146 mmol/l	(132–144)
	K	3·4 mmol/l	(3·1–4·8)
	Cl	106 mmol/l	(93–108)
	HCO_3	30 mmol/l	(21–32)
	Urea	3·8 mmol/l	(3·0–8·0)
	Creat	0·06 mmol/l	(0·06–0·12)
	Glu	7·1 mmol/l	(3·0–5·5)
	Osmol	304 mmol/kg	(281–297)

Comment

The initial electrolyte findings reflect the marked deficit of water that often occurs in these patients. Allowing for water shift, the corrected plasma sodium in the first blood sample is of the order of 168 mmol/l. Following normal saline infusion (osmolality of 306 mmol/kg), one would expect the plasma sodium and osmolality to fall. In fact, however, the corrected plasma sodium remained unchanged whilst the osmolality fell some 20 mmol/kg.

This anomaly is explained by reference to the blood glucose which had decreased to normal levels. As the glucose enters the cell, water accompanies the solute, and concentrates the ECF sodium. This increased concentration of sodium thus maintains a high ECF tonicity and does not allow excessive water to enter the cell, thereby decreasing the risk of cerebral oedema.

Although the insulin infusion was set at 2 u/h, exquisite sensitivity to the hormone was shown. For this reason, low-dose insulin therapy is recommended.

The initial metabolic alkalosis may have been the result of the diuretic therapy, or possibly due to the so-called 'contractional alkalosis'.

There appears to be an association between thiazide diuretic therapy and the development of hyperosmolar diabetic states. The mechanism of this association is unknown.

Further Reading

Adrogue N. J., Wilson H., Boyd III A. E. et al. (1982) Plasma acid-base patterns in diabetic ketoacidosis. *N. Engl. J. Med.* **307**, 1603–1610.

Cahill G. F. (1981) Ketosis. *Kid. Int.* **20**, 416–425.

Kreisberg R. A. (1978) Diabetic ketoacidosis: new concepts and trends in pathogenesis and treatment. *Ann. Int. Med.* **88**, 681–695.

National Diabetes Data Group (1979) Classification of diabetes mellitus and other categories of glucose intolerance. *Diabetes* **28**, 1039–1057.

10

Mineralocorticoids

The mineralocorticoids are steroid hormones which originate in the zona glomerulosa of the adrenal cortex and influence sodium and potassium homeostasis. The major natural hormone is aldosterone. An intermediate product of aldosterone synthesis, 11-deoxycorticosterone, also has significant mineralocorticoid activity ($\sim 6\%$ of aldosterone). Corticosterone, another precursor of aldosterone, and the major glucocorticoid, cortisol, both have minimal mineralocorticoid activity ($< 1\%$ of aldosterone). The major synthetic mineralocorticoid, used for therapeutic purposes, is fludrocortisone, which has 70–80% of the activity of aldosterone.

Physiology

Action

Aldosterone stimulates sodium uptake and potassium secretion by epithelial cells, particularly those of the distal nephron, the gut mucosae and the sweat and salivary glands. However, the major action is on the distal renal tubule and collecting duct cells where it effects Na^+ reabsorption and K^+ (and H^+) secretion.

This so-called Na^+–H^+ exchange at the renal tubule level is not a strict 1 : 1 cation exchange process but rather a secretion of K^+ and H^+ down an electrochemical gradient produced by active Na^+ reabsorption. Recent experimental work suggests that Na^+ is reabsorbed mainly in the proximal part of the distal tubule whilst K^+ is secreted chiefly by the distal portion. It has also been demonstrated that the amount of Na^+ reabsorbed by the distal renal tubule is usually greater than the combined amounts of K^+ and H^+ secreted. However, the end result of this distal cation interchange is conservation of Na^+ and excretion of K^+.

Aldosterone Synthesis

Progesterone, derived from cholesterol, is converted to aldosterone by a series of enzymatic reactions that take place in the zona glomerulosa of the adrenal cortex (*Fig.* 10.1).

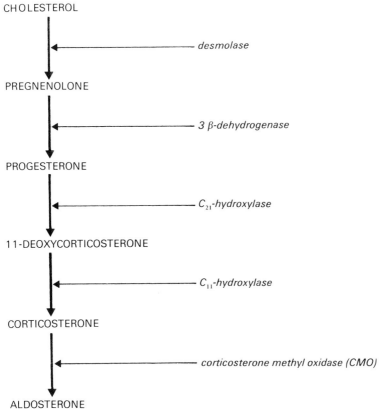

Fig. 10.1. Synthesis of aldosterone.

The mechanism of the final step in which corticosterone is converted to aldosterone, is uncertain, but is thought to involve two enzymes, corticosterone methyl oxidase (CMO) I and II, and the formation of an unstable intermediate product which may either decompose to 18-hydroxycorticosterone, or be converted to aldosterone, i.e.

1. Corticosterone $\longrightarrow$ 'intermediate product' (CMO I)
2. 'Intermediate product' $\longrightarrow$
 a. 18-Hydroxycorticosterone (spontaneous)
 b. Aldosterone (CMO II)

Control of Aldosterone Synthesis

The two major factors controlling aldosterone biosynthesis and secretion are the renin–angiotensin–aldosterone system and the plasma potassium concentration. ACTH normally plays a minor role.

ACTH

Aldosterone secretion, like that of cortisol, exhibits circadian rhythm and reflects the variations in pituitary ACTH release, and although pharmacological doses of

ACTH will increase aldosterone secretion rate this hormone does not appear to be an important regulator of aldosterone production. Diseases associated with high plasma levels of ACTH (e.g. Cushing's disease) do not show increased aldosterone secretion rates, and conversely the absence of ACTH (e.g. hypopituitarism) is not associated with decreased secretion.

Potassium

Hyperkalaemia stimulates aldosterone secretion (direct action on the zona glomerulosa) and hypokalaemia promotes the reverse action, i.e. aldosterone and potassium form a positive feedback loop:

$$\uparrow \text{plasma } [K^+] \longrightarrow \uparrow \text{aldosterone} \longrightarrow$$
$$\uparrow K^+ \text{ excretion} \longrightarrow \downarrow \text{plasma } [K^+] \longrightarrow \downarrow \text{aldosterone.}$$

Renin–angiotensin–aldosterone System (Fig. 10.2)

This system, as well as regulating potassium homeostasis through the action of aldosterone, also influences sodium balance, extracellular volume and blood pressure.

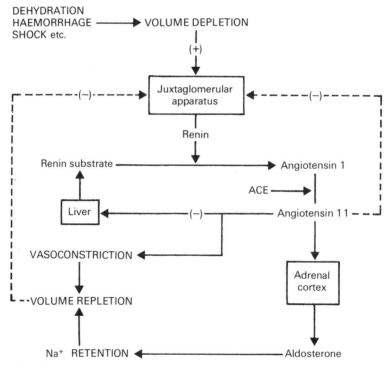

Fig. 10.2. The renin–angiotensin–aldosterone system. *ACE*, angiotensin converting enzyme.

Renin is released from the juxtaglomerular apparatus and reacts with a circulating glycoprotein (angiotensinogen, renin substrate), synthesized in the liver, to form angiotensin I. This product is converted, mainly in the lung capillaries, by angiotensin converting enzyme (ACE) to angiotensin II, which in turn stimulates the release of aldosterone. Angiotensin II is rapidly destroyed in the peripheral circulation by a number of peptidases (angiotensinase) present in tissues and blood. Recent work suggests that an early product of angiotensinase activity, a heptapeptide (angiotensin III), may also stimulate aldosterone synthesis and secretion, but with less activity than angiotensin II.

Angiotensin II has four major actions:

1. Arteriolar vasoconstriction
2. Aldosterone release from the adrenal cortex
3. Stimulation of hepatic synthesis of renin substrate
4. Inhibition of renin release (short feedback loop)

The major factor controlling renin secretion is the renal blood perfusion pressure (effective blood volume). Changes in renal perfusion are detected in the juxtaglomerular apparatus by baro- (stretch) receptors located in the afferent arterioles of the glomeruli. A decrease in renal blood perfusion (dehydration, hypotension, etc.) effects an increase in renin secretion, whilst an increased perfusion pressure decreases renin secretion.

Other factors that influence renin secretion are:

1. Sympathetic nervous system: This system acts through β-receptors and responds to postural changes (renin secretion increased in the ambulatory state), and possibly minimal changes in the extracellular volume (decreased volume produces increased renin output).
2. Sodium chloride transport across the macula densa of the distal convoluted tubule: It has been suggested, but not proven, that increased sodium perfusion at this level suppresses renin secretion. Recent evidence, however, suggests that the opposite may be true and that the mechanism responds to tubular luminal chloride concentration rather than that of sodium.
3. Potassium: Hyperkalaemia, although it stimulates aldosterone secretion, suppresses renin synthesis and release.
4. Angiotensin II: This peptide suppresses renin secretion and thus forms a short feedback loop.
5. Prostaglandins.

Metabolism of Aldosterone

Approximately 50–250 µg of aldosterone are produced daily, and transported in the blood bound to albumin, transcortin and aldosterone-binding globulin. The major site of aldosterone catabolism is the liver, where 90% is removed from the blood during a single passage, and inactivated by reduction to a tetrahydro form, then conjugated to glucuronic acid, and finally excreted in the urine. The term urinary aldosterone usually refers to this metabolic end-product rather than to 'free' aldosterone, which is present only in minute amounts.

Mineralocorticoid Excess

Consequences

Potassium Metabolism

Prolonged mineralocorticoid excess results in increased renal potassium excretion, potassium deficiency and hypokalaemia. The clinical manifestations of potassium depletion are: lethargy, cramps, muscle weakness, and if the deficit is severe, muscle paralysis. Polyuria can also occur due to the inability of a kidney depleted of potassium to reabsorb water.

Acid–base Metabolism

Mineralocorticoid excess, along with severe potassium depletion, induces renal H^+ excretion and bicarbonate generation (p. 112). This results in a metabolic alkalosis ($\uparrow$ plasma $[HCO_3^-]$).

Sodium and Water Metabolism

In primary hyperaldosteronism the increased renal retention of sodium and water results in an expanded extracellular volume. This increase does not progress beyond a certain stage because the sodium excretion rate eventually returns to a level which balances intake. The mechanism of this sodium 'escape' phenomenon is unclear, but involves a decreased proximal nephron sodium reabsorption. However, there are suggestions that the 'escape' may be due to the elaboration of natriuretic hormone in response to the increased extracellular volume.

Although there is sodium retention in primary hyperaldosteronism the plasma level is usually not raised to hypernatraemic levels as there is concurrent water retention, so that usually the plasma sodium concentration is at the upper limit of normal or, in occasional cases, only slightly above it.

Hypertension

Increased diastolic blood pressure is a feature of primary hyperaldosteronism. This is due in part to the salt and water retention, but there also appears to be other factors involved because:

1.   It is difficult to demonstrate hypertension in normal subjects given repeated doses of mineralocorticoids, although patients with treated Addison's disease may develop hypertension after several months of over-treatment with mineralocorticoids.
2.   Prolonged secondary hyperaldosteronism associated with oedematous states (cirrhosis, nephrosis, etc.) does not result in hypertension.

Causes

On the basis of the level of plasma renin activity (PRA) the mineralocorticoid excess syndromes can be divided into primary (low PRA), and secondary (high PRA) groups (*Table* 10.1). A rare syndrome (pseudohyperaldosteronism) associated with an abnormal renal tubular response to aldosterone constitutes a third group.

Table 10.1. Causes of mineralocorticoid excess syndromes

Primary (low PRA)
    Aldosterone
        Adrenal adenoma
        Adrenal hyperplasia
    Other steroids
        Adrenal enzyme defects: C_{11}-hydroxylase deficiency
                                    C_{17}-hydroxylase deficiency
        Cushing's syndrome: pituitary dependent
                              adrenal adenoma
                              adrenal carcinoma
        Ectopic ACTH syndrome
    Exogenous steroids
        Steroid therapy
        Liquorice ingestion (excessive)
        Carbenoxolone therapy
Secondary (high PRA)
    Physiological
        Volume depletion: dehydration
                        haemorrhage
                        diuretic therapy
                        renal tubular acidosis
    Oedema (normotensive)
        Congestive cardiac failure
        Nephrotic syndrome
        Liver cirrhosis
    Hypertension
        Renovascular
        Malignant hypertension
        Renin-secreting tumour
        Oestrogen therapy
    Bartter's syndrome
Pseudohyperaldosteronism
    Liddle's syndrome

PRA, plasma renin activity.

Evaluation/Diagnosis (*Fig.* 10.3)

The two major manifestations of mineralocorticoid excess, hypokalaemia and hypertension, are common clinical problems which can be associated with a wide variety of disorders. They may occur together not only in primary mineralocorticoid excess but also in the hypertensive varieties of secondary hyperaldosteronism (*Table* 10.1), and in essential hypertension managed with diuretic therapy.

Hypokalaemia

The differential diagnosis and investigation of hypokalaemia are considered elsewhere (p. 70). If the aetiology is obscure a spot urinary potassium estimation is often helpful, i.e. a low urinary $[K^+]$ (<20 mmol/l) suggests an extrarenal cause,

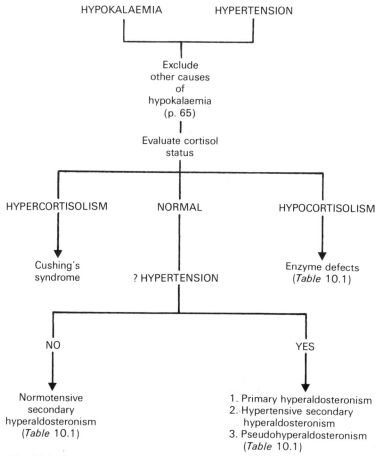

Fig. 10.3. Suggested scheme for the evaluation of suspected mineralo-corticoid excess.

e.g. diarrhoea, chronic purgation, and a high level (>20 mmol/l) suggests renal potassium-wasting, e.g. diuretic therapy, mineralocorticoid excess, etc.

Hypertension

Over 98% of hypertensive adults have idiopathic or essential hypertension. Less than 1% of hypertensive patients will have primary hyperaldosteronism. The characteristic biochemical features of this latter disorder are:

Hypertension
Usually mild, but can be severe and progressive.

Hypokalaemia
This feature is not always present, but the plasma potassium level is invariably below 4·0 mmol/l, and often less than 3·5 mmol/l.

Metabolic Alkalosis
A common but not invariable feature. Its presence depends on the severity of the concomitant potassium depletion. If the patient is hypokalaemic there is usually an accompanying metabolic alkalosis.

Hypernatraemia
A high plasma sodium level is unusual, but the level is always greater than 140 mmol/l, and sometimes slightly above the upper limit of normal.

High Urinary Potassium Excretion
A high urinary potassium concentration (>40 mmol/l) in association with hypo-kalamia is characteristic of primary hyperaldosteronism. This is a useful screening test for the disorder providing other causes (diuretic therapy, hypertensive secondary hyperaldosteronism) are excluded.

Increased Aldosterone (Plasma, Urinary)
Before a definitive diagnosis of primary hyperaldosteronism is made an increased plasma or urinary aldosterone level should be demonstrated.

Plasma Renin Activity (PRA)
The definite diagnosis of primary hyperaldosteronism rests on the demonstration of hypertension in the presence of an increased aldosterone secretion and a low PRA.

Diagnosis of Primary Hyperaldosteronism
The investigation of suspected primary hyperaldosteronism should be approached in three phases: screen, diagnosis, aetiology.

Screening
Primary hyperaldosteronism is a minor cause of hypertension ($<0.5–1.0\%$ of adult cases) and therefore diagnostic evaluation of these patients is a futile and costly exercise. Therefore an inexpensive procedure for selection of those patients requiring further investigation is necessary.

Although not all cases of primary hyperaldosteronism present with hypo-kalaemia it is reasonable, and cost effective, to limit for further investigation those hypertensive patients who fulfil the following criteria:
1.   Hypokalaemic (plasma potassium <3.5 mmol/l)
2.   Urinary potassium >40 mmol/l (spot urine)
3.   No drug therapy, especially diuretics
4.   On an unrestricted salt diet

Diagnosis
The first step in the diagnostic work up is to identify those patients with low plasma renin activity (PRA). A high PRA excludes primary hyperaldosteronism (*Fig.* 10.4). A low level may indicate low renin hypertension (LRH) or primary

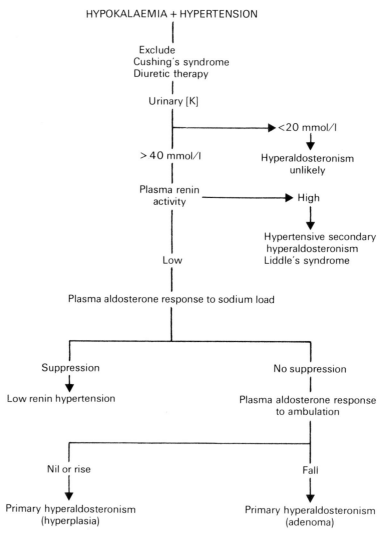

Fig. 10.4. Suggested scheme for the investigation of suspected primary hyperaldosteronism.

hyperaldosteronism. These latter two conditions can be separated on the basis of the plasma aldosterone response to a sodium load, e.g. plasma aldosterone measured before and after 2 litres of normal saline has been infused intravenously over a 4-h period.

In primary hyperaldosteronism the plasma aldosterone will initially be high and will not suppress below the upper limit of the reference range after saline infusion. In the case of LRH there is significant aldosterone suppression after the infusion.

Aetiology
Around 30% of patients with primary hyperaldosteronism have bilateral idiopathic adrenal hyperplasia, a condition which usually does not respond to adrenalectomy. On the other hand those cases due to adrenal adenoma usually respond to surgery. These two conditions may be distinguished by either of the following procedures:
1.   Aldosterone response to ambulation: Plasma aldosterone levels are estimated before and after 4–6 h of ambulation. Patients with an adenoma generally show a fall in the plasma aldosterone level, whereas those with hyperplasia show no change or an increased aldosterone level.
2.   Adrenal venous sampling: A patient with a unilateral adenoma will have a high aldosterone level in the blood draining the diseased gland, and a low level in the blood draining the other gland (suppression). In bilateral hyperplasia both adrenals secrete high levels of aldosterone.

Principles of Management
Specific management of the mineralocorticoid excess syndromes depends on the underlying pathology and is out of the range of a text of this size. Only the general principles of therapy are outlined below.

Primary Hyperaldosteronism

Adenoma
Surgical removal.

Hyperplasia
Spironolactone therapy (spironolactone is a competitive inhibitor of aldosterone action).

Enzyme Defects

C_{11}- and C_{17}-hydroxylase Deficiency
Suppress ACTH production by cortisol replacement therapy.

Cushing's Syndrome

Pituitary Dependent
Surgery (removal of pituitary tumour); pituitary irradiation.

Primary Adrenal Disease
Surgery (removal of adenoma or carcinoma); adrenolytic agents (*o,p'*DDD).

Ectopic ACTH Syndrome
Removal of primary tumour; bilateral adrenalectomy; metyrapone, *o,p'*DDD.

Secondary Hyperaldosteronism

1.   Removal of initiating cause, e.g. nephrectomy in renovascular hypertension, removal of a renin-secreting tumour, etc.
2.   Spironolactone therapy

Case Examples

Ectopic ACTH Syndrome: Carcinoma of the Lung

A 58-year-old male presented with a grand mal convulsion. He gave a history of recent weight loss, muscle weakness in legs and arms, and increasing fatigue. His plasma and urinary electrolyte values on admission are shown below.

Plasma	Na	137 mmol/l	(132–144)
	K	2·1 mmol/l	(3·2–4·8)
	Cl	89 mmol/l	(98–108)
	HCO_3	36 mmol/l	(23–33)
	Urea	3·8 mmol/l	(3·0–8·0)
	Creat	0·08 mmol/l	(0·06–0·12)
Urine	Na	26 mmol/l	
	K	37 mmol/l	

A routine chest X-ray on admission revealed a mass in the right hilar region which on bronchoscopy proved to be an oat-cell carcinoma. A plasma cortisol level on a sample taken on the day after admission was > 1600 nmol/l (RR 140–690) and the plasma ACTH level was 145 ng/l (RR < 60).

Comment

In the ectopic ACTH syndrome (ectopic production of ACTH by a non-endocrine tumour) there is bilateral adrenal hyperplasia and increased synthesis of cortisol and its precursors. There is also increased production of the aldosterone precursors, deoxycorticosterone and corticosterone. The aldosterone secretion rate may be increased, but is more often normal.

This mineralocorticoid excess syndrome may be due to the high concentration of circulating cortisol which at normal levels has minimal mineralocorticoid activity; or to increased secretion of deoxycorticosterone which itself has significant mineralocorticoid activity.

These patients usually present in the first instance with a hypokalaemic alkalosis, muscle weakness due to the hypokalaemia, and often also with an Addisonian type of pigmentation (↑ circulating β-lipotropin, formed along with the excess ACTH, which has melanocyte-stimulating hormone activity). The major manifestations of Cushing's syndrome (e.g. redistribution of adipose tissue) are unusual in this condition as the hypercortisolism is of rapid onset, and the patients usually succumb to the malignancy before the classic picture of this condition develops.

The ectopic ACTH syndrome has been described as being associated with many malignant tumours, particularly those of the bronchus, pancreas, thymus, oesophagus, stomach and larynx. In some of these tumours, especially carcinoma of the oesophagus and also some bronchial carcinomas, an increased circulating level of immunoreactive ACTH, but without clinical manifestations of hyper-cortisolism, has been noted.

Primary Hyperaldosteronism

A 47-year-old female presented with a blood pressure of 180/110 mmHg. She complained of tiredness, recurrent headache and weakness of the lower limbs. There was no family history of cardiovascular disorders and she was not on any medication. After intensive biochemical investigation she was diagnosed as having primary hyperaldosteronism. Subsequently a small adenoma (2·5 cm diameter) was removed from the left adrenal. Postoperatively her blood pressure fell to 145/90 mmHg and remained around this level. The admission electrolytes and endocrine studies are shown below.

Plasma	Na	143 mmol/l	(132–144)
	K	2·7 mmol/l	(3·2–4·8)
	Cl	98 mmol/l	(98–108)
	HCO$_3$	37 mmol/l	(23–33)
	Urea	6·6 mmol/l	(3·0–8·0)
	Creat	0·11 mmol/l	(0·06–0·12)
Urine	Na	25 mmol/l	
	K	56 mmol/l	

Plasma renin activity: 0·04 ng/ml/h (RR 0·1–0·4)

Plasma aldosterone: basal—3·6 nmol/l (RR 0·03–0·55); after a salt loading test the level was 3·3 nmol/l.

Comment

Hypertension is a common condition, whilst primary aldosteronism is rare. The latter classically presents as hypertension and hypokalaemic alkalosis; but there are many other causes of this clinical picture, the commonest being hypertension treated with diuretic therapy.

Causes of hypertension and hypokalaemic alkalosis include:

1. Diuretic (thiazide) therapy of essential hypertension
2. Primary hyperaldosteronism
3. Secondary hyperaldosteronism and hypertension (*Table* 10.1)
4. Cushing's syndrome

Mineralocorticoid Deficiency

Consequences

The clinical and biochemical features of the mineralocorticoid deficiency syndromes vary according to the aetiology of the disease and also the status of the other adrenocortical steroids.

The main manifestations of mineralocorticoid deficiency *per se* reflect abnormalities of potassium, acid–base and salt and water metabolism.

Potassium Metabolism

Hyperkalaemia, due to a decreased distal renal tubular potassium secretion, is a constant feature of mineralocorticoid deficiency. The plasma potassium concentration varies with the degree of mineralocorticoid deficiency, and very high levels (7–8 mmol/l) are not unusual, especially if the disease has been present for some time.

Acid–base Metabolism

Aldosterone deficiency is often, but not always, accompanied by a hyperchloraemic metabolic acidosis. This feature is often termed Type 4 renal tubular acidosis (p. 199), and is probably largely due to the resultant hyperkalaemia, which suppresses renal tubular ammonia production.

Salt and Water Metabolism

Decreased renal tubular sodium reabsorption results in renal sodium wasting, with consequent hyponatraemia, a low plasma osmolality and hypovolaemia. The urinary osmolality is usually high (greater than plasma osmolality), i.e. $\downarrow$ distal tubular Na^+ reabsorption $\longrightarrow \downarrow$ extracellular $[Na^+] \longrightarrow \downarrow ADH \longrightarrow \uparrow$ renal water excretion $\longrightarrow$ plasma $[Na^+]$ back to normal, but with hypovolaemia. Further loss of sodium repeats this process until there is moderate hypovolaemia which will now stimulate ADH release regardless of the plasma osmolality (p. 18). The presence of ADH will then increase renal water reabsorption and cause hyponatraemia (dilutional), a low plasma osmolality, and a high urine osmolality ($>$ plasma osmolality).

This situation should not be confused with the syndrome of inappropriate ADH secretion (SIADH, p. 42) which differs in that it is usually associated with both euvolaemia and normokalaemia.

Causes

For the purposes of evaluation and management the mineralocorticoid deficiency syndromes can be divided into those with isolated aldosterone deficiency, those which additionally have deficient secretion of cortisol, and those due to renal tubular dysfunction (*Table* 10.2).

Apart from pseudohypoaldosteronism (very rare disorder) other diseases and drugs which may result in an inadequate renal tubular response to aldosterone are:
1. Transplanted kidney
2. Renal amyloidosis
3. Systemic lupus erythematosus
4. Sickle-cell anaemia
5. Interstitial nephritis
6. Potassium-sparing diuretics—spironolactone, amiloride, triamterene (*see also* p. 259)

Table 10.2. Causes of mineralocorticoid deficiency syndromes

Cortisol and aldosterone deficiency
  Addison's disease
  Adrenal enzyme defects
    desmolase deficiency
    3β-ol-dehydrogenase deficiency
    C_{21}-hydroxylase deficiency

Isolated aldosterone deficiency
  Enzyme defects
    corticosterone methyl oxidase (1 and 11)
  Syndrome of hyporeninaemic hypoaldosteronism (SHH)
    diabetes mellitus
    tubulo-interstitial disease
  Heparin therapy

Attenuated tubular response
  Pseudohypoaldosteronism

Evaluation/Diagnosis (*see Fig.* 10.5)
Mineralocorticoid deficiency usually presents in one of two forms:
1. Adrenocortical failure
2. Persistent hyperkalaemia

Adrenocortical Failure

Adrenal failure (cortisol and aldosterone deficiency) may present either as an acute crisis or in a chronic form.

In the acute form there is anorexia, nausea, vomiting, abdominal pain, dehydration and circulatory collapse. This clinical picture when associated with Addisonian pigmentation, hyperkalaemia and hyponatraemia suggests the diagnosis and indicates the need for treatment with steroids and intravenous infusions of saline (or plasma expanders) immediately. Specific investigations (hormone studies) should be delayed until (*a*) the patient has been stabilized, and (*b*) the steroid therapy has been changed to dexamethasone, a synthetic glucocorticoid that does not interfere with the laboratory estimation of cortisol. An important point to remember about Addison's disease is that the typical pigmentation (buccal cavity, palmar creases, etc.) may not be present in all cases.

In the chronic form of Addison's disease there is an insidious onset with progressive weakness, weight loss, and pigmentation associated with vomiting, diarrhoea and postural hypotension. The biochemical features include hyponatraemia, hyperkalaemia and often a moderate normal anion gap metabolic acidosis (Type 4 renal tubular acidosis).

Adrenocortical failure due to various enzyme defects usually presents at birth. If there is a desmolase or 3β-ol-dehydrogenase deficiency the production of all adrenal steroids will be defective and survival is rare. In the case of C_{21}-hydroxylase deficiency there is failure to thrive, salt-wasting and hyperkalaemia. The increased levels of ACTH secretion, due to absence of the cortisol negative feedback, results in an increase in adrenal androgen production. This may result in the premature development of secondary sex characteristics in male infants and ambiguous genitalia and virilization in female infants.

Persistent Hyperkalaemia

An approach to the evaluation of patients with hyperkalaemia and suspected mineralocorticoid deficiency is shown in *Fig.* 10.5.

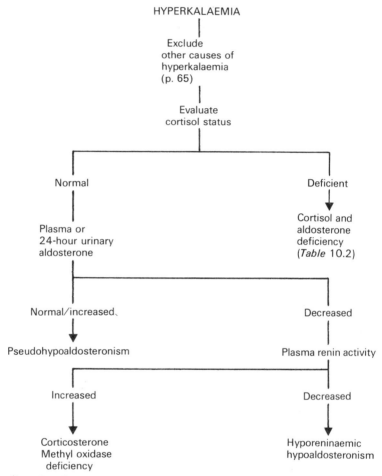

Fig. 10.5. Suggested scheme for the evaluation of suspected mineralo-corticoid deficiency.

Principles of Management

The management of the mineralocorticoid deficiency syndromes depends on the aetiology and the severity and acuteness of the disorder.

Acute Adrenal Failure

This is a medical emergency requiring immediate therapy, aimed at (*a*) replenishing and maintaining the plasma (and extracellular) volume, and (*b*) replacing adrenocortical hormones.

Restoration of Plasma Volume

Intravenous infusion of normal saline (with 5% glucose) should be started immediately. Up to 3–5 litres of fluid may be necessary over the first few hours. Noradrenaline infusions may be required if the blood pressure does not respond to saline.

Steroid Therapy

An immediate infusion of hydrocortisone (100–200 mg) should be given followed by 100 mg 6-hourly. When the patient's condition stabilizes the steroids may be given orally and the dose reduced to maintenance levels over the next 5–7 days.

Chronic Adrenal Failure

In the non-acute case of adrenal failure the patient should be commenced on 20 mg of hydrocortisone three times daily which may be reduced to a maintenance dose over 3–5 days. The maintenance dose is of the order of 20–30 mg of hydrocortisone daily. It should be administered to imitate the circadian rhythm of cortisol secretion, i.e. two-thirds of the daily dose in the morning and one-third at night.

Mineralocorticoid therapy is usually necessary and can be given as fludrocortisone, 0·1–0·2 mg daily.

C_{21}-hydroxylase Deficiency

This syndrome presents with salt depletion, glucocorticoid deficiency, mineralocorticoid deficiency and androgen excess. Therapy should therefore involve:

1. Salt and volume repletion: intravenous saline until the patient stabilizes
2. Hydrocortisone: glucocorticoid replacement and suppression of adrenal androgen production (suppression of ACTH)
3. Mineralocorticoid therapy: deoxycorticosterone acetate, fludrocortisone

The glucocorticoid replacement should be finely balanced so that overdosage does not occur on the one hand (leads to growth retardation), and underdosage (leads to accelerated bone maturation) on the other hand. The dosage may be controlled by keeping a careful watch on the rate of growth and on one of the following biochemical parameters: urinary oxosteroids, plasma 17-hydroxyprogesterone, plasma ACTH.

Isolated Hypoaldosteronism

Replacement therapy in this situation is achieved with fludrocortisone (0·05–0·1 mg/day). In the case of the syndrome of hyporeninaemic hypoaldosteronism large amounts of fludrocortisone (0·2–0·4 mg/day) may be required before there is any response to therapy; another feature of this condition is that replacement therapy may take up to 7 days to have any effect.

Case Examples

Addison's Disease

A female aged 40 years presented with a 6–9 month history of weight loss, muscle weakness, 'dizzy spells' and mental depression. On examination she showed evidence of recent weight loss, had a mild postural drop in blood pressure; and it was noted that she was well 'sun-tanned' but was not thought to have pigmentation typical of Addison's disease. After an inspection of the admission electrolyte results a short Synacthen test was performed and she was diagnosed as having primary Addison's disease. The plasma electrolyte values below are those found on admission and 4 days later after 3 days' treatment with hydrocortisone. Intravenous normal saline was commenced on day 1 (3 litres in 12 h).

Date		01/02	05/02	
Plasma	Na	127	139 mmol/l	(132–144)
	K	5·3	3·2 mmol/l	(3·2–4·8)
	Cl	97	101 mmol/l	(98–108)
	HCO$_3$	21	25 mmol/l	(23–33)
	Urea	15·5	4·5 mmol/l	(3·0–8·0)
	Creat	0·11	0·08 mmol/l	(0·06–0·12)
Urine	Na	45	— mmol/l	
	K	17	— mmol/l	

Short Synacthen test: The basal plasma cortisol level of 70 nmol/l rose to 96 and 85 nmol/l at 30 min and 60 min respectively after an intramuscular injection of 250 μg of Synacthen. In the normal adult subject the baseline cortisol should be greater than 140 nmol/l (lower limit of reference range) and at least one post-Synacthen sample should rise by at least 200 nmol/l, and also exceed an absolute value of 550 nmol/l.

Comment

The presenting features of this patient which suggested mineralocorticoid deficiency were:

1. Postural hypotension—suggests hypovolaemia
2. Hyponatraemia
3. High urinary sodium—> 20 mmol/l
4. Hyperkalaemia
5. Mild, normal anion gap, metabolic acidosis

(2)+(3) = renal salt wasting

(4)+(5) = possible Type 4 renal tubular acidosis (p. 199)

Any clinical picture similar to this indicates that adrenocortical deficiency must head the provisional diagnosis list and be excluded without delay. In this respect a dynamic function test (e.g. short Synacthen test) should be performed immediately rather than waiting for the results of a random plasma cortisol estimation. It is not unusual, in adrenocortical failure, to find a cortisol level within the normal range, i.e. the diseased adrenal gland may be secreting cortisol at its maximum rate which is sufficient to maintain a normal plasma level but lacks any reserve capacity to provide enough cortisol for the body to deal with stress situations.

Further Reading

Schambelan M., Sebastian A. and Hulter H. N. (1978) Mineralocorticoid excess and deficiency syndromes. In: Brenner B. M. and Stein J. H. (ed.) *Contemporary Issues in Nephrology*, Vol. 2. New York, Churchill–Livingstone, pp. 232–268.

Vaughan N. J. A., Jowett T. P., Slater J. D. H. et al. (1981) The diagnosis of primary hyperaldosteronism. *Lancet* 1, 120–125.

Weinberger M. H., Grim C. E., Hallifield J. W. et al. (1979) Primary hyperaldosteronism: diagnosis, localization, and treatment. *Ann. Intern. Med.* **90**, 386–395.

11

Drugs affecting water and electrolyte homeostasis

Ion and water metabolism can be adversely affected by a wide range of therapeutic agents. Comprehensive information on these effects can be found in the publication edited by Young D. S., Pestaner L. C. and Gibberman V. (1975) Effects of drugs on clinical laboratory tests. *Clinical Chemistry* **21**, 1D–432D. The following discussion looks at diuretics in some detail as these commonly used therapeutic agents can produce a wide variety of electrolyte disorders. The remainder of the chapter deals with other drugs, and their effects, in a shorter synoptic manner.

Diuretics

The clinically useful diuretics act by blocking Na^+ reabsorption in the renal tubules, resulting in increased sodium and water excretion (sodium diuresis). In the following discussion the diuretic drugs are classified according to their site of action in the nephron, i.e.:

Proximal tubule: carbonic anhydrase inhibitors
Ascending limb of loop of Henle: 'loop' diuretics
Cortical diluting segment: thiazides
Distal tubule and collecting duct: potassium-sparing diuretics.

Proximal Tubule

Diuretics
Acetazolamide, dichlorphenamide, ethoxzolamide

Action
Carbonic anhydrase inhibition.

A major portion of the Na^+ reabsorbed in the proximal tubule is linked to H^+ secretion and HCO_3^- conservation. This mechanism is dependent on the action of the enzyme carbonic anhydrase.

Within the tubule cell H_2O and CO_2 react in the presence of carbonic anhydrase to form first H_2CO_3 and then H^+ and HCO_3^-. The H^+ is secreted into the lumen in exchange for Na^+, which is then secreted back into the blood along with the cell-generated HCO_3^-. The secreted H^+ reacts in the lumen with filtered HCO_3^- to form H_2CO_3 and then CO_2 (this reaction is catalysed by carbonic anhydrase which is located in the tubule cell brush border). This tubule-generated CO_2 diffuses into the tubule cell and re-enters the H^+/HCO_3^- generation process (p. 91).

The carbonic anhydrase inhibitors suppress the action of this enzyme in the proximal tubule, resulting in:

1.   ↓ Na^+ reabsorption
2.   ↓ HCO_3^- reabsorption

Although these drugs can inhibit 25–30% of proximal Na^+ reabsorption they are poor diuretics (excrete only 2–3% of filtered Na^+) because a large amount of these sodium ions will be reabsorbed in the normally functioning distal nephron. Bicarbonate ions on the other hand are poorly reabsorbed distally and are excreted in the urine.

The increased delivery of Na^+ (and HCO_3^-) to the distal tubule results in an increased tubular flow rate which stimulates K^+ secretion; the resulting kaliuresis may lead to potassium depletion (p.55).

These drugs also inhibit carbonic anhydrase in other parts of the body, including the eye where they decrease the formation of aqueous humour; thus their use in some types of glaucoma.

Biochemical Consequences

Prolonged use of these drugs may result in:

1.   Bicarbonaturia and a low plasma [HCO_3^-], i.e. renal tubular acidosis type 2 (*see* p. 196)
2.   Potassium depletion and hypokalaemia

The metabolic acidosis is self-limiting because as the plasma [HCO_3^-] falls, less of this ion is delivered in the glomerular filtrate to the proximal tubule. Eventually a stage is reached when the proximal tubule, although compromised, can reabsorb all the HCO_3^- presented to it. The plasma bicarbonate level rarely falls below 15 mmol/l during carbonic anhydrase inhibition therapy (*see* p. 200 for a case example).

Ascending Limb of Loop of Henle

Diuretics

'Loop' diuretics (frusemide, ethacrynic acid), and organomercurials.

Action

In the ascending limb of the loop of Henle sodium ions are thought to be reabsorbed passively following active chloride reabsorption. The 'loop' diuretics act by preventing Cl^- reabsorption. The increased Na^+ presented to the distal tubule results in an increased flow rate and consequently increased renal K^+ excretion.

Biochemical Consequences

1. Natriuresis
2. Kaliuresis. This may result in potassium depletion and hypokalaemia, especially in patients with oedematous conditions who may have an associated secondary hyperaldosteronism, e.g. nephrotic syndrome, hepatic cirrhosis
3. Calciuresis. The 'loop' diuretics increase renal calcium excretion by suppressing Ca^{2+} reabsorption in the ascending limb of the loop of Henle. This property, although not resulting in hypocalcaemia in the normal patient, is used to advantage in the treatment of hypercalcaemia (p. 142)

Cortical Diluting Segment

Diuretics

Thiazides, e.g. chlorothiazide.

Action

In the normally functioning renal diluting segment, which is impermeable to water, reabsorption of sodium results in tubular fluid dilution, hence the ability of the kidney to produce a dilute urine (to $\sim 50\,mmol/kg$). Sodium ion reabsorption in this part of the tubule is, like that in the thin ascending loop of Henle, thought to be secondary to active Cl^- reabsorption. The thiazide group of drugs produce natriuresis by preventing Na^+ reabsorption in this area. The resulting increased delivery of Na^+ and water to the distal tubule will result in kaliuresis, and possible potassium depletion.

The thiazide group of drugs also have minimal carbonic anhydrase inhibition activity.

Biochemical Consequences

1. Natriuresis
2. Occasional dilutional hyponatraemia (*see below*)
3. Hypokalaemia. The association of thiazide therapy and hypokalaemia is common, and tends to occur in patients who are treated for oedema rather than those treated for hypertension (*see below*)
4. Hypocalciuria. This is a fairly common feature of thiazide therapy and may be associated, rarely, with hypercalcaemia (p. 140). The decrease in renal calcium excretion is probably related to an increased proximal tubule Na^+ reabsorption as a consequence of hypovolaemia
5. Hyperuricaemia. Thiazides decrease the urinary excretion of urate, and are often associated with hyperuricaemia. The mechanism of this action is unclear but is possibly due to an increased proximal tubule reabsorption as a result of hypovolaemia (hypovolaemia increases the proximal renal tubular reabsorption of urate and calcium as well as that of sodium)

Distal Tubule and Collecting Ducts

Diuretics
'Potassium-sparing'—spironolactone, triamterene, amiloride.

Action
These three drugs act by different mechanisms.

Spironolactone
This diuretic competes with aldosterone, and other mineralocorticoids, for the binding sites of the distal tubular cells. This action can be overcome by high level, of mineralocorticoid, and will not occur if mineralocorticoids are absent, e.g. Addison's disease.

Triamterene
The diuretic mechanism of this drug is unclear, but it appears to act at a site of sodium reabsorption (and potassium secretion) which is independent of mineralocorticoid activity, i.e. it is active in the absence of mineralocorticoids.

Amiloride
This drug blocks distal tubular Na^+ reabsorption by interfering with the reabsorptive site on the luminal side of the tubular cell.

Biochemical Consequences
These three diuretics are all mild natriuretic agents but potent inhibitors of potassium secretion, and therefore their use may result in severe hyperkalaemia. These two actions reflect the functions of the distal tubule, i.e. a minor site of sodium absorption (2–8% of filtered sodium reabsorbed); a major site of potassium excretion. Hydrogen ion excretion is also suppressed by all three drugs. Metabolic acidosis is an uncommon complication of therapy, although severe acidaemia has been described in a number of patients on prolonged therapy.

Diuretics and Potassium Metabolism
The commonest side effect of diuretic therapy is the potential for disturbing potassium homeostasis.

Hypokalaemia
All diuretics, with the exception of the potassium-sparing variety, increase renal K^+ excretion and thus have the potential to produce potassium depletion and hypokalaemia.

The percentage of patients on diuretic therapy who develop hypokalaemia is small (<5% of 1294 patients in one large survey), however the number of patients on diuretic therapy is large and thus diuretic-induced hypokalaemia is a common occurrence. The patients mainly at risk are the oedematous group (nephrosis, cirrhosis, cardiac failure). These subjects usually also have a degree of secondary hyperaldosteronism which would also increase the possibility of potassium depletion. Non-oedematous patients, e.g. hypertensives treated with diuretics, rarely develop potassium depletion. In this group mild hypokalaemia has been shown to occur in the presence of a normal total body potassium. This may be due to a diuretic-induced imbalance of the potassium gradient between the intracellular and extracellular fluids.

The metabolic alkalosis often associated with the diuretic-induced hypo-kalaemia is the result of increased H^+ excretion and bicarbonate generation due to potassium depletion and hypovolaemia (p. 112).

Hyperkalaemia

The potassium-sparing diuretics (spironolactone, triamterene, amiloride) all have the potential to produce severe hyperkalaemia as a consequence of decreased renal K^+ excretion. This hyperkalaemia may be associated with a metabolic acidosis of the normal anion gap variety (see Type 4 renal tubular acidosis, p. 199).

Example

A 74-year-old female, on treatment for cardiac failure which included amiloride (5 mg three times daily), presented with nausea, vomiting and muscle weakness. The plasma electrolyte results obtained on admission, and 4 and 12 days after cessation of amiloride therapy are shown below.

Date	16/02	20/02	23/02	
Plasma Na	142	141	140 mmol/l	(132–144)
K	6·2	4·9	4·2 mmol/l	(3·2–4·8)
Cl	123	113	108 mmol/l	(98–108)
HCO_3	13	21	24 mmol/l	(23–33)
Creat	0·13	0·12	0·09 mmol/l	(0·06–0·12)
AG	12	12	12 mEq/l	(7–17)

Comment

As stated above severe hyperkalaemia and metabolic acidosis may complicate potassium-sparing diuretic therapy. In the case of amiloride distal tubular secretion of cation (H^+, K^+) is diminished because of suppressed Na^+ reabsorption, i.e. the normal electrochemical gradient, due to Na^+ reabsorption (negative potential difference on luminal side of the cell membrane), is diminished and therefore cations are retained. When the above patient's amiloride therapy was discontinued her plasma electrolyte picture, as expected, slowly returned towards normal.

Diuretics and Water Homeostasis

As noted above the diuretics act by decreasing the renal tubular reabsorption of Na^+ which results in an osmotic (sodium) diuresis. The patient therefore becomes depleted of both sodium and water in the ratio of around 140 mmol of sodium to 1 litre of water and thus remains normonatraemic. Occasionally patients on thiazides or frusemide may develop hyponatraemia which, in some cases, may be severe.

Example

A female of 72 years presented at the Accident and Emergency Department complaining of tiredness and muscular weakness. She had been prescribed bendrofluazide (10 mg daily) 3 weeks previously for hypertensive cardiac failure. Clinically she did not appear to be dehydrated but had postural hypotension. On the strength of the history of thiazide therapy, the postural hypotension, and the mildly raised plasma urea and creatinine, the patient was considered to be hypovolaemic. The thiazide medication was ceased and 3 litres of 'normal' saline and 8 g of KCl (~ 104 mmol of K^+) were given over the next 24 h. The laboratory results given below are those found on admission and after 24 h of i.v. therapy.

Date		17/11	18/11	
Plasma	Na	121	131 mmol/l	(132–144)
	K	2·1	3·5 mmol/l	(3·2–4·8)
	Cl	78	95 mmol/l	(98–108)
	HCO_3	35	28 mmol/l	(23–33)
	Urea	10·5	4·8 mmol/l	(3·0–8·0)
	Great	0·13	0·08 mmol/l	(0·06–0·12)
	Osmol	256	276 mmol/kg	(281–295)
Urine	Na	37	— mmol/l	
	K	12	— mmol/l	
	Osmol	395	— mmol/l	

Comment

The association of diuretic therapy and hyponatraemia is not unusual. Affected patients often have several features in common:
1.   Usually occurs in the elderly
2.   Associated with moderate to severe hypokalaemia
3.   The diuretic involved is usually a thiazide
4.   Biochemical abnormalities improve when the diuretic is discontinued, but sometimes potassium may be required before any improvement occurs.

The pathophysiology of this syndrome is unclear but appears to be related to an increased secretion of antidiuretic hormone (note the low plasma osmolality and the high urine osmolality in the above case) as a possible consequence of:
1.   A diuretic-induced decrease in circulating blood volume (stimulation of baroreceptors)
2.   Exaggerated ADH baroreceptor response ($\uparrow$ ADH) as a result of potassium deficiency

This syndrome shows biochemical features that are similar to those of the syndrome of inappropriate ADH secretion (p. 42) except that in the latter situation the plasma potassium concentration is usually normal and there are no signs of hypovolaemia.

Antidiuretic Drugs

There is a large (and increasing) number of drugs which, through antidiuretic action, may be responsible for mild to severe water retention (*Table* 11.1). These

Table 11.1. Drugs associated with antidiuresis

Drugs stimulating ADH secretion
  Narcotics: morphine, other opiates
  Hypnotics: barbiturates
  Oral hypoglycaemics: chlorpropamide, tolbutamide
  Anticonvulsants: carbamazepine
  Antineoplastics: cyclophosphamide, vinblastine, vincristine
  Antidepressants: amitryptiline
  Miscellaneous: clofibrate, isoprenaline, nicotine derivatives
Drugs potentiating ADH action
  Chlorpropamide
  Paracetamol
  Indomethacin

---

drugs decrease the kidney's ability to excrete water and can result in chronic dilutional hyponatraemia (p. 35).

The mechanism for the water retention could be due to a direct stimulation of ADH secretion, or a potentiation of ADH action on the renal collecting ducts. The biochemical syndrome produced is identical to that of the syndrome of inappropriate ADH secretion (p. 42), but treatment usually only requires that the drugs be withdrawn. Occasionally, especially if the patient is on i.v. fluid therapy, severe hyponatraemia may occur and require further intervention.

Drugs Associated with Diabetes Insipidus

Drug-induced diabetes insipidus is rare. It has been reported to have occurred with each of the following drugs:

1.   Lithium carbonate
2.   Demethylchlortetracycline (demeclocycline)
3.   Methoxyflurane
4.   Phenytoin sodium

The first three drugs listed interfere with the action of ADH at the level of the renal collecting duct, whilst phenytoin sodium suppresses the release of ADH by the posterior pituitary. Lithium and demethylchlortetracycline have been used as therapeutics agents in the treatment of the syndrome of inappropriate secretion of ADH (p. 41).

Drugs affecting Potassium Homeostasis

The drugs that can commonly result in disturbances of the plasma potassium concentration are the diuretic group (discussed above). There are also a number of other agents that may interfere with potassium homeostasis, resulting in hyper- or hypokalaemia.

Hyperkalaemia
1. Abnormal internal distribution
   a. Succinylcholine—cell membrane depolarization
   b. Digitalis—inhibition of the Na^+-K^+ ATPase pump
2. Decreased renal excretion
   a. Potassium-sparing diuretics (*see above*)
   b. Heparin infusin—depresses adrenal aldosterone synthesis
   c. Indomethacin—depresses renin production by suppression of prostaglandin synthesis

Hypokalaemia
1. Altered internal distribution
   a. Insulin therapy
   b. Salbutamol/adrenaline—stimulates β-receptors
   c. ?Thiazide diuretics
2. Increased renal excretion
   a. Diuretics (*see above*)
   b. Mineralocorticoids/liquorice—mineralocorticoid-like action
   d. Oestrogen therapy—increased production of renin substrate —(angiotensinogen)
   e. Carbenicillin—large doses are excreted by the kidney as poorly absorbable anions $\longrightarrow$ ↑ tubular flow
   f. Gentamicin—direct tubule toxicity

Drugs affecting Acid–base Homeostasis

Respirctory Acidosis
Drugs overdose—narcotics/hypnotics (suppress respiration)

Respiratory Alkalosis
Salicylates—(overdose stimulates respiratory centre)

Metabolic Acidosis
1. Lactic acidosis—ethanol, methanol, salicylate, biguanides
2. Ketoacidosis—ethanol
3. Renal tubular acidosis
   Proximal (Type 2)—carbonic anhydras inhibitors, outdated tetracyclines
   Distal (Type 1)—amphotericin B, lithium, analgesics
4. Potassium-sparing diuretics (*see above*)

Metabolic Alkalosis
1. Diuretics (*see above*)
2. Carbenicillin/penicillin—poorly absorbable anion presented to distal renal

tubule $\longrightarrow$ ↑ tubular flow $\longrightarrow$ ↑ K^+ excretion $\longrightarrow$ K^+ depletion $\longrightarrow$ ↑ H^+ excretion and HCO_3^- generation

3. Mineralocorticoids (*see* p. 238)

Mixed Respiratory Alkalosis and Metabolic Acidosis
Salicylate (p. 127)

Drugs affecting Calcium Metabolism

Hypercalcaemia
1. Vitamin D overdose— ↑ gut reabsorption
2. Thiazides— ↑ renal reabsorption, ?PTH stimulation
3. Vitamin A overdose—? ↑ bone resorption
4. Alkali and calcium—milk alkali syndrome (p. 140)

Hypocalcaemia
1. Anticonvulsants—phenytoin sodium—interference with vitamin D metabolism
2. Phosphate therapy—sequestration of insoluble calcium phosphates

Hypercalciuria
Frusemide—decreases Ca^{2+} reabsorption in ascending limb of loop of Henle

Hypocalciuria

Thiazides
Reabsorption of Ca^{2+} in the proximal tubule is closely linked to Na^+ reabsorption, and factors that increase Na^+ reabsorption also increase Ca^{2+} reabsorption. Possible sequence of events is: thiazides $\longrightarrow$ natriuresis $\longrightarrow$ hypovolaemia $\longrightarrow$ ↑ proximal Na^+ and Ca^{2+} reabsorption $\longrightarrow$ ↓ urinary Ca^{2+} excretion.

Further Reading
Miller M. and Moses A. M. (1976) Drug-induced states of impaired water excretion. *Kid. Intern.* **10**, 96–103.
Young D. S., Pestaner L. C. and Gibberman V. (1975) Effects of drugs on clinical laboratory tests. *Clin. Chem.* **21**, 1D–432D.

Index

Acetoacetic acid, 220, 225
Acetone, 220, 225
Acid, definition of, 84
Acidaemia, definition of, 84
Acid–base, 84
  abnormal homeostasis, 93
  acute renal failure and, 189
  carbon dioxide and, 92
  chronic renal failure and, 180
  compensation, 86
  definitions, 84
  diabetes mellitus and, 225
  diarrhoea and, 109, 211
  drugs and, 263
  evaluation of, 97
  gut obstruction and, 213
  homeostasis, 87
  hydrogen ion metabolism, 87
  hyperkalaemia and, 57
  liver disease and, 214
  metabolic acidosis, 94, 104
  metabolic alkalosis, 94, 111
  metabolic component, 86
  mineralocorticoid deficiency and, 199, 250
  mineralocorticoid excess and, 116, 242
  mixed disorders of, 95, 124
  plasma electrolytes and, 97
  potassium and, 53, 98
  renal function and, 89, 175
  renal tubular acidosis, 194
  respiratory acidosis, 94, 117
  respiratory alkalosis, 95, 121
  respiratory component, 86
  salicylate toxicity and, 127
  units, 84
  vomiting and, 114, 208
Acidosis (*see also* Metabolic acidosis,
    Respiratory acidosis, Mixed acid-base
    disorders)
  definition of, 84

Acidosis (*cont.*)
  diarrhoea and, 109
  drugs and, 263
  high anion gap and, 105
  hyperkalaemia and, 4, 53, 57
  metabolic, 94, 104
  metabolic acidosis and alkalosis, 97,
    128
  metabolic acidosis and respiratory alkalosis,
    96, 127
  normal anion gap and, 105
  renal disease and, 180, 189, 193
  renal tubular acidosis and, 194
  respiratory, 95, 117
  respiratory acidosis and metabolic acidosis,
    95, 124
  respiratory acidosis and metabolic alkalosis,
    96, 126
Acromegaly, hyperphosphataemia and, 156
ACTH (adrenocorticotropic hormone) ectopic
    production of, 32, 248
Acute tubular necrosis (ATN), 187
  acid–base and, 189
  calcium and, 189
  case example, 192
  causes of, 187
  consequences of, 188
  diagnosis of, 187
  hypercalcaemia and, 140
  potassium and, 189
  sodium and, 188
  water and, 188
Addison's disease
  case examples, 40, 201, 254
  hyperkalaemia and, 40, 63
  hyponatraemia and, 35, 40, 63
  potassium and, 63
  renal tubular acidosis and, 199, 201
  sodium and, 41
ADH (*see* Antidiuretic hormone)